Anorexia Nervosa: Diagnosis and Treatment

Anorexia Nervosa: Diagnosis and Treatment

Editor: Christopher Schneider

AMERICAN
MEDICAL PUBLISHERS
www.americanmedicalpublishers.com

AMERICAN
MEDICAL PUBLISHERS
www.americanmedicalpublishers.com

Cataloging-in-Publication Data

Anorexia nervosa : diagnosis and treatment / edited by Christopher Schneider.
p. cm.
Includes bibliographical references and index.
ISBN 978-1-63927-876-3
1. Anorexia nervosa. 2. Anorexia nervosa--Diagnosis. 3. Anorexia nervosa--Treatment.
4. Psychology, Pathological. 5. Psychiatry. I. Schneider, Christopher.
RC552.A5 A56 2023
616.852 62--dc23

American Medical Publishers,
41 Flatbush Avenue,
1st Floor, New York,
NY 11217, USA

ISBN 978-1-63927-876-3 (Hardback)

Contents

Preface

Over the recent decade, advancements and applications have progressed exponentially. This has led to the increased interest in this field and projects are being conducted to enhance knowledge. The main objective of this book is to present some of the critical challenges and provide insights into possible solutions. This book will answer the varied questions that arise in the field and also provide an increased scope for furthering studies.

Anorexia nervosa is an eating disorder characterized by extreme food restriction and an intense fear of gaining weight. The signs and symptoms of anorexia nervosa can be classified into emotional, physical, and behavioral aspects. Some emotional and behavioral symptoms are social withdrawal, insomnia, irritability, and frequent checks in the mirror for perceived flaws. Thin appearance, abnormal blood counts, fatigue, dehydration and swelling in the body are some common physical symptoms of anorexia nervosa. The diagnosis of this condition includes physical examination by a doctor followed by some tests. Blood tests, urine tests, electrocardiogram, thyroid function tests, imaging tests such as computed tomography (CT) scan, and bone density scan are commonly used to diagnose anorexia nervosa. The treatment for anorexia is aimed at overcoming both psychological and physical symptoms. It includes medications, counseling, and therapies. This book outlines the diagnosis and treatment for anorexia nervosa in detail. It will serve as a valuable source of reference for graduate and post graduate students.

I hope that this book, with its visionary approach, will be a valuable addition and will promote interest among readers. Each of the authors has provided their extraordinary competence in their specific fields by providing different perspectives as they come from diverse nations and regions. I thank them for their contributions.

Editor

1

User satisfaction with family-based inpatient treatment for adolescent anorexia nervosa: retrospective views of patients and parents

Inger Halvorsen[1*] and Øyvind Rø[1,2]

Abstract

Background: Research is scarce on patient and parent satisfaction with family-based treatment for adolescent anorexia nervosa (AN), especially family-based treatment adapted to inpatient settings. The purpose of this study was to describe and compare patient and parent satisfaction with an inpatient family-based treatment program for adolescent AN, and to investigate whether the level of satisfaction with treatment was associated with eating disorder outcome.

Methods: Former patients and their parents were contacted approximately five years (4.5 ± 1.7, range: 1.3–7.0) after discharge from family-based inpatient treatment. Ninety-four participants (patients: $n = 34$, mothers: $n = 40$, fathers: $n = 20$) from 46/58 (79.3%) families took part in the study. Former patients and both parents completed treatment satisfaction questionnaires. Outcome at follow-up was assessed by the Eating Disorder Examination Questionnaire and body mass index (kg/m^2).

Results: Overall, mothers and fathers reported a high level of satisfaction with treatment, while the former patients' satisfaction was moderate. There were no significant differences between treatment satisfaction scores for mothers and fathers. However, the former patients' treatment satisfaction scores were significantly lower than the parents' scores on several of the items. Correlations between eating disorder outcome parameters and treatment satisfaction were small, except for fathers' satisfaction with treatment and weight outcome at follow-up.

Discussion: Family-based treatment adapted to inpatient settings is a novel treatment approach for adolescents with AN that require hospitalization. Inclusion and empowerment of parents are considered crucial in outpatient family-based treatment, but may be just as important in inpatient programs. Mothers and fathers alike reported high levels of satisfaction with treatment, which may constitute an important factor in the success of family-based treatment.

Conclusion: Family-based inpatient treatment for adolescents with severe AN who have failed to respond to outpatient treatment seemed to be highly valued by parents and viewed by adolescents as acceptable. Parental satisfaction with their child's treatment is likely to be an important factor for treatment implementation and adherence both in outpatient and inpatient settings.

Keywords: Patient satisfaction, Parent satisfaction, Family-based treatment, Inpatient treatment, Anorexia nervosa

* Correspondence: inger.halvorsen@uus.no
[1]Regional Department for Eating Disorders, Division of Mental Health and Addiction, Oslo University Hospital - Ullevål Hospital, P.O. Box 4956, Nydalen, N-0424 Oslo, Norway
Full list of author information is available at the end of the article

Plain English summary

Knowledge of patients' and parents' satisfaction with treatment is important to improve treatment for families affected by serious illnesses such as adolescent anorexia nervosa. The most effective treatment for adolescents with anorexia nervosa is family-based, with a high level of parental involvement. Thus, the parents' experiences with treatment are particularly important in family-based treatment. However, knowledge of patients' and parents' satisfaction with family-based treatment for anorexia nervosa is scarce, particularly in cases when the patient requires hospitalization.

In this study, we investigated the experiences of former patients and their parents following discharge from a family-based, specialized treatment program. Parents physically accompany their child during hospitalization and participate intensively in the treatment. Patients, mothers, and fathers completed treatment satisfaction questionnaires approximately 5 years following discharge. Upon reflection, mothers and fathers expressed high levels of satisfaction with the treatment received. However, as is reflected in other studies on adolescent anorexia nervosa, the parents tended to be more satisfied with treatment than former patients themselves.

Introduction

Assessment of patient experiences is important for the evaluation and improvement of health services [1–3]. Satisfaction with health services is likely to influence the patient's engagement in treatment and collaboration with the staff, as well as treatment adherence. Ambivalence to treatment is a major challenge in anorexia nervosa (AN). Patients often report negative treatment experiences [4–6] and have a high dropout rate [7, 8]. However, dropout from family therapy for AN has been found to be much lower than from individual therapy [8]. Because the parents have a crucial role in ensuring that their children seek and adhere to treatment, the parents' views and satisfaction with treatment may be more important for a successful delivery and implementation than the patients' own satisfaction [9, 10].

Family-based treatment (FBT) [11, 12] is the most well-documented treatment for adolescent AN [13, 14]. Originally, FBT was developed as an outpatient intervention. However, many adolescents with AN need to be hospitalized due to severe physical complications, failure to respond to outpatient FBT, or lack of access to adequate outpatient treatment. When outpatient FBT is insufficient, FBT adapted to more intensive levels of care might be beneficial for adolescents with AN [15–19].

An important challenge when adapting outpatient FBT to inpatient settings is to combine FBT's strong focus on empowering the parents with the highly structured framework in inpatient programs that may be deemed necessary to manage the patient's medical condition [15]. During family-based hospital admissions, the parents are included in the daily care and intensive treatment and are able, therefore, to get more extensive coaching and support than what is possible in outpatient settings [16, 17]. As in outpatient FBT, the staff will support the parents' authority, but, typically, the inpatient staff will assume more responsibility for monitoring the patient's medical condition and for the framework in the treatment program. Adolescents with AN who require hospitalization will be expected to have a more severe prognosis than those in outpatient care, but family-based inpatient treatment may be associated with better outcomes than individual admissions [16, 18]. For instance, one study that compared outcome after an inpatient FBT intervention for medical stabilization in youths with AN with "treatment as usual" (TAU) hospitalization, found that those who received the FBT intervention were 2.84 times more likely than the TAU-group to achieve at least 95% of treatment goal weight at 6 months post-discharge [16]. Also, parental self-efficacy increased significantly in caregivers who participated in the FBT intervention [16]. The close collaboration with parents in family-based inpatient treatment may be important to reduce dropout.

Despite the parents' key role in the treatment, only a few studies have investigated parental satisfaction with their child's ED treatment [20–24], or with interventions aimed at parents [24, 25]. None of these studies has investigated parental satisfaction with family-based inpatient treatment. A study from the United Kingdom, for example, investigated patients' and parents' satisfaction with three types of services for adolescent AN [20]. Results showed that parental satisfaction was highest for specialized outpatient services, intermediate for specialized inpatient services, and lowest for unspecialized child and adolescent mental health services [20]. Research on family-based treatment for EDs have generally found high levels of parental satisfaction with treatment for adolescent AN, and interestingly, parents tend to be more satisfied than the patients themselves [20, 21]. Supporting parents' efforts to help their child is often underscored as an important aspect of care related to greater satisfaction [24, 25].

A core aspect of FBT involves the inclusion of both parents in treatment, provision of support, and close collaboration in helping their child to overcome the ED [11, 26]. In addition to a high level of maternal involvement, the extent of fathers' participation in FBT has been found to predict better outcome at the end of treatment [27]. Also, the agreement between mothers and fathers in their perceptions of treatment may influence their collaboration in coping with the ED. To our knowledge, only one previous study has compared mothers' and fathers' perceptions of their child's AN treatment [21]. In that study, both fathers and mothers reported an overall positive perception of their child's treatment, with a high level of parental agreement.

Knowledge is scarce and inconsistent as to whether patient and/or parent satisfaction with treatment for adolescent AN is associated with better ED outcome. In a study by Paulson-Karlsson et al. [23], there was no statistically significant difference in treatment satisfaction between recovered and not-recovered patients. However, the parents of recovered patients reported significantly higher treatment satisfaction than parents of non-recovered patients. A study by Halvorsen & Heyerdahl [21] found that patient and parental treatment satisfaction was not significantly associated with whether the patient still suffered from an ED at follow-up assessment.

The primary aim of the current study was to describe and compare how former patients, mothers, and fathers perceived and experienced family-based inpatient treatment for adolescent AN following discharge. Specifically, areas covered included the effectiveness or perceived benefit of treatment, perceptions of the therapists, and fulfillment of treatment goals at follow-up. Furthermore, a secondary aim was to investigate whether outcome (i.e., weight gain (kg) from admission to follow-up, BMI, and eating disorder psychopathology at follow-up) were related to patient and parent treatment satisfaction.

Methods

This was a sub-study of a larger follow-up of families who received family-based inpatient treatment for adolescent AN at the Regional Department for Eating Disorders at Oslo University Hospital during the period 2008–2014 [17]. Patients were referred from specialized mental health services and all had received previous inpatient and outpatient treatment at their local child- and adolescent mental health services. This had included family-based interventions, typically focusing on parental support to eat, but usually not manualized FBT. At the child and adolescent inpatient unit (for patients up to 18 years old), the standard treatment program is family-based treatment [11, 12] which has been adapted for delivery at an inpatient setting. This approach was selected based upon evidence supporting the effectiveness of FBT for adolescent AN in outpatient settings [13]. The unit has beds for a maximum of five patients to be admitted with their parents (and siblings when applicable).

Children under 18 years of age in Norway have the right to be accompanied by a parent during hospital stays because proximity to primary caregivers is considered important for the health and well-being of sick children and adolescents [28]. Parents/guardians in Norway receive financial benefits to stay with children under 18 years of age during hospitalization, which is usually equivalent to full salary. All families who participated in the present study had at least one parent who agreed to stay at the hospital with their child during the admission.

Participants and procedure

All former patients ($n = 58$) and parents ($n = 104$) who received family-based inpatient treatment at the unit during the period May 2008–June 2014 were contacted via a letter of invitation sent to each family member asking them to participate in the study. Non-responders were reminded by mail and/or telephone. In the case of re-admissions to the same unit, the focus of the follow-up was based upon the initial family admission. Only one family discontinued treatment against recommendations from the medical treatment team. At admission, all patients had a diagnosis of AN, with the exception of one patient who was admitted with a bulimia nervosa diagnosis despite a past history of AN. Mean age at admission was 15.8 ± 1.8 years, mean BMI percentile (for age and sex) 4.9 ± 15.4, and mean duration of illness 2.8 ± 1.8 years. Mean duration of the family admission was 20.3 ± 12.9 weeks, mean weight gain during the admission 7.1 ± 4.5 kg and mean discharge BMI percentile 20.9 ± 20.6.

The sample included 34 former patients, 40 mothers, and 20 fathers from 46 (79%) of the 58 eligible families. There were 31 mother/patient pairs, 18 mother/father pairs and 12 father/patient pairs available for the analyses. The number of participants from each family ranged from one to three. When the participants had provided written consent, they completed the follow-up assessment packet at home and brought it along to an interview conducted by an experienced clinician. No statistically significant differences existed between the 46 participating and the 12 non-participating families for the following background variables: duration of ED before admission, age at admission, admission BMI percentile, weight gain during the admission, discharge BMI percentile, age at the time of the follow-up study, and time between discharge to follow-up.

Treatment

Treatment principles from the Maudsley FBT [11, 12, 29] were adapted and modified for delivery on an inpatient setting. As in FBT-adapted day treatment programs [18] and traditional day treatment, the inpatient program was intensified compared to outpatient care to meet the needs of patients with severe medical conditions and/or unsatisfactory response to outpatient treatment. While day treatment, or partial hospitalization, programs may be delivered from a few hours to several days a week, and parents usually attend only part of that time [18], inpatient family-based treatment entails that one or both parents would stay at the hospital during the entire period to take part in the intensive daily care and treatment of their child [16, 17].

If the parents lived together ($N = 31$, 66% of the families), both parents were encouraged to stay at the unit to facilitate parental communication and to develop cooperative skills in managing the illness. Typically, both of the parents stayed at the unit during the first phase of the treatment, and thereafter alternated between staying at the hospital versus at home with siblings. If the parents did not live together ($N = 15$, 33%), one of the parents stayed at the hospital at a time, while both participated in treatment meetings, parental counseling, and family sessions. In nine (20%) of the families, only one parent was able to participate in treatment, typically due to health problems affecting the other parent or in the case of sole custody.

Most of the inpatient admission corresponds to the first phase of the Maudsley approach, where the main focus is on helping the parents take charge of their child's weight restoration. In our inpatient setting, the staff assumed more responsibility than in outpatient FBT to provide a structured regime for weight gain, i.e., by providing meal plans, prescribing supplemental nutritional drinks, or in seldom cases tube-feeding, if the patient did not finish her/his meal, and recommending how much activity and rest the child needed. The more extensive support was provided to help ensure adequate weight gain, as previous inpatient and outpatient treatment had not led to remission. Treatment was administered in close collaboration with the parents, and with a clear goal to support the parents' role in caring for their child both emotionally and with overcoming the ED.

The family ate all meals together in a designated family room or at a family table in the dining room. The parents were responsible for helping their child to eat sufficiently, while the staff's role was to support the parents to accomplish this task rather than taking over the responsibility for the child's eating. If the parents needed help during the meal, one of the staff members would encourage them to trust in themselves, to not give up and to support each other, but also offer consultation and specific advice, for example, on how to articulate and repeat the message that the food must be eaten. Milieu therapy staff aimed to support the whole family in coping with the ED, reducing conflicts, promoting cooperation and facilitating positive relationships between family members, and empowering parents to support their sick child. During the last phase of hospitalization, when most patients had regained normal body weight, the focus gradually shifted toward encouraging the adolescent to assume greater responsibility for eating and exercise with continued parental supervision, that is, to help themselves to food from the buffet or negotiate how to resume physical activities. This transition corresponds to the second phase in Maudsley FBT.

Physical health was closely monitored, and a weekly weight gain of approximately one kg was recommended. The individual treatment plan was reviewed and adjusted at weekly treatment meetings. Both parents attended treatment meetings, and occasionally, staff members from the referring local child- and adolescent mental health services also attended. The family spoke with the staff on a daily basis to review progress and attended joint family sessions once or twice a week. The family sessions included core elements from outpatient FBT/Maudsley approach, but was adapted to our inpatient setting and to the families' situation, which was characterized by long duration and severity of AN as well as previously unsuccessful treatment. Parents also attended weekly group sessions for parents, where they could share experiences and support one another, and meetings alone with staff members. Supportive individual sessions were offered weekly to patients if requested. During some periods, group sessions for patients and a sibling group was also offered. Finally, weekend leaves from the hospital were integrated into treatment to encourage patients and parents to practice and transfer skills to the home environment, with longer leaves granted toward the end of hospitalization. At discharge, the patients were referred to further outpatient treatment at their local mental health services. Thirty (88%) had received outpatient treatment, and 13 (38%) had been rehospitalized, during the follow-up period.

Data from the treatment phase were collected from patient records.

Assessment at follow-up

ED diagnoses and body weight were assessed by an experienced clinician at the patient interview [17].

Body weight and height

Body mass index (BMI, kg/m^2) was calculated from either measured ($n = 16$) or self-reported ($n = 18$) weight and height. Self-reported weight and height were used if the participant did not want to be weighed and when the interview took place at home or by telephone. Mean BMI based on measured weight/height (19.8 ± 3.3) did not differ from that based on self-report (19.9 ± 2.9, n.s.) in the group with only self-reported BMI.

Assessment of ED symptoms

The Eating Disorder Examination Questionnaire 6.0 (EDE-Q) [30] is a widely-used 28-item self-report measure of ED psychopathology based on the EDE interview. The EDE-Q focuses on core ED symptoms and behaviors, including binge eating and purging, during the past

28 days. It is comprised of four subscales: dietary restraint, eating concern, weight concern, and shape concern. The mean of the subscale scores comprises a global EDE-Q score. An EDE-Q global score $\leq$ 2.5 has been demonstrated as the clinical threshold to optimally distinguish non-cases from cases in a sample of Norwegian women [31]. The Norwegian version of the EDE-Q has shown adequate psychometric properties in community and clinical samples, with good convergent validity between the EDE and EDE-Q, and good internal consistency (Cronbach's Alpha coefficients 0.76–0.90) and inter-rater reliability (0.70–0.97) for the four subscales [32].

Assessment of treatment satisfaction

The following questionnaires were administered to former patients, mothers and fathers:

General satisfaction with treatment: The Norwegian Generic Short Patient Experiences Questionnaire (GS-PEQ) [1, 33] covers important aspects of user experiences across a range of specialist health services and is widely used in Norwegian health services. The questionnaire consists of 14 items with five response categories ranging from "not at all satisfied" to "very satisfied" (see Table 1). The GS-PEQ has shown good evidence for validity and reliability, good internal consistency (Cronbach's Alpha coeffiecient > 0.70) and good test-retest reliability (intraclass correlations between 0.62–0.85 for the different items) [34].

Perceived benefit of treatment: One item from the GS-PEQ on overall benefit of treatment was administered (Table 1, a). The test-retest reliability of this single item was found to be 0.73 [33]. Additionally, two items were designed by the authors to assess overall usefulness of treatment for other family members (Table 1, b and c) as well as items on the perceived utility of 19 different treatment aspects, with five response categories ranging from "no benefit" to "very large benefit".

Table 1 The family members' general experiences with, and benefit of, family inpatient treatment

General experiences with the treatment[a]	Mean score ± SD			Patients /moth.[b]		Patients./fath.[c]		Moth./fath.[d]	
	Patients N = 34	Mothers N = 40	Fathers N = 20	P-value[e]	Effect size[f]	P-value[e]	Effect size[f]	P-value[e]	Effect size[f]
Mean general experiences with treatment score (item 1–12)	3.2 ± 1.0	3.7 ± 0.7	3.9 ± 0.5	0.001	0.6	0.029	0.9	0.457	0.3
1. Did you have confidence in the clinicians' professional competence?	3.3 ± 1.4	4.1 ± 0.8	4.2 ± 0.5	0.006	0.7	0.117	0.9	0.718	0.1
2. Did the clinicians talk to you in a way that was easy to understand?	3.8 ± 1.0	4.4 ± 0.7	4.1 ± 0.6	0.001	0.7	0.236	0.4	0.579	0.5
3. Did you get sufficient information about the illness/ diagnosis?	3.6 ± 1.1	3.9 ± 0.9	3.9 ± 0.8	0.008	0.3	0.242	0.3	0.651	0.0
4. Did you perceive the treatment as suited to your situation?	2.9 ± 1.4	3.5 ± 1.2	3.9 ± 0.9	0.009	0.5	0.034	0.8	0.311	0.4
5. Were you involved in decisions regarding your/your child's treatment?	2.9 ± 1.2	3.7 ± 1.1	3.5 ± 0.9	0.038	0.7	0.191	0.7	0.529	0.3
6. Did you perceive the institution's work as well organized?	3.4 ± 1.3	3.9 ± 1.0	3.9 ± 0.7	0.055	0.4	0.223	0.5	0.632	0.0
7. Was the staff aware of siblings' situation?[g]	2.4 ± 1.2	3.2 ± 1.0	3.7 ± 0.8	0.003	0.7	0.120	1.3	0.510	0.6
8. Did the staff collaborate well with the parents?	3.4 ± 1.4	4.1 ± 0.8	4.1 ± 0.6	0.021	0.6	0.296	0.6	0.632	0.0
9. Did the staff collaborate well among themselves?	3.6 ± 1.2	4.0 ± 0.9	4.0 ± 0.5	0.131	0.4	0.312	0.4	0.458	0.0
10. Did the staff cooperate well with other public services?	3.2 ± 1.1	3.4 ± 1.0	3.8 ± 0.7	0.282	0.2	0.082	0.7	0.111	0.5
11. Did you perceive that the institution prepared you for the time after discharge?	2.6 ± 1.4	3.0 ± 1.1	3.3 ± 0.9	0.142	0.3	0.468	0.6	0.718	0.3
12. Overall, was the help and treatment you/ your child received satisfactory?	2.9 ± 1.3	3.7 ± 1.0	4.1 ± 0.9	< 0.001	0.7	0.001	1.3	0.333	0.6
Mean score on overall benefit of the treatment for family members (a-c)[h]	3.1 ± 1.0	3.3 ± 1.1	3.5 ± 1.1	0.019	0.2	0.046	0.4	0.913	0.2
a) Overall benefit for the patient	3.0 ± 1.1	3.6 ± 1.1	3.6 ± 1.2	< 0.001	0.5	0.016	0.5	0.333	0.0
b) Overall benefit for the parents	3.5 ± 1.1	3.6 ± 1.1	3.7 ± 1.0	0.147	0.1	0.795	0.2	0.331	0.1
c) Overall benefit for siblings[g]	2.7 ± 1.3	2.4 ± 1.3	3.0 ± 1.2	0.843	0.2	0.457	0.2	0.305	0.5
Mean score on benefit of 19 different treatment elements[g]	3.0 ± 0.9	3.4 ± 0.9	3.4 ± 0.8	0.042	0.4	0.218	0.5	0.128	0.0

[a)]Reply options: not at all, to a small extent, to a moderate extent, to a large extent, to a very large extent. Possible range:1–5, more satisfied the higher score, [b)] 31 pairs, [c)] 12 pairs, d)18 pairs, [e)]paired samples t-tests, [f)]Cohen's d (small: 0.2. medium: 0.5, large: 0.8), [g)]applicable for $n = 25$ patients, $n = 35$ mothers and $n = 19$ fathers, [h)]reply options: no benefit, little benefit, some benefit, large benefit, very large benefit. Possible range:1–5, more satisfied the higher score

Perception of therapists (POT): A treatment satisfaction questionnaire from the Swedish National Quality Register on EDs [21, 35] was translated into Norwegian by the first author. The instrument consists of 11 items on the perceptions of the therapists, which in this context was defined as all staff members who participated in the treatment, plus two items for parents that were added for this study (Table 2). The instrument has six response categories ranging from "never" to "always".

Treatment goals: Another questionnaire from the same Swedish National Quality Register [21, 35] was used, and was translated into Norwegian by the first author. The instrument includes ten goals for ED treatment that were rated according to the degree to which each goal was perceived as fulfilled (four response categories ranging from "not at all" to "yes, completely") (Table 3). The original instrument also had questions about each goal's relevance and importance, but these were not used in the present study.

Statistical analyses

Data were fairly normally distributed and parametric analyses were used. Independent t-tests were used to investigate differences in background variables between participants and non-participants. Differences between former patients, mothers, and fathers on the treatment satisfaction measures were investigated using paired samples t-tests. Bivariate associations between continuous variables were investigated with Pearson's correlations. All analyses were two-tailed. When multiple analyses were used, the alpha level was set at $p \leq .01$.

The study was approved by the Regional Medical Ethics Committee.

Results

The average time between discharge and follow-up was 4.5 ± 1.7 years (range 1.3–7.0). Mean age of the former patients was 20.4 ± 2.7 years. Twenty-one (62%) of the participants were weight recovered (i.e., BMI ≥ 18.5) and 13 (38%) fully recovered (i.e., normal eating attitudes and behavior defined as an EDE-Q global score ≤ 2.5, no binge eating/purging during the past three months, and BMI ≥ 18.5).

General experience with treatment

Overall, parents reported a high level of satisfaction with all central aspects of treatment, including perceived competence of the therapists, communication and collaboration (Table 1). There were no significant

Table 2 Perception of the contact with the therapists/staff members who participated in the treatment (POT) by patients and their parents

	Mean score ± SD			Patient/mother[c]		Patient/father[d]		Mother/father[e]	
	Patient N = 34	Mother N = 40	Father N = 20	P-value[f]	Effect size[g]	P-value[f]	Effect size[g]	P-value[f]	Effect size[g]
Mean POT[a] score (item 1–11)	3.6 ± 1.2	4.6 ± 0.9	4.8 ± 0.7	< 0.001	0.9	< 0.001	1.2	0.227	0.2
Do you think that the therapist(s)[b]:									
1. Understood your problems?	3.3 ± 1.4	4.5 ± 1.0	4.5 ± 0.6	< 0.001	1.0	0.007	1.1	0.751	0.0
2. Received you well?	4.1 ± 1.4	4.8 ± 0.9	4.9 ± 0.8	0.002	0.6	0.001	0.7	0.261	0.1
3. Respected you as a person?	4.2 ± 1.5	4.9 ± 1.1	5.2 ± 0.8	0.002	0.5	0.003	0.8	0.264	0.3
4. Let you to talk about what was important to you?	4.1 ± 1.6	4.7 ± 1.1	5.0 ± 0.6	0.018	0.4	0.013	0.7	0.164	0.3
5. Listened to you?	4.1 ± 1.5	4.6 ± 1.2	5.0 ± 0.7	0.103	0.4	0.002	0.8	0.188	0.4
6. Were able to help you/your daughter/son?	3.6 ± 1.6	4.1 ± 1.3	4.2 ± 1.3	0.022	0.3	0.017	0.4	0.751	0.1
7. Gave your parents/you enough help to support you/your daughter/son in overcoming the ED?	3.0 ± 1.4	4.6 ± 1.2	4.7 ± 0.9	< 0.001	1.2	0.001	1.4	0.387	0.1
8. Agreed with you on the treatment goal?	2.9 ± 1.5	4.8 ± 1.0	4.7 ± 1.0	< 0.001	1.5	< 0.001	1.4	0.721	0.1
9. Agreed with you on how the treatment should be?	2.9 ± 1.4	4.4 ± 1.0	4.5 ± 0.9	< 0.001	1.2	< 0.001	1.4	0.586	0.1
10. Had sufficient knowledge of ED and knew what they were doing?	3.8 ± 1.6	4.9 ± 1.1	4.9 ± 1.0	< 0.001	0.8	0.002	0.8	1	0.0
11. Valued your own efforts in overcoming the ED?	3.6 ± 1.7	4.7 ± 1.2	4.8 ± 1.0	0.001	0.7	0.001	0.9	0.301	0.1
For parents only:									
12. Were able to help you as a mother/father?		4.1 ± 1.2	4.3 ± 0.8					0.818	0.2
13. Gave you enough help to support each other as parents?		3.9 ± 1.4	4.5 ± 1.1					0.302	0.5

[a] Perception of therapists, [b]reply options: never, seldom, sometimes, often, very often, always. Possible range:1–6, more satisfied the higher score, [c] 31 pairs, [d] 12 pairs: $n = 24$, e) 18 pairs,, [f]paired samples t-tests, [g]Cohen's d (small: 0.2, medium: 0.5, large: 0.8)

Table 3 Fulfillment of treatment goals

	Mean score ± SD			Patients /moth.[b]		Patients./fath.[c]		Moth./fath.[d]	
	Patients N = 34	Mothers N = 40	Fathers N = 20	P-value[e]	Effect size[f]	P-value[e]	Effect size[f]	P-value[e]	Effect size[f]
Mean goal fulfillment score (mean of the 10 potential goals)	2.1 ± 0.7	2.4 ± 0.6	2.6 ± 0.6	0.006	0.5	0.019	0.8	0.527	0.3
Potential treatment goals: Was the goal fulfilled?[a]									
1. To learn more about eating disorders	2.4 ± 0.9	2.8 ± 0.7	2.9 ± 0.6	0.094	0.5	0.045	0.7	0.775	0.2
2. To get help talking about painful experiences	2.3 ± 1.1	2.4 ± 0.7	2.6 ± 0.7	1.000	0.1	0.799	0.3	0.336	0.3
3. Learn to eat normally	2.3 ± 1.0	2.4 ± 0.9	2.4 ± 0.8	0.326	0.1	0.760	0.1	0.720	0.0
4. Learn to cope with unreasonable notions about food and body size	1.8 ± 0.7	2.3 ± 0.8	2.4 ± 0.9	0.008	0.7	0.081	0.7	0.190	0.1
5. Become more satisfied with myself and my body	1.5 ± 0.7	2.1 ± 0.8	2.3 ± 0.9	< 0.001	0.8	0.019	1.0	0.426	0.2
6. To get help to stand up for what I feel / she or he feels	2.0 ± 1.0	2.4 ± 0.7	2.6 ± 0.6	0.036	0.5	0.104	0.7	0.336	0.3
7. Reduce guilt and self-blame	1.7 ± 0.8	2.2 ± 0.7	2.3 ± 0.9	0.002	0.7	0.021	0.7	0.793	0.1
8. To get support in crisis situations	2.6 ± 1.1	2.8 ± 0.9	2.8 ± 1.0	0.231	0.2	0.321	0.2	0.613	001
9. Get help to cope with difficult feelings such as sadness, anxiety and anger	2.2 ± 1.0	2.4 ± 0.8	2.4 ± 0.7	0.183	0.2	0.563	0.2	1.000	0.0
10. To reduce conflicts in the family related to difficulties with eating	2.1 ± 0.9	2.5 ± 0.8	2.6 ± 0.8	0.004	0.5	0.049	0.6	0.673	0.1

[a)] Range: 1–4, the higher score the more fulfilled. Reply options: 1 = not at all, 2 = only to some extent, 3 = yes, mostly, 4 = yes, absolutely, [b)] 31 pairs, [c)] 12 pairs, [d)]18 pairs, [e)]paired samples t-tests, [f)]Cohen's d (small: 0.2, medium: 0.5, large: 0.8)

differences between mothers and fathers in their general experience of treatment. Former patients had significantly lower scores than mothers and fathers on the items, "Did you perceive the treatment as well-suited to your situation?" and "Overall, was the help and treatment you/your child received satisfactory?" In addition, former patients had significantly lower mean scores on the 12 general experience items. Effect sizes indicated moderate to large differences in scores between parents and former patients (Table 1). The mean score for former patients' "general experience with treatment" was 3.2 (±1.0), reflecting a medium level of satisfaction. All family members had the lowest scores on the item: "Did you perceive that the institution prepared you for the time after discharge?"

Five percent of mothers and fathers replied that they thought their child had "in any way received the wrong treatment", in contrast to 15% of the former patients.

Benefit of treatment

The former patients rated their own overall benefit from treatment significantly lower than the parental ratings of the overall benefit for their child (medium effect sizes, Table 1). However, former patients and parents had similar views on the overall benefit of treatment for parents. Parents and former patients also had similar, but lower, ratings on the overall benefit for siblings (Table 1). Table 1 illustrates the mean scores for the perceived benefit of 19 different treatment elements.

Perception of the contact with the therapists/staff members

Mothers and fathers alike reported a similarly high level of satisfaction with therapist contact (Table 2). The former patients, however, perceived the contact with therapists more negatively than mothers or fathers, with medium-to-large effect sizes. The former patients gave the highest ratings to being well-received, respected, allowed to talk about what was important to her/him, and being listened to (> 4, corresponding to "often"). The lowest scores (≤ 3, corresponding to "sometimes") related to agreement on treatment goals, agreement on treatment structure/content, and the help their parents had received to support their recovery from an ED.

Fulfillment of treatment goals

Ten possible goals for ED treatment were rated according to the extent to which the goal was perceived as fulfilled (Table 3). Former patients had a significantly lower overall mean goal fulfillment score than mothers and fathers (medium-large effect sizes) as well as poorer ratings for several of the specific goals. Receiving "help in crisis situations" and "learning more about EDs" were perceived by all participants (former patients, mothers, and fathers) as the most fulfilled goals. Increased satisfaction with body/self, reduction of guilt/shame, and learning to cope with unrealistic beliefs regarding food and body weight/shape were perceived as the least fulfilled goals by all groups.

Correlations between treatment satisfaction measures and outcome variables

As shown in Table 4, correlations were performed to investigate associations between the various aspects of treatment satisfaction and the three ED outcome variables (weight gain from admission to follow-up, BMI and EDE-Q global score at follow-up). Among former patients, all correlations between treatment satisfaction and the ED outcome variables were low ($r \leq 0.17$, n.s.). Among mothers, all correlations were low except the correlation between mothers' average goal fulfillment score and the two outcome variables weight gain from admission to follow-up ($r = 0.49$, $p = 0.008$) and BMI at follow-up ($r = 0.56$, $p = 0.002$). In contrast, for the fathers, all the treatment satisfaction measures showed large correlations with weight gain from admission to follow-up and BMI at follow-up, but not with the EDE-Q global score (Table 4).

Discussion

Despite the crucial role that parents play in treatment engagement and adherence for their child, research is scarce on how parents perceive and experience treatment for adolescent AN. This study investigated patient and parental satisfaction with family-based inpatient treatment for adolescent AN as assessed retrospectively at approximately five years (4.5 ± 1.7 years) following discharge.

Several main conclusions can be derived from our findings. First, mothers and fathers alike reported similar and overall positive experiences with treatment, whereas the former patients were significantly less satisfied than parents, reporting a medium level of overall satisfaction. Second, we found no strong support for the notion that treatment satisfaction was associated with outcome of the ED. Eating disorder symptomology as measured by the EDE-Q demonstrated very low correlations ($r < 0.2$, n.s.) with the various aspects of treatment satisfaction rated by patients and parents.

Our finding that parents reported a higher level of satisfaction with their child's AN treatment than the patients themselves is in accordance with three other studies comparing parents' and patients' treatment satisfaction [20, 21, 23]. The very low dropout rate from treatment in the present study (1/58 families) may be related to the high level of parental satisfaction. Overall, mothers and fathers reported rather similar perceptions of treatment, which might be a positive factor for collaboration and consistency between the parents in their efforts to help their child. In terms of perceived benefit of treatment for the child, former patients showed lower ratings than parents, however, all family members rated the overall benefit for parents as good (Table 1). FBT emphasizes that the parents, not the patient, must take charge of their child's weight restoration, and, thus, the parents' benefit of treatment may be an important factor for outcome. One reason for FBT's superiority compared to individually-based treatment for adolescent AN may be that the treatment is less affected by the young patient's own ambivalence and fear of weight gain.

Table 4 Correlations between treatment satisfaction variables and ED outcome variables[a]

		ED outcome variables		
		Weight gain from admission to follow-up	BMI At follow-up	EDE-Q global score At follow-up
Weight gain from admission to follow-up		1		
BMI at follow-up		0.82*	1	0.02
EDE-Q global score at follow-up		0.10	0.02	1
Mean general experiences with treatment score (see Table 1)	Patient	0.08	0.11	0.09
	Mother	0.28	0.19	0.10
	Father	0.66	0.68	0.20
Mean score on overall benefit of the treatment for family members (see Table 1)	Patient	0.16	0.17	0.03
	Mother	0.20	0.16	0.16
	Father	0.72*	0.62	−0.03
Mean Perception of therapist (POT) score (see Table 2)	Patient	0.06	0.17	−0.07
	Mother	0.17	0.15	0.07
	Father	0.67	0.72	−0.08
Mean goal fulfillment score (see Table 3)	Patient	−0.05	0.05	−0.07
	Mother	0.49*	0.56*	−0.07
	Father	0.84*	0.85*	0.15

[a]Pearson's correlations. Number of pairs: between patient variables: 34, patient/mother: 31, patient/father: 12

*$p < 0.001$

Studies of patient satisfaction with health services tend to find that most patients report a high level of satisfaction [33, 36], which is consistent with the present findings for parents, but not the patients. AN is a highly ego-syntonic disorder for those personally afflicted by the illness, but not for parents, and this may differentially influence patients' and parents' perceptions of treatment [37, 38]. Extreme fear of eating and weight gain are core symptoms of AN, and the patients usually experience particularly strong ambivalence to treatment components directly aiming to restore a healthy body weight [38]. Weight restoration is a main overarching goal for hospitalization and, thus, it may be natural that patients, even in retrospect, might experience their ED treatment as difficult and challenging, with lower treatment satisfaction ratings than their parents.

Lower patient scores were observed for items related to agreement with treatment goals and treatment content/structure, with average scores of 2.9 (corresponding to "sometimes"). As several aspects of treatment were non-negotiable, such as the amount of food, amount of rest and physical activity, this finding is perhaps expected. Unfortunately, we do not know whether former patients desired greater influence on their treatment plan, or if they retrospectively felt that parents and therapists needed to manage these aspects of treatment.

Various aspects of the therapeutic relationship, such as being well-received, respected, listened to, and having the freedom to discuss personally important topics received the highest treatment satisfaction ratings from former patients. This finding is consistent with other studies that have found that patients with AN tend to be satisfied with their relationship with therapists [39], but less satisfied with treatment goals relating to restoration of a healthy body weight, which are goals typically viewed as essential by healthcare professionals [38, 40]. Suffering from AN during adolescence is inarguably extremely difficult and distressing, and it is encouraging that the majority of former patients retrospectively perceived their relationship with the therapists positively, despite the lower rating given for other aspects of treatment.

Inpatient treatment has been shown to be effective in achieving weight gain, but less effective in improving psychological symptoms [41, 42]. Consistent with these findings, our sample of former patients, mothers, and fathers reported the lowest goal fulfillment scores for reducing psychological ED symptoms, e.g., body dissatisfaction, and intermediate scores for the item "learning to eat normally". Outcome studies of FBT for adolescent AN have found that the majority of the patients successfully achieved weight recovery by the end of treatment and/or follow-up, but that a lower proportion achieved normal eating attitudes [13]. For instance, in a randomized treatment study by Lock et al. [43] only 34% of participants who had received FBT, and 20% that had received individual therapy, had achieved both EDE-Q global scores in the normal range and full weight-restoration at one year follow-up. Consistent with other studies [13], a minority (38%) was shown to meet the criteria for full recovery at follow-up in our study despite the rather long follow-up time (4.5 years) [17].

It might have been expected that patients with a favorable ED outcome and their parents would be comparatively more satisfied with treatment. However, in line with two other studies [21, 23], we did not find any strong evidence to support this assertion. Our results suggested no clear picture of the relationship between treatment satisfaction and degree of improvement or outcome at follow-up. Some were satisfied with treatment despite having a poor ED outcome, while others were less satisfied despite having a favorable outcome, perhaps believing they had managed to overcome the illness despite unsatisfactory treatment. It is possible that patients tend to value the therapeutic relationship, while aspects of treatment that directly tackle weight-restoration, despite being necessary to recover from AN, are associated with ambivalence and reluctance.

Parental therapeutic alliance in FBT has been found to be associated with weight gain, which parents have control over in FBT, but less associated with cognitive improvement that parents have less control over [44]. Unlike mothers and former patients, the fathers' ratings of treatment satisfaction correlated strongly with the patients' weight outcome. Thus, weight recovery may have contributed to treatment satisfaction among fathers, or, vice versa, that fathers with high levels of treatment satisfaction contributed to effective weight restoration [44]. Further research should investigate whether fathers emphasize the importance of achieving a healthy body weight to a greater extent than mothers or patients. This would be consistent with a study on fathers' views on parental interventions which found that fathers tended to prefer a focus on measurable outcomes [45]. It is possible that fathers may experience even stronger feelings of helplessness than mothers when their child is affected by AN and that they particularly appreciated the focus on strengthening specific parental skills in helping their underweight child gain weight during the family-based treatment. Fathers may also feel that mental health services are focused on the mother and perhaps consider the mother's competence and ability to provide care as more important [45]. One study found that the mothers' attendance in FBT-sessions for adolescent AN was much higher than fathers', but that a higher rate of attendance by fathers predicted better outcome [27], suggesting the importance of extensive involvement of both mothers and fathers in AN treatment.

The present study provides insight into patient and parental satisfaction with family-based inpatient treatment for adolescent AN, which is a novel treatment approach with comparatively less research attention. Moreover, studies of patient and parental satisfaction for treatment of adolescent AN is scarce, despite the importance to improve available health services. The inclusion of both parents is considered essential in FBT, but there is a lack of studies on how mothers and fathers experience treatment. The present study included several measures of treatment satisfaction, and compared satisfaction between former patients, mothers, and fathers.

Nevertheless, this study had several limitations that should be noted. The number of participants was small, rendering statistical power low. The number of participants from the same families varied, which limited the numbers of available pairs to investigate mean differences or correlations. In particular, the available patient-father pairs were low ($n = 12$ pairs), which renders uncertainty about the representativeness of the results. Thus, these findings should be considered preliminary and require replication. Treatment satisfaction was assessed at follow-up, following an average of 4.5 years after discharge, which is likely to have affected how the participants recalled the treatment. The majority of the patients had received further treatment during the follow-up period, which also might have influenced their retrospective perceptions of the family inpatient program. "General satisfaction with treatment" was assessed with an instrument with well-established psychometric properties, although data on reliability or validity were unavailable for two of the treatment satisfaction questionnaires ("Perception of the contact with the therapists" and "Treatment goals"). Furthermore, the study was conducted at the institution that had delivered the treatment, which might have influenced the family members' responses.

Family admissions are demanding both for health service providers and parents, and the generalizability of findings related to this treatment approach may be limited by a lack of social welfare systems to compensate for parents' loss of income during their child's illness. However, individual admissions also demand extensive resources from families and the health services. If individual admissions are shown to be less effective than family admissions, resulting in prolonged parental distress and burden of care [46, 47], this could adversely affect parents' health and work ability, surpassing the financial toll incurred during a family admission. When an adolescent with AN fails to remit despite receiving outpatient FBT, the parents need extensive support to regain trust in their own ability to help their child [48]. Individual admissions might be less beneficial for the parent-child relationship, mother-father collaboration, and their ability to cope with the ED, both during and after the hospital stay. Thus, greater knowledge is warranted about inpatient approaches that include parents in the treatment of adolescents with AN.

Caring for siblings was an important dilemma encountered during the family admissions, and parents found it often challenging to determine whether siblings should stay at the hospital to maximize treatment participation, or remain at home to maintain regular contact with their school, friends, and activities. Although the unit emphasized awareness of siblings' needs, parents and patients alike perceived the overall benefit of the treatment for siblings as small to moderate. Adolescent AN greatly affects siblings' family situation and daily life [49–51], and concern for the welfare of siblings was especially prominent in our study, owing to the severity and chronicity that characterized the patient sample. More research on the perspectives of the siblings of adolescents with AN is important, and in particular, how parents and health services should accommodate the needs of siblings.

Clinical implications and conclusion

A clinical implication from this study is that family-based inpatient treatment for adolescents with AN may be a useful option when outpatient treatment has proven insufficient. We found that parents, and to some degree former patients, were satisfied with this treatment approach, which supports its feasibility. All families agreed that one or both of the parents would stay at the hospital for the full length of the admission, and dropout was very low (1/58), which also supports the acceptability of the treatment. Although the participation of both parents is crucial in FBT, fathers' participation level is often low. Our finding that fathers reported a similar, and equally high, level of satisfaction as mothers indicates that the treatment approach was perceived as useful for fathers as well as for mothers, which is likely to promote fathers' participation.

Abbreviations

AN: Anorexia nervosa; ED: Eating disorder; EDE-Q: The eating disorder examination questionnaire; FBT: Family-based treatment; GS-PEQ: The Norwegian generic short patient experiences questionnaire; POT: Perception of therapists; TAU: Treatment as usual

Acknowledgements

We wish to thank the participants for their time and effort in helping enhance our knowledge of how families experience treatment. We thank our leaders and colleagues for their valuable contributions to the study, and Selma Øverland Lie and Deborah L. Reas for language editing.

Authors' contributions

The first author has had the main responsibility for planning the study, data collection, data analyses and writing the paper. The second author's contribution has been consultation on all parts of the study, and particularly on data analyses and the writing of the paper. Both authors read and approved the final manuscript.

Competing interests

The author declares that he has no competing interests.

Author details
[1]Regional Department for Eating Disorders, Division of Mental Health and Addiction, Oslo University Hospital - Ullevål Hospital, P.O. Box 4956, Nydalen, N-0424 Oslo, Norway. [2]Division of Mental Health and Addiction, Institute of Clinical Medicine, University of Oslo, Oslo, Norway.

References

1. Sjetne IS, Bjertnaes OA, Olsen RV, Iversen HH, Bukholm G. The generic short patient experiences questionnaire (GS-PEQ): identification of core items from a survey in Norway. BMC Health Serv Res. 2011;11:88. https://doi.org/10.1186/1472-6963-11-88.
2. Peterson CB, Becker CB, Treasure J, Shafran R, Bryant-Waugh R. The three-legged stool of evidence-based practice in eating disorder treatment: research, clinical, and patient perspectives. BMC Med. 2016;14:69. https://doi.org/10.1186/s12916-016-0615-5.
3. Escobar-Koch T, Banker JD, Crow S, Cullis J, Ringwood S, Smith G, et al. Service users' views of eating disorder services: an international comparison. Int J Eat Disord. 2010;43(6):549–59. https://doi.org/10.1002/eat.20741.
4. Clinton D, Bjorck C, Sohlberg S, Norring C. Patient satisfaction with treatment in eating disorders: cause for complacency or concern? Eur Eat Disord Rev. 2004;12(4):240–6. https://doi.org/10.1111/j.1365-2702.2004.00943.x.
5. Offord A, Turner H, Cooper M. Adolescent inpatient treatment for anorexia nervosa: a qualitative study exploring young Adults' retrospective views of treatment and discharge. Eur Eat Disord Rev. 2006;14:377–87. https://doi.org/10.1002/erv.687.
6. Bell L. What can we learn from consumer studies and qualitative research in the treatment of eating disorders? Eat Weight Disord. 2003;8:181–7.
7. Kahn C, Pike KM. In search of predictors of dropout from inpatient treatment for anorexia nervosa. IntJ Eat Disord. 2001;30(3):237–44. https://doi.org/10.1002/eat.1080.
8. Dejong H, Broadbent H, Schmidt U. A systematic review of dropout from treatment in outpatients with anorexia nervosa. IntJEatDisord. 2012;45(5):635–47. https://doi.org/10.1002/eat.20956.
9. Thomson S, Marriott M, Telford K, Law H, McLaughlin J, Sayal K. Adolescents with a diagnosis of anorexia nervosa: parents' experience of recognition and deciding to seek help. Clin Child Psychol Psychiatry. 2014;19(1):43–57. https://doi.org/10.1177/1359104512465741.
10. Pereira T, Lock J, Oggins J. Role of therapeutic alliance in family therapy for adolescent anorexia nervosa. IntJ Eat Disord. 2006;39(8):677–84. https://doi.org/10.1002/eat.20303.
11. Lock J, le Grange D. Treatment Manual for Anorexia Nervosa. A Family-Based Approach. 2. New York: Guilford Press; 2012 Aug. 24, 2012. ISBN 978-1-4625-0676-7.
12. Blessitt E, Voulgari S, Eisler I. Family therapy for adolescent anorexia nervosa. CurrOpinPsychiatry. 2015;28(6):455–60. https://doi.org/10.1097/YCO.0000000000000193.
13. Couturier J, Kimber M, Szatmari P. Efficacy of family-based treatment for adolescents with eating disorders: a systematic review and meta-analysis. IntJEatDisord. 2013;46(1):3–11. https://doi.org/10.1002/eat.22042.
14. NICE Guideline. Eating disorders: recognition and treatment. NG69. London: National Institute of Clinical Excellence; 2017.
15. Murray SB, Anderson LK, Rockwell R, Griffiths S, Le Grange D, Kaye WH. Adapting family-based treatment for adolescent anorexia nervosa across higher levels of patient care. EatDisord. 2015;23(4):302–14. https://doi.org/10.1080/10640266.2015.1042317.
16. Matthews A, Peterson CM, Peugh J, Mitan L. An intensive family-based treatment guided intervention for medically hospitalized youth with anorexia nervosa: parental self-efficacy and weight-related outcomes. Eur Eating Disord Rev. 2019;27(1):67–75. https://doi.org/10.1002/erv.2632.
17. Halvorsen I, Reas DL, Nilsen J-V, Rø Ø. Naturalistic outcome of family-based inpatient treatment for adolescents with anorexia nervosa. Eur Eat Disord Rev. 2018;26(2):141–5. https://doi.org/10.1002/erv.2572.
18. Richards IL, Subar A, Touyz S, Rhodes P. Augmentative approaches in family-based treatment for adolescents with restrictive eating disorders: a systematic review. Eur Eat Disord Rev. 2018;26(2):92–111. https://doi.org/10.1002/erv.2577.
19. Wallis A, Alford C, Hanson A, Titterton J, Madden S, Kohn M. Innovations in Maudsley family-based treatment for anorexia nervosa at the Children's Hospital at Westmead: a family admission programme. J Fam Ther. 2013;35:68–81. https://doi.org/10.1111/j.1467-6427.2012.00604.x.
20. Roots P, Rowlands L, Gowers SG. User satisfaction with services in a randomised controlled trial of adolescent anorexia nervosa. EurEatDisordRev. 2009;17(5):331–7. https://doi.org/10.1002/erv.944.
21. Halvorsen I, Heyerdahl S. Treatment perception in adolescent onset anorexia nervosa: retrospective views of patients and parents. IntJEatDisord. 2007;40(7):629–39. https://doi.org/10.1002/erv.2191.
22. Krautter T, Lock J. Is manualized family-based treatment for adolescent anorexia nervosa acceptable to patients? Patient satisfaction at the end of treatment. J Fam Ther. 2004;26(1):67–82. https://doi.org/10.1111/j.1467-6427.2004.00267.x.
23. Paulson-Karlsson G, Nevonen L, Engström I. Anorexia nervosa: treatment satisfaction. J Fam Ther. 2006;28:293–306. https://doi.org/10.1111/j.1467-6427.2006.00353.x.
24. Zucker NL, Marcus M, Bulik C. A group parent-training program: a novel approach for eating disorder management. Eat Weight Disord. 2006;11(2):78–82.
25. Pasold TL, Boateng BA, Portilla MG. The use of a parent support group in the outpatient treatment of children and adolescents with eating disorders. Eat Disord. 2010;18(4):318–32. https://doi.org/10.1080/10640266.2010.490121.
26. Forsberg S, Lock J. Family-based treatment of child and adolescent eating disorders. Child Adolesc Psychiatr Clin N Am. 2015;24(3):617–29. https://doi.org/10.1016/j.chc.2015.02.012.
27. Hughes EK, Burton C, Le Grange D, Sawyer SM. The participation of mothers, fathers, and siblings in family-based treatment for adolescent anorexia nervosa. J Clin Child Adolesc Psychol. 2017:1–11. https://doi.org/10.1080/15374416.2017.1390756.
28. van der Horst FCP, van der Veer R. Changing attitudes towards the care of children in hospital: a new assessment of the influence of the work of Bowlby and Robertson in the UK, 1940–1970. Attach Hum Dev. 2009;11(2):119–42. https://doi.org/10.1080/14616730802503655.
29. Eisler I, Simic M, Blessitt E, Dodge L. Maudsley Service Manual for Child and Adolescent Eating Disorders. https://www.national.slam.nhs.uk/.../Maudsley-Service-Manual-for-Child-and-Adolescen... King's Health Partners. Kings's College Hospital. South London and Maudsley. London; 2016. p. 1–164.
30. Fairburn CG, Beglin SJ. Assessment of eating disorders: interview or self-report questionnaire? Int J Eat Disord. 1994;16(4):363–70. https://doi.org/10.1002/1098-108X(199412)16:4<363::AID-EAT2260160405>3.0.CO;2-#.
31. Ro O, Reas DL, Stedal K. Eating disorder examination questionnaire (EDE-Q) in Norwegian adults: discrimination between female controls and eating disorder patients. Eur Eat Disord Rev. 2015;23(5):408–12. https://doi.org/10.1002/erv.2372.
32. Reas DL, Wisting L, Kapstad H, Lask B. Convergent validity of the eating disorder examination and the eating disorder examination-questionnaire among university women in Norway. EurEatDisordRev. 2011;19(4):357–61. https://doi.org/10.1002/erv.1068.
33. Bjertnaes OA, Sjetne IS, Iversen HH. Overall patient satisfaction with hospitals: effects of patient-reported experiences and fulfilment of expectations. BMJ Qual Saf. 2012;21(1):39–46. https://doi.org/10.1136/bmjqs-2011-000137.
34. Pettersen KI, Veenstra M, Guldvog B, Kolstad A. The patient experiences questionnaire: development, validity and reliability. Int J Qual Health Care. 2004;16(6):453–63. https://doi.org/10.1093/intqhc/mzh074.
35. Lago C, Norring C, Engström I. Rikssät. ional Quality Register for Eating Disorders Treatment (Nationellt kvalitetsregister för ätstörningsbehandling, Rikssät). Center for Psychiatry Research (Psykiatriskt forskningscentrum). Örebro läns landsting. Sweden; 1998.
36. Williams B, Coyle J, Healy D. The meaning of patient satisfaction: an explanation of high reported levels. Soc Sci Med. 1998;(9):47, 1351–1349. https://doi.org/10.1016/S0277-9536(98)00213-5.
37. Bravender T, Elkus H, Lange H. Inpatient medical stabilization for adolescents with eating disorders: patient and parent perspectives. Eating and weight disorders. EWD. 2017;22(3):483–9. https://doi.org/10.1007/s40519-016-0270-z.
38. Westwood LM, Kendal SE. Adolescent client views towards the treatment of anorexia nervosa: a review ofthe literature. J Psychiatr Ment Health Nurs. 2012;19(6):500–8. https://doi.org/10.1111/j.1365-2850.2011.01819.x.
39. Hannon J, Eunson L, Munro C. The patient experience of illness, treatment, and change, during intensive community treatment for severe anorexia nervosa. Eat Disord. 2017;25(4):279–96. https://doi.org/10.1080/10640266.2017.1318626.
40. de la Rie S, Noordenbos G, Donker M, van Furth E. Evaluating the treatment of eating disorders from the patient's perspective. Int J Eat Disord. 2006;39:11. https://doi.org/10.1002/eat.20317

41. Goddard E, Hibbs R, Raenker S, Salerno L, Arcelus J, Boughton N, et al. A multi-Centre cohort study of short term outcomes of hospital treatment for anorexia nervosa in the UK. BMC Psychiatry. 2013;13:287. https://doi.org/10.1186/1471-244X-13-287.:287-13.
42. Hartmann A, Weber S, Herpertz S, Zeeck A. Psychological treatment for anorexia nervosa: a meta-analysis of standardized mean change. PsychotherPsychosom. 2011;80(4):216–26. https://doi.org/10.1159/000322360.
43. Lock J, le Grange D, Agras WS, Moye A, Bryson SW, Jo B. Randomized clinical trial comparing family-based treatment with adolescent-focused individual therapy for adolescents with anorexia nervosa. ArchGenPsychiatry. 2010;67(10):1025–32. https://doi.org/10.1001/archgenpsychiatry.2010.128.
44. Isserlin L, Couturier J. Therapeutic alliance and family-based treatment for adolescents with anorexia nervosa. Psychotherapy(Chic). 2012;49(1):46–51. https://doi.org/10.1037/a0023905.
45. Sicouri G, Tully L, Collins D, Burn M, Sargeant K, Frick P, et al. Toward father-friendly parenting interventions: a qualitative study. Aust N Z J Fam Ther. 2018;39(2):218–31. https://doi.org/10.1002/anzf.1307.
46. Raenker S, Hibbs R, Goddard E, Naumann U, Arcelus J, Ayton A, et al. Caregiving and coping in carers of people with anorexia nervosa admitted for intensive hospital care. Int J Eat Disord. 2013;46(4):346–54. https://doi.org/10.1002/eat.22068.
47. Anastasiadou D, Medina-Pradas C, Sepulveda AR, Treasure J. A systematic review of family caregiving in eating disorders. Eat Behav. 2014;15(3):464–77. https://doi.org/10.1016/j.eatbeh.2014.06.001/1471-0153.
48. Wufong E, Rhodes P, Conti J. "We don't really know what else we can do": Parent experiences when adolescent distress persists after the Maudsley and family-based therapies for anorexia nervosa. J Eat Disord. 2019;7:5. https://doi.org/10.1186/s40337-019-0235-5.
49. Halvorsen I, Ro O, Heyerdahl S. Nine-year follow-up of girls with anorexia nervosa and their siblings: retrospective perceptions of parental bonding and the influence of illness on their everyday life. EurEatDisordRev. 2013;21(1):20–7. https://doi.org/10.1002/erv.2191.
50. Dimitropoulos G, Freeman VE, Bellai K, Olmsted M. Inpatients with severe anorexia nervosa and their siblings: non-shared experiences and family functioning. EurEatDisordRev. 2013;21(4):284–93. https://doi.org/10.1002/erv.2230.
51. Fjermestad KW, Ro AE, Espeland KE, Halvorsen MS, Halvorsen IM. "Do I exist in this world, really, or is it just her?" Youths' perspectives of living with a sibling with anorexia nervosa. Eat Disord. 2019:1–16. https://doi.org/10.1080/10640266.2019.1573046.

2

"As long as they eat"? Therapist experiences, dilemmas and identity negotiations of Maudsley and family-based therapy for anorexia nervosa

Jessica Aradas[1*], Diana Sales[1], Paul Rhodes[2] and Janet Conti[1*]

Abstract

Background: Maudsley Family Therapy and its manualised version Family-Based Therapy for Anorexia Nervosa (FBT-AN) have accrued the most significant research evidence-base for the treatment of adolescent Anorexia Nervosa (AN). A tradition of seeking augmentations for this treatment has also been established to enhance efficacy. There exists, however, a gap in the uptake of this form of manualised treatment into the "real world" of clinicians who work with adolescent AN.

Aims: This research study investigated the key experiences and identity negotiations of a group of nine Australian clinicians who were interested in contributing to research into ways that Maudsley and FBT-AN might be improved.

Methods: Nine clinicians, who at the time of the interview practised or had previously practised, FBT-AN participated in a semi-structured interview. A critical discursive analysis of interview transcripts generated a thematic map of these therapists' experiences and identity negotiations in their practice of FBT-AN.

Results: These therapists experienced the structure of FBT-AN as both a secure map for therapy, yet also constraining at times, in their work with adolescents and their families. Additionally, their professional identities were both invested and troubled by the identity position of themselves as evidence-based practitioners, particularly where evidence-based practice (EBP) meant strict fidelity to the manual and restrained them from tailoring a broader range of therapeutic interventions to an individual adolescent and their family. Within their narratives, these therapists refashioned alternative identity positions around what it meant to be an evidence-based practitioner through listening to and drawing on their clinical expertise of what works in therapeutic practice with an individual adolescent and their family.

Conclusions: These therapists narratives highlight the power of the dominant discourse of EBP that works to privilege the research evidence over other forms of evidence that include clinician expertise and client preferences. The dilemmas faced by these therapists questioned not only the strict application of FBT-AN for adolescent AN across diverse therapeutic contexts, but also the effects of supervisory practices that paralleled this strict fidelity to the model. Further research is needed into therapeutic interventions and supervisory practices that give greater scope for clinicians to draw on their expertise in the flexible tailoring of treatments to the unique needs and preferences of the individual adolescent and their family.

Keywords: Anorexia nervosa, Maudsley, Family-based therapy, Evidence-based practice, Therapist, Identity

* Correspondence: jessica.aradas@hotmail.com; j.conti@westernsydney.edu.au
[1]University of Western Sydney, Locked Bag 1797, Penrith 2751, Australia
Full list of author information is available at the end of the article

Plain English summary

FBT-AN is currently the most prominent approach to the treatment of AN in young people and is supported by a range of empirical studies. Many studies have also been conducted on augmentations to the approach, with care taken not to contravene its core principles. While there is evidence that this approach works for some families, little is known about how clinicians negotiate their identities as both evidence-based clinicians and therapists who rely on their own clinical expertise and values. This study demonstrates that clinicians can feel secure in the knowledge that the model they are using is supported by research, but also troubled when strict adherence contradicts their own judgements about how to best support young people and families.

Background

Maudsley Family Therapy [1] and its subsequent manualised version Family-Based Therapy for Anorexia Nervosa[1] [2, 3] (FBT-AN), are considered to be one of the few efficacious treatments for adolescent Anorexia Nervosa (AN) [4–7]. The core principles of the therapy include: externalisation of the illness, positioning of families as the best resource to fight the AN and postponing individual and family issues until weight restoration has been achieved. Therapists are asked to "insist that the parents remain relentless until they are convinced that the patient clearly understands that she will not be able to return to anorexic behaviour while a part of the parents' household" ([3], p., 126). A substantive body of augmentations to this approach have also been developed and studied, including integration with inpatient and outpatient programs, multiple family therapy, and the inclusion of exposure techniques and cognitive-behavioural therapy for perfectionism [8]. Augmentations have been designed so not to alter the core principles of the original model and there is limited guidance as to how clinicians might decide on which enhancement to use for which situations [8].

The research evidence for FBT-AN has largely been in the form of randomized controlled trials (RCT's) [6, 7, 9, 10] and systematic reviews [11, 12]. Not including those who dropout from treatment, these family interventions have been found to have good long-term outcomes (including in establishing weight gain and improved eating disorder (ED) symptomatology) for approximately half of medically stable adolescents with a shorter duration of AN and aged between 12 and 18 years [13–15]. More specifically, 40% of adolescents are remitted after FBT-AN (i.e. meeting "high bar" recovery definitions based on symptom remission), however, clinical improvement has been found in around double this number ([16], p., 482). Furthermore, a recent randomised multi-centre trial has found good or intermediate outcomes (on the Morgan-Russell scales) in 60% of adolescents treated with single family FBT and 75% treated with multi-family therapy FBT [17]. On the other hand, when psychological distress has been measured more comprehensively in addition to ED symptom improvement in one RCT, around 40% of the adolescents reported (either themselves or by their parents) at 4 years post FBT-AN to be experiencing "considerable on-going psychological and psychiatric difficulty" ([18], p., 672)

A recent systematic review [11] has highlighted the need for future research into the implementation of FBT-AN into clinical practice in the context of research that has identified barriers to its translation. The research to date has also lacked (1) Comparison with individual psychological interventions; and (2) Usable outcome data of general and family functioning post AN treatment [19]. Furthermore, in the proliferation of research that has augmented FBT-AN with other interventions, only two out of 26 studies have received a strong quality rating at systematic review [8].

Manualised treatments play an important role in standardising and disseminating empirically-supported therapies (EST's) that may be applied more broadly into clinical contexts [20]. However, Sackett and colleagues' model of evidence-based practice (EBP) constitites three arms that, in addition to the resesarch evidence, also includes clinician expertise and client preference and values [21]. There contines to be limited guidance on, and continued debate about, the extent by which therapists have scope to draw on their clinical expertise to tailor FBT-AN to an individual adolescent, their family and within a potentially complex social environment [22, 23]; particularly when this expertise takes them away from fidelity to the FBT-AN manual. Discourse analysts believe that "facts" and "evidence" are most heatedly drawn upon when there is a sensitive issue at stake [24]. So where and how do ED clinicians position themselves in this debate as they seek to provide manualised FBT-AN for adolescent AN?

Qualitative research provides scope for a comprehensive and nuanced understanding of patient and clinician experiences, therefore elucidating the components of EBP that are less accessible by RCT's and manualised treatments [25]. Qualitative research into clinicians' experiences of FBT-AN has focused on factors that have increased or decreased therapists' willingness to practise FBT-AN [26] and some of the ways that therapists adapt FBT-AN for older adolescents to prioritize the adolescent and family needs [27]. While this research is helpful in exploring some of the ways therapists navigate the research-practice gap [28], it tends to be unidirectional in focus on processes by which clinicians make the decision whether or not to practice or adapt the model. What is less understood are questions such as how a clinician's professional identity (e.g. experiences, values) shapes their uptake or non-uptake of FBT-AN, how they negotiate a sense of professional identity (or who they understand themselves to be as therapists) when drawing on FBT-AN and how they navigate working within and outside the manualised FBT-AN model. These questions are significant, given that there are a number of factors that may increase the rates of burnout for therapists who work with EDs [29] and there is need to more richly understand how ED therapists negotiate and sustain their professional identities in their work with adolescents and their families.

Methods

Participants

Nine Australian clinicians who self-identified themselves as a practitioner (either past or present) in FBT-AN participated in this study. This sample was recruited through two research advertisements in 2016 and 2017 distributed through Australian associations relevant to the practice of psychology or within the ED field. The research advertisement invited clinicians who had worked as FBT-AN therapists to talk about their experiences and to generate constructive feedback through asking them: "How we can improve Maudsley Family Therapy for adolescent anorexia?"

The final sample consisted of seven female and two male therapists: five clinical psychologists, two psychologists, one psychotherapist, and one dietitian. Their years of working within ED's ranged between 5 and 23 years, and they identified themselves as FBT-AN practitioners for between 1 and 10 years. They had all attended Maudsley and/or FBT-AN training and received supervision by experienced FBT-AN practitioners in Australia. For reasons of confidentiality, this demographic information has not been linked to individual participant narratives.

At the time of the interviews, three clinicians indicated they had discontinued both working within FBT-AN and with adolescent AN, although continued to work with adult EDs (Joy, Gloria and Glenda). The remaining six therapists identified as continuing to use some form of FBT-AN to treat adolescent AN. Table 1 summarises how these therapists reported varying their work from the FBT-AN manual [2, 3].

Procedure and materials

The research study was approved by the University of Western Sydney Human Research Ethics Committee. On consenting for this research study, participants completed a brief demographic and clinical background questionnaire (Additional file 1).

Data was generated through individual semi-structured interviews. The interview questions (Additional file 2) were drawn from the therapeutic paradigm of narrative therapy [30] and were interested both in the way clinician's practised FBT-AN as well as the ways they ascribed meaning and negotiated their identities in the context of these experiences.

Two researchers (DS and JA) conducted the 45–60 min individual interviews with participants either in person or over the phone between May 2016 and June 2017. The audio-recordings were then transcribed verbatim using light transcription [31], including the use of pauses, in order to better capture shifts in both language and flow. The transcripts were identifiable only by the participant's chosen pseudonym. The clinicians were also invited to read through their transcripts to remove further potentially identifying information for reasons of their confidentiality.

Analysis

Analysis aimed to generate understandings of therapists' experiences, perspectives and the positioning of their work as FBT-AN practitioners, the language forms that they used to ascribe meaning to these experiences, and some of the ways that they negotiated and preserved their identities within these contexts. Initially, open and focused coding [32] was conducted by two researchers (JA and DS) line-by-line using the qualitative research software program Nvivo 11© [33], with the intention of generating multiple perspectives [34] from which themes were constructed. This was followed by memo-writing, conducted by the researchers (JA and DS) and with a group of qualitative researchers (including JC and PR), that analysed the data through a critical discursive paradigm [35, 36]. This included the identification of some of the discursive resources used by participants to piece together their narratives and negotiate personal meanings and social identities. These discursive resources included first, interpretative repertoires or culturally inherited patterns of speech (or small "d" discourse) that the participants used to piece together a range of positions and arguments [36, 37]; and second, positioning in discourse that constitutes the diverse locations within which the participants were both positioned and positioned themselves in discourse. These discourse positionings provided a platform from which the therapists constructed and negotiated a sense of professional identity within a social context [38]. Analysis traced how these therapists' accounts of their experiences were continually (re)constructed, (re)negotiated, and (re)formed through argument, addressing ideological dilemmas and rhetoric [37, 39].

The clinician participants were invited to read a draft of this paper, in particular to member-check the validity

Table 1 Therapists' reported utilisation of specific FBT-AN manual protocols and use of other therapeutic modalities

Therapists	Always weigh every session?	Always postpone all issues till weight restoration?	Always conduct family meal?	Always externalize "AN"?	Use other models for treating EDs?
Marmot	YES	YES	YES	YES	YES
Josh	YES	YES	NO	YES	YES
Francesca	YES	YES	YES	YES	YES
Anja	YES	NO	NO	YES	YES
Sebastian	NO	NO	NO	YES	YES
Paige	YES	NO	YES	YES	YES
Glenda[a]	YES	NO	YES	YES	YES
Gloria[a]	YES	NO	NO	YES	YES
Joy[a]	YES	NO	YES	YES	YES

[a]No longer practising FBT-AN at time of interview

of the analysis of their transcripts in interpreting their experiences.

Results

Interview data was constructed into four themes, each with two subthemes, that highlighted clinician investments in the FBT-AN intervention, therapeutic dilemmas and professional identity negotiations in working within and outside FBT-AN. Figure 1 depicts the themes and associations generated in the analysis of interview data.

Theme 1: Clinician investments in FBT-AN

The therapists rationalised and justified their therapeutic implementation of FBT-AN by taking up the position that it is EBP and a window into early intervention in the prevention of AN running a chronic course.

The "best evidence"

All of the currently practising FBT-AN therapists were invested in the model and justified this positioning through a scientific discourse that elevated the knowledge of research evidence whereby EBP became reduced to the application of manualised ESTs.

Extracts 1

Anja: *I guess what matters to me is feeling that people get [...] best evidence sort of care. [...] that I don't just go with my gut feeling or [...] on a personal perspective, but more from a professional perspective.*

Josh: *I see myself as a therapist who deliberately chooses and adheres to evidence-based treatments, then I go and vary an evidence-based treatment [...] maybe I'm falling into the kind of hubris [...] It causes what we'll call cognitive dissonance and some doubt about whether [...] I am indeed an evidence-based therapist or not, because that is part of my identity.*

Francesca: *I do strongly believe in evidence-based practice. Eating disorders are very complex illnesses and I don't profess to know any better than the next person.*

Within these stretches of text, these clinicians' identities were invested in being "evidence-based" practitioners. These therapists' positioning on FBT-AN was built on a scientific repertoire [40] that constructed the research evidence as fact, and the implementation of FBT-AN was understood as synonymous with EBP. Nevertheless, the certainty of this position was also implicitly questioned through use of qualifiers such as "sort of" (Anja).

These therapists expressed concern not to elevate their clinical expertise over the model. Within some accounts research evidence was assumed to be "good" knowledge, thereby marginalising therapists' expertise as a lesser knowledge ("personal perspective") that, if relied on too heavily, was an unacceptable elevation of a therapist's expertise ("hubris"). Implicit in these dilemmas were these therapists' commitment to accountability in their work as practitioners who provide effective treatment interventions to adolescents and their families.

Prevention of "the revolving door"

Six of the nine therapists derived a sense of meaning and purpose in their work through being part of the broader project of preventing "the revolving door" (Francesca) of AN.

Extracts 2

Francesca: I felt extremely disheartened by the revolving door [...] my sense is like there has to be some other way. So, what it has meant for me over the years, I guess, is something about feeling more effective as a clinician.

Glenda: I don't have to bang my head against a wall for six years. So, I suppose it meant to me that I was part of a new edge of treatment [...] that I was joining.

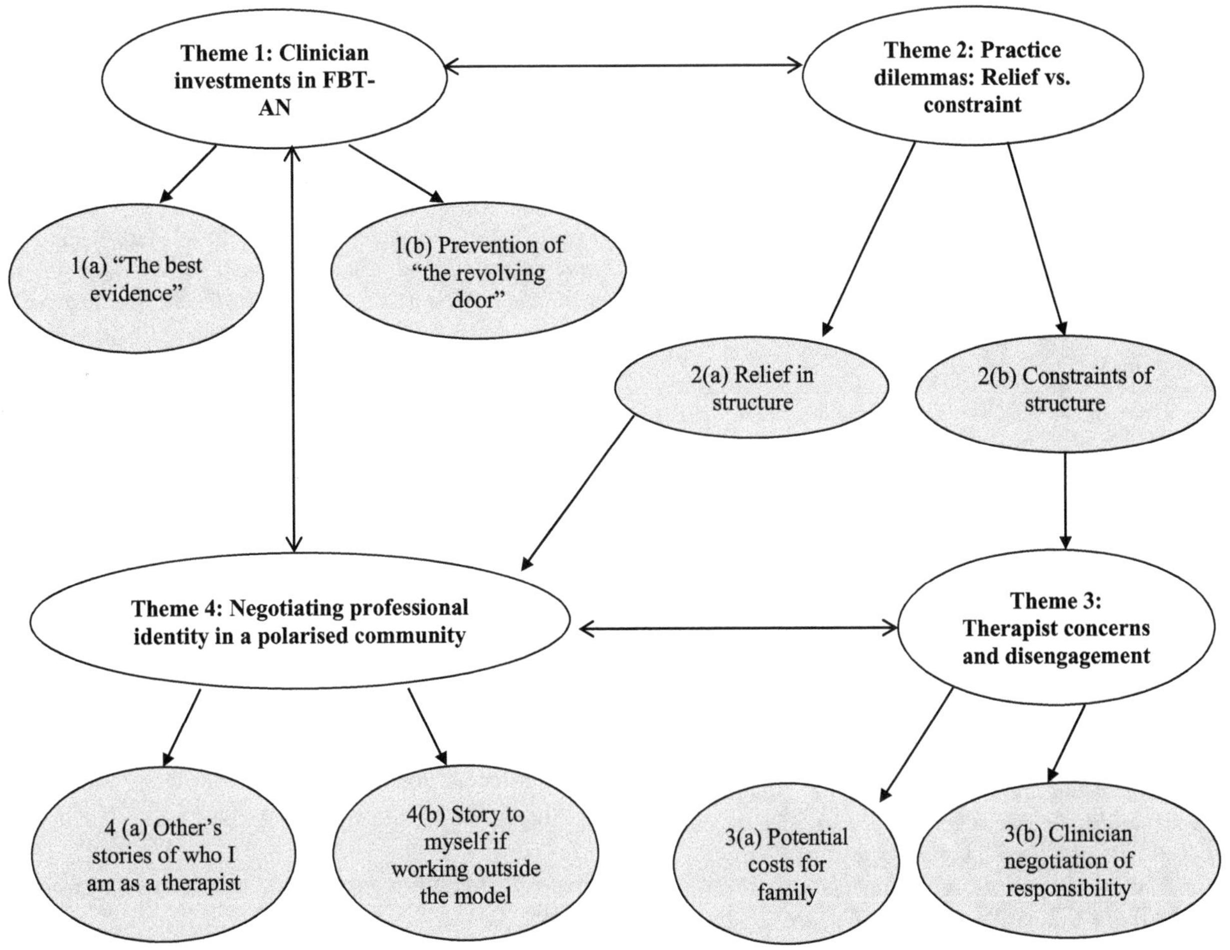

Fig. 1 Thematic map of therapist engagement with FBT-AN

Marmot: I've got school-aged girls, and so it means a lot to me, personally [...] girls having a strong sense of themselves, and not being railroaded into viewing themselves in a very narrow way [...].

These therapists' identities were supported in being part of a community that stood against adolescent AN running a chronic course. Working as an FBT-AN therapist contributed to a sense of oneself as engaging in effective therapeutic practice (Francesca), aligning oneself with cutting edge therapeutic practices (Glenda) and standing with young women in the development of durable and diverse identities (Marmot).

Theme 2: Practice dilemmas: relief vs. constraint by the structured intervention

The therapists were both comforted and constrained by the structured manualised approach that, in the earlier phases of therapy, strategically narrowed therapeutic conversations to prioritise focus on the adolescent's eating and weight gain.

Relief in a structured approach to adolescent AN

Seven of the nine therapists experienced relief in, and justified, the structured approach of the FBT-AN manual.

Extracts 3

Anja: I find really helpful that it's a very clear structured approach [...] [Giving] families [...] [a] focus on which is re-feeding rather than you know, going into the depths of why, what and how.

Paige: My initial reaction to it [FBT-AN] was fantastic, like, this is something where we get lots of containment [...] I felt confident that I could manage all these different things that were going to come up.

Francesca: Working with families initially wasn't (pause) I wouldn't say it was overwhelming, but it was like just how do you manage that? Many voices and personalities in the room? I think having the structure of something like FBT gives you a sense of confidence in the room.

Anja understood the structured approach of the FBT-AN script as a way of shifting the focus from questions for which there may not be a clear answer. Paige and Francesca found that, particularly when they were inexperienced therapists, the structure of FBT-AN provided containment of a parallel process of anxiety between the adolescent, their family and themselves as therapists.

Constraints of a structured approach to adolescent AN

Eight of the nine therapists recounted feeling constrained by the structured approach of FBT-AN and both implicitly and explicitly questioned rigid adherence to the model.

EXTRACTS 4a

Paige: You're being really directive [...] And it feels like actually harming [...] but I know that's what's going to get the patient well.

Glenda: Everybody knows exactly where they are at any one time. Now of course that also had downsides too. Because you were sacrificing important conversations for staying on track.

Josh: The treatment, necessarily, comes at the expense of talking about the adolescent's emotional state and individual needs, [...] and that's what makes it work, quite frankly.

Anja: Ideally, I'd like them to be engaged with me [...] but they hate me, that's alright. As long as they eat.

These therapists expressed concerns about FBT-AN, particularly in the earlier phases, being "really directive" (Paige), and that this ultimately led to "sacrificing important conversations" (Glenda) such as the "adolescent's emotional state" (Josh) or undermining an "ideal" therapeutic engagement (Anja). These therapists were caught in an ideological dilemma that was generated in contexts where the FBT-AN script was elevated over their own clinical expertise and their clients' preferences ("they hate me", Anja). These negotiations were built on a moral discourse that adopted a consequentialist ethical framework [41] whereby these therapists were able to justify their temporary neglect of the adolescent's "emotional state and individual needs" (Josh) to keep "on track" (Glenda) in the service of saving lives.

EXTRACT 4b

Francesca: I think having a model that you could kind of rest into reasonably confidently, I think that gives you confidence as a clinician as well. Obviously, as you become more experienced you can become more flexible with use of the model.

One of the therapists did not experience FBT-AN as constraining in her work but rather as a model to "rest into" (Francesca, extract 4b) with augmentations assumed ("obviously") to arise out of a therapist's growing expertise and confidence.

Extracts 5

Marmot: She says to her parents when she's not feeling well [...] "I'm not learning anything about looking after myself, because you tell me what to do with what I eat and exercise." And you know, she's got a point; but the problem is, if they didn't, she'd just be back in hospital.

Paige: I think the way I've been trained has been very rigid, it's almost like 'give a man a fish, he'll eat for a day, teach a man to fish and he can feed himself'. I almost feel like I've been given fish with this model.

Within these stretches of text, there existed a parallel process between adolescents and the clinicians who treat them where they were both told what to do through FBT-AN ("given a fish") that had the effect of impeding the development of their own sense of competence around tailored formulation-based treatment ("teach a man to fish").

Overall, the status of the FBT-AN manual as "good" or a more valid form of knowledge risked disempowering adolescents and the clinicians who treat them through the marginalisation of their own knowledge and expertise in AN interventions and recovery.

Theme 3: Therapist concerns and disengagement from FBT-AN

FBT-AN became increasingly dilemmatic for some therapists in contexts where the adolescent did not progress to weight restoration. At these points in their narratives, they negotiated questions of responsibility and blame, and their role as therapist became increasingly burdensome.

Therapists' concerns for the potential costs for families

Seven of the nine therapists expressed concern about the expectations and lack of resources for parents within this therapeutic intervention.

Extracts 6

Sebastian: We had [hospital] staff [...] highly knowledgeable, very specialized [...] eight hours work with these patients and they're drained [...] I appreciate that one of the tenants of Maudsley is that parents have the ability to re-feed their child [...] But what we're asking them to do is outside of the realms of normal parenting.

Gloria: The families where it worked either very well or well enough, they gave up huge income to do it [...] This is what we need to do to save our daughter's life.

Paige: Probably we underestimate how difficult it is for parents to treat their young person.

These clinicians were troubled by the core FBT-AN premise that it is reasonable to ask parents to take on primary responsibility for refeeding their child and the emotional and material effects of this. Implicit in these clinicians' arguments is the extent by which the FBT-AN model risks under-acknowledging and underestimating emotional and material cost on parents who are asked to take responsibility for re-feeding their child in the early phases.

Extract 7

Francesca: I can't say that putting parents in charge is unhelpful to kids [...] I think it is very challenging, but I think it's extremely helpful. [...] I think that the families who don't go well are the families in which mum and dad struggle to take charge.

In contrast, Francesca positioned the task asked of parents as "challenging" but necessary. Drawing on the discourse of structural family therapy [42], she argued the families who do not do well with the intervention are those where the parents struggle to "take charge" and that "this doesn't mean they're to blame, it means this treatment may not be for them".[2] A number of questions following on from this position, including how do therapists discern that FBT-AN intervention may not be appropriate for an individual and their family and how are alternative treatment options navigated?

Clinician negotiation of responsibility

In contexts where FBT-AN did not work, the question of responsibility was raised by eight of the nine therapists..

Extracts 8

Francesca: I'm not responsible for change, like if the kid doesn't get well or a family doesn't respond to the treatment, and I need to remember that it's not going to work for everybody.

Anja: I guess that's just a value of therapy. Therapies never work out how we want them to.

Paige: The feedback that I've been given is keep going within the model but just always try harder [...] it undermines my confidence because I think I'm not doing it right or not doing it well enough.

Josh: Whenever any client isn't doing well [...] I go through quite a deliberate, conscious process of thinking [...] That's a conscious self-doubting, self-examination, but I'm in favour of that.

In order to sustain themselves in the context of therapeutic challenges, Francesca and Anja negotiated the causal discourse of responsibility and blame through reminding themselves that outcomes are complex and collaborative. On the other hand, feedback from her supervisor to "keep going within the model" and "try harder" eroded a sense of professional competence for Paige. Josh preserved a sense of professional identity when a client was "not doing well" through positioning self-doubt as a form of self-examination that was aligned with his professional values.

The theme of responsibility also arose when the therapists narrated some of the more troubled experiences that contributed to their decision to ultimately cease working as FBT-AN therapists.

Extracts 9

Gloria: It's the therapist's job to sit with that distress and help them sit with their distress and get their thinking back so that they can keep their child alive and help them get well. That is a lot to hold [...].

Glenda: [...] I wanted so badly to be a good Maudsley practitioner and I'd had good experiences [with adolescents and their families with FBT-AN] *and I wanted to follow the encouragements my supervisors were giving me, but in my heart I thought I don't think this is right. [...] The manual did not then, I don't know if it has changed, address any sort of concept of window of tolerance of the young person. [...] In my FBT training and ongoing supervision I was not taught or invited to be aware of when the distress may be so impactful it becomes a new set of problems –* i.e. *trauma. Looking back [...]I would have challenged my supervisor and stated that in my opinion there is a limit to the distress that I would be willing to normalise within FBT. [...] I have left behind the dogmatic culture of FBT, which I believe cloaked my capacity to act on what felt uneasy because it was not adhering to the model. I am somewhat haunted by the sense the model was used to 'justify the unjustifiable'.*[3]

These therapists recounted their struggles to "sit with" and "hold" (Gloria) the distress of an adolescent and their family in the FBT-AN treatment. An experience that contributed to Glenda's decision to cease practising as a FBT-AN therapist was the implicit risk of an intervention that heavily relies on parents to engage in home-based refeeding of their child in the early stages of treatment with less focus or consideration of the level of distress that this may invoke for the adolescent and within the family system. This approach, where the ends justifies the means, reduced Glenda's personal agency as an early career FBT clinician in the field and she experienced a parallel process [43] of distress that was unable to be contained by the ongoing strict adherence to the model in supervision.

Theme 4: Negotiating professional identity in the context of a polarised community

All the therapists expressed reticence in working outside the framework of FBT-AN. How they ascribed meaning to working with adolescents and their families outside FBT-AN was shaped by the stories they believed others might tell about them as a therapist and the stories they told themselves to preserve an identity sourced in their values.

Others' stories of who I am as a therapist

The therapists' stories of self, when working outside FBT-AN, were shaped by the broader professional context.

Extracts 10

Josh: My supervisor says [...] I should work harder to make sure that everybody's there, all the time, in fact, they say I'm not really doing Maudsley, if the siblings aren't in the room.

Sebastian: One of the comments that stands out for me is one of the trainers saying if Maudsley's not working then the clinician's not doing their job.

Joy: So, I feel like I just don't have the capacity or the interest really to be carrying [...] "She's someone who works with adolescents in a non-evidenced based way."

These therapists talked about the power of the supervisors' gaze overseeing and evaluating their work, particularly when departing from FBT-AN. Josh described an obligation to adhere to the model as his supervisor construed any deviation, even implicitly, as not working hard enough. Sebastian was troubled by his supervisor's assumption that if FBT-AN was not working then the therapist was to blame. Joy decided she did not want to carry other's label of her as a therapist who works "in a non-evidenced based way" and the material effects of this were her decision to cease seeing adolescent's and their families.

Extracts 11

Joy: The Boys' Club, I just feel like there's quite a lot of bullying, like not in a really - in a covert sort of way [...] Some of the phrases that they use, which when I've had supervision, by them; [...] "You've got to pull them in before you punch them."

Glenda: I know of people who have been challenged by Maudsley cultists almost. They say, "well we want to know what you're doing seeing adolescents if you're not going to offer this."

These therapists, who had ceased using FBT-AN, expressed concern about rigid and strict adherence to the model. Joy exaggerated these concerns to the level of "Maudsley cultist almost" to highlight the investments in the rigid application of the model within the broader context of a gendered profession ("the boys club"). These terms capture the implicit effects of extreme fidelity to FBT-AN that work to marginalise and de-legitimise those who offer treatments through other frameworks of care. The real effects of these power dynamics between therapists in the field of ED's led to three of the therapists in this research to not only cease working within the model but to also abandoning work with adolescent AN. For these therapists, the fear and risks of not working within the model and being recruited into the identity of non-evidence-based practitioners were too great.

Five of the six therapists who continued their work as FBT-AN practitioners at the time of the interview remarked on the effects of a split treatment community.

Extracts 12 *Josh: The ones that are rigid [...] are the ones that aren't educated, and don't use it [FBT-AN] at all. I've got a couple of colleagues, psychiatrists that will even tell their patients, "Oh, don't do Maudsley, that's just a fad."*

Francesca: My job becomes infinitely harder because it's very hard to hold a bottom line in treatment with a young patient when there is no sort of medical review or support in place [...] so I would like more support, more awareness dissemination.

Josh positioned the divide between those who are "educated" and practise FBT-AN, and those who are "rigid" and firmly oppose it. Being part of a community where some professionals were resistant to the potential benefits of FBT-AN also was experienced as presenting risks to client safety. Francesca's commitment to "hold a bottom line in treatment" in standing for the adolescent's medical safety in a community that was not informed of FBT-AN was experienced as isolating and unsupported.

Story to myself: who I am as a therapist if I work outside the model?

The "choice" to work outside of the script of FBT-AN was dilemmatic for the majority of the therapists as they engaged in identity negotiations and justifications as to why.

Extracts 13

Sebastian: I think you've got to sort of draw a line in the sand and say okay well do we just keep doing what we're doing, knowing that the weight's not going on and the parents are getting stressed and the relationships are disintegrating, or do we start looking at other options.

Joy: I feel it's a bit disrespectful to the clients.... to build rapport before you hit them with something that's going to shatter them. [...] I feel uncomfortable with the way that they [FBT-AN trainers/supervisors] talk [...] just disrespectful, actually.

Sebastian argued that his choice to work within the model involved the adolescent and their family. Drawing on the metaphor of "a line in the sand", he highlighted the point at which a therapist is faced with giving the adolescent and their family more of the same intervention or switching direction to draw on other therapeutic interventions. Joy's concerns with the model were centred upon a values clash where she no longer wanted to participate in therapeutic practices that she experienced at times as disrespectful and holding the potential to "shatter" the adolescent and their family.

All the therapists were also faced with what it meant to them if they were to draw on other therapeutic interventions when working with adolescents who experience AN and their families.

Extracts 14

Josh: The families and the kids find it (pause), they kind of go, "That's frustrating!", and it's one of the things that leads to drop out rates. They say, "You're not talking about what's really going on".

Marmot: I would find it very difficult to just follow a manual, because I would feel that I was compromising on my clinical ability – and my values. I was just kind of forcing people through something, when in my head, my clinical experience is going, "This isn't right; this isn't going to be as effective if I do it in this way." [...] I don't know if that's actually true, but that's my sense.

Joy: I mean I feel torn because there's a part of me that would like to see a bit more capacity for people to work freely according to their clinical judgment, but then I see that there's a lot of danger in that as well.

Implicit in each of these stretches of text were these therapists' values including authenticity ("talking about what's really going on"; Josh), accountability (not "forcing people through something" that "isn't going to be as effective"; Marmot) and flexibility (Joy). These therapists' professional identities were sourced in their values yet also troubled by a fear that drawing on their clinical expertise risked "danger" (Joy).

Discussion

This study highlights some of the commitments and professional identity negotiations of therapists who practise or have practised FBT-AN. These therapists were committed to adhering to FBT-AN and frequently experienced themselves as engaging in therapeutic processes that were effective and created positive change for adolescents and their families. These experiences contributed to their identity investments as evidence-based practitioners. On the other hand, eight of the nine clinicians highlighted a range of difficulties in negotiating their professional identities and sustaining themselves in this work that became increasingly burdensome in contexts where they took up personal responsibility for the adolescent's eating and behaviour change. One clinician derived a durable and relatively untroubled sense of identity through her practice as a FBT-AN therapist. Three of the practitioners had ceased working not only with the FBT-AN model but also with adolescents who experience AN.

The script of FBT-AN was experienced as a relief and justified through the prioritisation of the adolescent's medical safety and in the prevention of AN running a chronic course. However, these commitments became morally dilemmatic in contexts that included when the intervention did not work, witnessing the burden placed on parents in taking on the role of refeeding their child, the adolescents' loss of voice and marginalisation of their emotional distress to focus on eating and weight restoration in the earlier phases of treatment, and when adolescents and families dropped out of treatment.

These therapists' identities were invested in being "evidence-based practitioners", which was often self-evidenced by adherence to the FBT-AN manual [2, 3]. This knowledge was positioned as "good" knowledge [44] through a scientific repertoire that elevated research evidence over the therapists' clinical knowledge and expertise. The power of the scientific discourse was evident by the swift assumption made by clinicians that strict fidelity to the manual was a required component of EBP. The uptake of this discourse was evident where clinicians were troubled by departures from the FBT-AN script and in the marginalisation of their own knowledge and expertise of what intervention/s might work better at a particular time in treatment for an individual adolescent and their family.

Previous research has found that therapists do not fully ascribe to FBT-AN for a range of pragmatic and ideological reasons, including the belief that "one size does not fit all" ([26], p., 182). What is less known is how their negotiations and actions to modify this intervention shape their sense of professional identity. These therapists ascribed a range of meanings to deviations from the model when relying on their clinical intuition, including feeling burdened by doubt, and fear they were biased and inflating their self-importance. One clinician was untroubled by drawing on her own expertise to augment the FBT-AN model and argued that this may at times be of greater therapeutic benefit to the adolescent and their family. All the therapists, however, were reticent to draw on their clinical expertise to question to basic tenets of the model or to transform (rather than merely augment) its structure when working with adolescent AN.

This research also highlights the divisive effects of a polarised community of practitioners where therapists were recruited into "choosing" between "us and them" within different contexts. Those who no longer practised FBT-AN experienced themselves as outsiders to the ED community. This marginalisation was experienced by some as an act of power through the assumption that

FBT-AN was the only means to engage with EBP, thereby disqualifying those clincians who drew from different therapeutic modalities for adolescent AN. On the other hand, those who practised FBT-AN experienced themselves as misunderstood and unsupported by the broader community of health professionals, thereby posing a risk to collaborative care.

These "us and them" debates in the clinicians' narratives paralleled those within the broader ED community, such as those who argue for the effectiveness of the intervention [45] and those who argue that FBT-AN is "overvalued" ([23]: p. 264) and that AN treatments should be formulated and treated by a more complex reasoning process than by prescribing a single manualised EST. These debates also highlight the issues of power and masculinity in the neoliberal distribution of EST's as a "product", rather than promoting a process that embodies the original conceptualisations of EBP that draw on clinician expertise to tailor clinical interventions to the needs, preferences and values of the client [21].

Implications

This research highlights that the polarisation of the ED community through the uptake of the dominant discourse of EBP risks therapists being isolated, undermined, confused or scrutinized about their treatment decisions, whether they adhere to FBT-AN, implement alternative therapeutic modalities or make augmentations to the model. This research makes transparent this research-practice gap and considers how the subjective experiences of clinicians may inform future practice.

These clinician narratives highlight some key areas to bridge this research-practice gap that include:

1) The establishment of more comprehensive guidelines and ongoing assessment of "the appropriateness and efficacy of FBT(-AN)" ([46], p., 298) in therapeutic contexts including for example, when:
   a. The adolescent's emotional distress (including in their eating and weight restoration) is too great and the intervention risks being traumatising;
   b. The burden on a family is too great and what might be the next steps in the care of the adolescent and their family; and
   c. There exists a risk of child emotional abuse and family violence, thus highlighting the need for therapists who practice FBT-AN to have comprehensive training in responding to child emotional abuse and family violence [46].
2) Drawing on therapist expertise to both inform clinical practice guidelines [25] and future research into how to effectively tailor manualised treatments to the adolescent and family needs and preferences through reflective practice in supervision [43].
3) Addressing the pressing need for the development and evaluation of more diverse treatment interventions for adolescent AN, including those that have scope to be flexibly tailored by clinicians to the needs and preferences of the adolescent and their family. These treatments need to prioritise approaches that give the adolescent a voice and scope for choice [47] alongside treatment "non-negotiables" such as weight gain [48].
4) Further development of supervision methods for FBT-AN that cultivate an awareness of some of the implicit messages that clinicians may take up when the focus is on strict fidelity to the model and where any therapeutic departures are scrutinised and interrogated and how this may disempower therapists and risk burnout.
5) Researching ways reflective practice in supervision [43] might empower ED therapists to strengthen their connection with their preferred identities, sustain themselves in clinical practice, and to continue to develop expertise in the discernment of ways to effectively tailor therapeutic interventions including through prioritising the voice of the adolescent and their families [49].

While there is a proliferation of studies exploring augmentations to FBT-AN, this does not address the gap between therapist adherence to the manual and when and how to draw on their clinical wisdom. These augmentations tend to accommodate other interventions onto the model and are reluctant to corrupt the core principles of FBT-AN [50] that include allocation of responsibility of re-feeding the adolescent to parents in the early phases of treatment. Furthermore there continues to be a reluctance to engage in transformative models of care in adolescent AN and a paucity of research into such other treatment paradigms [8].

Scope of the study

This research is an in-depth analysis of the views of nine Australian clinicians. It is possible that the research advertisement for recruitment of participants that put forward an interest to explore ways to "improve" FBT-AN shaped the study participants such that those who were troubled by the model were more likely to participate. Nevertheless, there was a broad range of experiences and positionings articulated by these nine practitioners. It would be valuable to explore whether clinician views differ, particularly in the context of diverse cultures, countries and healthcare systems.

While the interview questions were intended to investigate both the helpful and unhelpful aspects of FBT-AN, it is possible that the telling or analysis may not have equally captured both, for example due to a retrospective bias on accounts that have more emotional valence. As well as this, as the interviewees themselves could not be anonymous to the interviewers, it is possible this may have limited their disclosure in an effort to protect aspects of their professional identity. Lastly, it is worth noting this paper has drawn on Sackett et al.'s model [21] of EBP, which rather than elevating research evidence over clinician and client expertise construes it as an interplay between these different forms of knowledge. This positioning may diverge from those who argue that "scientific evidence must be accorded priority" ([51]: p.886) when there is doubt in clinical decision-making.

Conclusions

This research provides a unique insight into the experiences of therapists who practise FBT-AN, and the meaning making processes that they negotiate to sustain themselves in their work. While FBT-AN is an effective treatment for many adolescents, greater focus needs to be accorded to the role of clinician expertise in the tailoring of therapeutic interventions to client preferences rather than the strict application one EST, which for the majority of these therapists was dilemmatic. Through developing a two-way relationship between research and practice, there exists scope to expand therapeutic interventions for adolescent AN that embody the intended meaning of EBP that is, to provide clinicians with scope and a more comprehensive map to tailor the best possible treatment interventions to the needs, preferences and values of the individual adolescent/family [21].

Endnotes

[1]Although Maudsley Family Therapy (Family therapy for eating disorders originating from the Maudsley London Hospital under the Eisler group) (Russell, 1987); is not exclusively synonymous with Family-Based Therapy for Anorexia Nervosa (the manualised treatment based on the Maudsley treatment by Lock and Le Grange in the USA), this article will refer to these interventions with the term FBT-AN, acknowledging that some of the therapists who had worked for a longer period of time with the model would have been trained in either or both of Maudsley Family Therapy and FBT interventions.

[2]This quote was ascertained from a member-check correspondence.

[3]This quote was ascertained from a member-check correspondence

Abbreviations

AN: Anorexia Nervosa; EBP: Evidence-Based Practice; ED: Eating Disorder; EST: Empirically Supported Therapy; FBT-AN: Maudsley and Family-Based Therapy; RCT: Randomized Controlled Trial

Acknowledgements

The authors would like to acknowledge Emma Sheens (Sydney University), Sara Cibralic (formerly WSU) and Tanya Meade (WSU) in their support of this research.

Authors' contributions

DS initially interviewed eight of the nine participants, analysed and interpreted these interviews, and wrote a master's thesis based on this data. JA interviewed the remaining participant and wrote a master's thesis specifically focused on the data of those practising FBT-AN at the time of the interview. JA wrote this final paper that included the re-analysis of all of the interview data and generation of the thematic map. JC was the supervisor of both DS and JA and contributed to the data analysis and writing of this paper. PR provided consultation and read and approved the final paper.

Competing interests

The authors declare that they have no competing interests.

Author details

[1]University of Western Sydney, Locked Bag 1797, Penrith 2751, Australia.
[2]University of Sydney, Penrith, Australia.

References

1. Eisler I, Simic M, Blessitt E, Dodge L & team. Maudsley Service Manual for Child and Adolescent Eating Disorders (Revised). Child and Adolescent Eating Disorders Service. London: South London & Maudsley NHS Foundation Trust; 2016. Available at: https://eur04.safelinks.protection.outlook.com/?url=http%3A%2F%2Fwww.national.slam.nhs.uk%2Fservices%2Fcamhs%2Fcamhs-eatingdisorders%2Fresources%2F&data=02%7C01%7C%7Caf3a2b0e805f4af1f11608d67e6c623d%7C84df9e7fe9f640afb435aaaaaaaaaaaa%7C1%7C0%7C636835401315612419&sdata=eejab5pQXvaBUhL9ZcS4DMlhGxVN1KSYUtRh9%2BXac8c%3D&reserved=0
2. Lock J, DI G, Agras WS, Dare C. Treatment manual for AN: a family-based approach. New York: Guilford Press; 2001.
3. Lock J, Le Grange D. Treatment manual for AN: a family-based approach. 2nd ed. New York: Guilford Press; 2012.
4. Eisler I, Dare C, Hodes M, Russell G, Dodge E, Le Grange D. Family therapy for adolescent AN: the results of a controlled comparison of two family interventions. J Child Psychol Psychiatry Allied Discip. 2000;41(6):727–36.
5. Eisler I, Dare C, Russell GF, Szmukler G, le Grange D, Dodge E. Family and individual therapy in AN: a 5-year follow-up. Arch Gen Psychiatry. 1997; 54(11):1025–30.
6. Lock J. Evaluation of family treatment models for eating disorders. Curr Opin Psychiatry. 2011;24(4):274–9.
7. Russell GF, Szmukler GI, Dare C, Eisler I. An evaluation of family therapy in AN and bulimia nervosa. Arch Gen Psychiatry. 1987;44(12):1047–56.
8. Richards IL, Subar A, Touyz S, Rhodes P. Augmentative approaches in family-based treatment for adolescents with restrictive eating disorders: a systematic review. Eur Eat Disord Rev. 2018;26(2):92–111.
9. Eisler I, Dare C, Hodes M, Russell G, Dodge E, Le Grange D. Family therapy for adolescent AN: the results of a controlled comparison of two family interventions. J Child Psychol Psychiatry. 2000;41(6):727–36.
10. Eisler I, Simic M, Russell GF, Dare C. A randomised controlled treatment trial of two forms of family therapy in adolsecent anorexia nervosa: a five-year follow-up. J Child Psychol Psychiatry. 2007;48(6):552–60.
11. Couturier JL, Kimber MS. Dissemination and implementation of manualized family-based treatment: a systematic review. Eat Disord. 2015;23(4):281–90.
12. Bulik CM, Berkman ND, Brownley KA, Sedway JA, Lohr KN. AN treatment: a systematic review of randomized controlled trials. Int J Eat Disord. 2007;40(4):310–20.
13. Eisler I, Simic M, Hodsoll J, Asen E, Berelowitz M, Connan F, Ellis G, Hugo P, Schmidt U, Treasure J, et al. A pragmatic randomised multi-Centre trial of multifamily and single family therapy for adolescent AN. BMC Psychiatry. 2016;16(1):422.
14. Le Grange D, Hughes EK, Court A, Yeo M, Crosby RD, Sawyer SM. Randomized clinical trial of parent-focused treatment and family-based treatment for adolescent AN. J Am Acad Child Adolesc Psychiatry. 2016; 55(8):683–92.
15. Lock J, Le Grange D, Agras WS, Moye A, Bryson SW, Jo B. Randomized clinical trial comparing family-based treatment with adolescent-focused

individual therapy for adolescents with AN. Arch Gen Psychiatry. 2010; 67(10):1025–32.
16. Lock J, Le Grange D. Family-based treatment: where are we and where should we be going to improve recovery in child and adolescent eating disorders. Int J Eat Disord. 2018;52(4):481–7.
17. Eisler I, Simic M, Hodsoll J, Asen E, Berelowitz M, Connon F, Ellis G, Hugo P, Schmidt U, Treasure J, Yi I, Landau S. A pragmatic randomised multi-Centre trial of multifamily and single family therapy for adolescent anorexia nervosa. BMC Psychiatry. 2016;16(1):422.
18. Lock J, Couturier J, Agras WS. Comparison of long-term outcomes in adolescents with anorexia nervosa treated with family therapy. J Am Acad Child Adolesc Psychiatry. 2006;45(6):666–72.
19. Fisher CA, Skocic A, Rutherford KA, Hetrick SE. Family therapy approaches for anorexia nervosa. Cochrane Database of Systematic Reviews; 2019;(5): CD004780. https://doi.org/10.1002/14651858.CD004780.pub4
20. Eisler I, Wallis A, Dodge E. What's new is old and what's old is new: the origins and evolution of eating disorders family therapy. In: Le Grange D, Lock J, Loeb KL, Le Grange D, Lock J, editors. Family therapy for adolescent eating and weight disorders: new applications. Loeb KL. New York: Routledge/Taylor & Francis Group; 2015. p. 6–42.
21. Sackett DL, Rosenberg WM, Gray JM, Haynes RB, Richardson WS. Evidence based medicine: what it is and what it isn't. Br Med J. 1996;312:71–2.
22. Hay PJ. Avoid being 'tyrannised' by the evidence: reflections on family-based treatment in adolescent anorexia nervosa. Aust N Z J Psychiatry. 2012;46(11):1102–3.
23. Strober M, Johnson C. The need for complex ideas in AN: why biology, environment, and psyche all matter, why therapists make mistakes, and why clinical benchmarks are needed for managing weight correction. Int J Eat Disord. 2012;45(2):155–78.
24. Potter J, Edwards D, Wetherell M. A model of discourse in action. Am Behav Sci. 1993;36(3):383.
25. Kazdin AE. Evidence-based treatment and practice: new opportunities to bridge clinical research and practice, enhance the knowledge base, and improve patient care. Am Psychol. 2008;63(3):146–9.
26. Couturier J, Kimber M, Jack S, Niccols A, Van Blyderveen S, McVey G. Understanding the uptake of family-based treatment for adolescents with AN: therapist perspectives. Int J Eat Disord. 2013;46(2):177–88.
27. Dimitropoulos G, Freeman VE, Allemang B, Couturier J, McVey G, Lock J, Le Grange D. Family-based treatment with transition age youth with AN: a qualitative summary of application in clinical practice. J Eat Disord. 2015;3(1):1.
28. Cha CB, DiVasto KA. Introduction: applying clinical psychological science to practice. J Clin Psychol. 2017;73(5):504–10.
29. Warren CS, Schafer KJ, Crowley ME, Olivardia R. A qualitative analysis of job burnout in eating disorder treatment providers. J Treat Prev. 2012;3:175–95.
30. White M. Maps of narrative therapy. Adelaide: Dulwich Centre; 2007.
31. Edley N. Analysing masculinity: interpretative repertoires, ideological dilemmas and subject positions. In: Wetherell M, Taylor S, Yates SJ, editors. Discourse as data: a guide for analysis edn. London: Sage; 2001. p. 189–224.
32. Charmaz K. Constructing grounded theory: a practical guide through qualitative analysis. London: Sage; 2006.
33. NVivo © Qualitative Data Analysis Software; QSR International Pty Ltd. Version 11, 2015.
34. Charmaz K. The power of constructivist grounded theory for critical inquiry. Qual Inq. 2017;23(1):34–45.
35. Potter J, Wetherell M. Discourse and social psychology: beyond attitudes and behaviour. London: Sage; 1987.
36. Wetherell M, Potter J. Discourse analysis and the identification of interpretative repertoires. In: Antaki C, editor. Analysing everyday explanation a casebook of methods. London: Sage; 1988. p. 168–83.
37. Burr V. Social constructionism. 3rd ed. New York: Routledge; 2015.
38. Davies B, Harré R. Positioning: the discursive production of selves. J Theory Soc Behav. 1990;20(1):43–63.
39. Billig M. Ideological dilemmas: a social psychology of everyday thinking. London: Sage; 1988.
40. Mulkay M, Gilbert G. Opening Pandora's box: a sociological analysis of scientists' discourse. Cambridge: Cambride University Press; 1984.
41. Crockett MJ. Models of morality. Trends Cogn Sci. 2013;17(8):363–6.
42. Minuchin SR, Baker L. Psychosomatic families: AN in context. Cambridge: Harvard University Press; 1978.
43. Hewson D, Carroll M. Reflective practice in supervision: companion volume to the reflective supervision toolkit. Hazelbrook: Moshpit; 2016.
44. Sampson EE. Identity politics: challenges to psychology's understanding. Am Psychol. 1993;48(12):1219.
45. Lock J, Le Grange D. Proposition: family-based treatment is overvalued. Position: opposed. Adv Eat Disord. 2014;2(3):284–95.
46. Kimber M, McTavish JR, Couturier J, Le Grange D, Lock J, MacMillan HL. Identifying and responding to child maltreatment when delivering family-based treatment—a qualitative study. Int J Eat Disord. 2019;52(3):292–8.
47. Dring G. Finding a voice: family therapy for young people with anorexia. London: Karnac Books; 2015.
48. Geller J, Srikameswaran S. Treatment non-negotiables: why we need them and how to make them work. Eur Eat Disord Rev. 2006;14(4):212–7.
49. Norcross JC. Psychotherapy relationships that work: evidence-based responsiveness. 2nd ed. New York: Oxford University Press; 2011.
50. Rhodes P, Gosbee M, Madden S, Brown J. 'Communities of concern' in the family-based treatment of anorexia nervosa: towards a consensus in the Maudsley model. Eur Eat Disord Rev. 2005;13(6):392–8.
51. Lilienfeld SO, Ritschel LA, Lynn SJ, Cautin RL, Latzman RD. Why many clinical psychologists are resistant to evidence-based practice: root causes and constructive remedies. Clin Psychol Rev. 2013;33(7):883–900.

3

Accuracy of self-reported physical activity in patients with anorexia nervosa: links with clinical features

Louise Bezzina[1], Stephen Touyz[1], Sarah Young[1], Nasim Foroughi[2], Stacy Clemes[3], Caroline Meyer[4], Jon Arcelus[5], Sloane Madden[1], Evelyn Attia[6], Kathleen M. Pike[6] and Phillipa Hay[7*]

Abstract

Background: High levels of physical activity (PA) have long been described in patients with Anorexia Nervosa (AN). Despite the importance of measuring PA in this population, there are two important factors that remain unknown. First, it is not clear how accurate self-report measures of PA are among patients. Second, little is known about how clinical characteristics are associated with the accuracy of self-reported PA. Therefore, this study aimed to examine the accuracy of self-reported PA compared to an objective measure of PA in patients with AN. It also investigated whether levels of accuracy/inaccuracy were associated with compulsive exercise, motivation to change, and psychological distress.

Method: Data were analysed from 34 adult outpatients with AN. Patients wore an accelerometer device (ActiGraph) for 4 days and completed a retrospective self-report measure of exercise (Exercise Participation Screening Questionnaire). They also completed measures of compulsive exercise (Compulsive Exercise Test), motivation to change (The Anorexia Nervosa Stages of Change Questionnaire), and psychological distress (Kessler-10).

Results: On the self-report measure, patients accurately reported their time spent in moderate and vigorous intensity PA, however, they significantly under-reported their light physical activity (compared to the accelerometer data). Accurate reporting of total PA was positively associated with higher levels of compulsive exercise. There was evidence to suggest that clinical features, such as motivation to change and psychological distress, may be associated with inaccurate reporting at some levels of PA intensity and not others.

Conclusions: Results indicate that patients with AN are likely to under-report their light intensity PA. We also found preliminary evidence for how compulsive exercise, motivation to change, and distress are associated with self-reported PA accuracy. Clinical implications and directions for future research are considered.

Keywords: Anorexia nervosa, Physical activity, Self-report, Accelerometry, Compulsive exercise, Anxiety, Depression, Motivation to change

* Correspondence: p.hay@westernsydney.edu.au
[7]Translational Health Research Institute, School of Medicine, Western Sydney University, Locked Bag 1797, Penrith, South NSW 2715, Australia
Full list of author information is available at the end of the article

Plain English summary

High levels of physical activity are common in people with anorexia nervosa and are associated with poorer physical and psychological outcomes. It is important to measure the amount of activity or exercise a person is engaging in as part of assessment and treatment. This study looked at whether a self-report questionnaire (answering a survey) would be accurate in measuring physical activity. We compared the patient's self-reported physical activity to that estimated from an accelerometer (pedometer) device worn around the person's waist. We found that people under-reported their light activity on the self-report questionnaire (e.g. walking), but did not under-report their moderate or vigorous activity. We then looked at whether the accuracy of self-reported activity was related to a tendency to be compulsive about exercise, motivation to recover from anorexia nervosa, and psychological distress. We found that people whose exercise was more compulsive had more accurate self-reported total exercise. There was weak evidence to suggest that motivation to change and psychological distress may be associated with inaccurate reporting at different levels of exercise intensity. The results may help us better understand the usefulness of self-report exercise measures, and when accelerometer devices may be more appropriate. Results may also help the development of more accurate self-report measures and treatment programs for people with anorexia nervosa.

Background

Anorexia nervosa (AN) is a psychological illness characterised by low body weight, body image distortion and an intense fear of gaining weight [1]. Fear of weight gain often manifests through dietary restriction and often coincides with increased levels of physical activity (PA). High levels of PA have long been described in patients with AN [2], and studies have found that 31–80% of patients with AN engage in high levels of PA [3–5]. High levels of PA in patients with AN have been associated with further negative physical [6–8] and psychological [8, 9] implications.

There is increasing recognition that measuring an individual's level of PA is an important aspect of assessment and treatment in patients with AN [10]. In clinical settings, PA is typically measured either using observation or self-report measures including: observation by clinical experts [11], questionnaires [12], semi-structured interviews [13], and activity diaries [14]. However, there has been concern that these measures may not accurately reflect the level of PA engaged in due to dependence on factors such as patients' recall and accuracy of patient reporting [15]. The potential for bias in self-report measures has led to a suggested shift towards measuring PA using direct or objective measures that do not rely on the patient's self-report [15, 16]. The most commonly used direct methods for studying PA in patients with AN has been accelerometry [15]. Accelerometer devices are typically attached to the wearer at the wrist or hip, and measure activity using acceleration signals. These signals can then be converted to units of energy expended, and / or summarised as time spent in different intensities of PA, using standardised cut points such as sedentary, light, moderate, and vigorous PA [17].

Research has explored the extent to which self-report measures reliably measure PA, compared to accelerometer data, across various populations and contexts [18]. Indeed, a recent systematic review found that non-clinical samples tended towards overestimating their PA on self-report measures compared to accelerometer devices [18]. Although this trend was apparent in both genders, it was particularly strong among females who self-reported 138% more PA than was recorded on accelerometer devices [18]. It has also been found that when stratified by intensity of activity, non-clinical samples are most accurate when reporting time in light intensity PA (such as slow walking) and least accurate when reporting higher intensity PA (such as brisk walking, jogging or running) [18].

There are mixed findings regarding the accuracy of self-report measures of PA in patients with AN. To date, four have compared self-report measures to objective measures of PA in patients with AN. One such study compared self-reported PA levels over three days on a visual analogue scale (0–10) to an accelerometer (Actiwatch) in 18 patients with AN [16]. It was found that patients under-reported their PA on self-report measures and there was no correlation between self-reported PA and accelerometer data. Similarly, a study by Bratland-Sanda [19] asked seven inpatients with AN to record the type, frequency, duration (minutes / session), and intensity (using Borg's 6–20 rating of perceived exertion scale) of their PA. It was shown that patients significantly under-reported their moderate-vigorous physical activity on the self-report diary compared to an accelerometer (ActiGraph MTI model 7164; Manufacturing Technology, Fort Walton Beach, FL) over a seven-day period. There was no significant difference between self-report and objective measures in the nonclinical control group. Finally, Alberti et al. [20] demonstrated that 52 inpatients with AN significantly under-estimated PA on a self-administered format of the International Physical Activity Questionnaire (IPAQ) compared to an accelerometer device (Actiheart) over a seven-day period.

In contrast, Keyes and colleagues [21] found that patients with AN were more likely than controls to report higher PA on self-report measures compared to accelerometer data. In this study, self-reported PA on the IPAQ was compared to accelerometer data (Actiwatch AW4; Cambridge Neurotechnology, Cambridge, UK) in patients with AN [both inpatients ($n = 18$] and outpatients ($n = 37$)] and healthy controls over seven days. Accelerometer data indicated that patients with AN exercised for similar periods of time, and with a similar intensity, to healthy controls. However, patients with AN self-reported that they had engaged in more exercise than healthy controls. The authors hypothesised that in AN, self-report may overestimate PA due to differences in perception related to their eating disorder psychopathology [21]. Thus, while the research suggests that patients with AN are inaccurate in their self-reported PA compared to accelerometer data, evidence is conflicting as to whether they overestimate or underestimate their PA on self-report measures.

Limited research to date has investigated why patients with AN are inaccurate in their self-reported PA. One factor that may contribute to the accuracy of self-reported PA may be the nature of the PA itself. According to Adkins and Keel [22], dysfunctional exercise in eating disorders may have two dimensions. The first is the quantitative dimension, such that exercise is excessive as defined by its frequency, intensity and duration. The second is the qualitative dimension, or the compulsive nature of the exercise. Compulsive exercise is defined as a rigid and highly driven urge to exercise, and there is a perceived inability to cease despite the risk of harmful consequences [23]. Meyer and colleagues [24] developed a model of compulsive exercise in eating disorders, wherein compulsive exercise is maintained by factors including perfectionism, rigidity, eating disorder pathology, compulsivity, and psychological dependence. High levels of compulsive exercise have also been found to be positively associated with record keeping [25]. As such, it is important to understand whether patients with higher levels of compulsive exercise may be more accurate on self-report measures, as they may be more rigidly adhering to their goals, and therefore more aware, of their PA levels.

Another factor that might be related to the accuracy of self-reported PA is an individual's motivation to change and recover from anorexia nervosa. For instance, in a study by Bratland-Sanda and colleagues [19] one participant reported "I am not physically active – I only go for walks", while also reporting that she walked one hour daily. The authors hypothesised that under-reporting may be deliberate and occur due to fear of mandatory increase of energy intake/ restriction of PA in the hospital/treatment program. As such, patients may not report light exercise as they would under-report their exercise participation [19]. Similar findings were described in an interview study by Kolnes [26]. Specifically, patients under-reported and rephrased descriptions of their engagement with exercise, often implying that their activity (e.g. walking) would not necessarily be counted as exercise. Kolnes [26] reported that participants articulated a clear understanding of the need to reduce PA as part of their treatment program, but at the same time engaged in long periods of light activity. Thus, they suggested that a patient's tendency to underreport their PA may be a way to convey adherence with treatment while still expending energy contributing to weight loss. It has been established that a key feature of AN is that it is ego-syntonic in nature, leading to poor insight and low motivation to change [27]. In general, lower motivation to change has been found to be associated with poorer patient outcomes in eating disorder treatment including lower BMI [28], slower weight gain [29], higher rates of compulsive exercise [8], and poorer quality of life [30]. The trans-theoretical model of motivation to change [31] has been used within the eating disorder field and suggests that patients may move between six stages of change. These stages include precontemplation, contemplation, preparation, action, maintenance and termination. As such, it may be expected that patients in the early stages of change may be more likely to under-report their PA. However, this hypothesis has not yet been tested.

Level of psychological distress may be another factor related to the accuracy of self-report measures of PA. Depression and anxiety symptoms are frequently comorbid with AN [32, 33]. The lifetime prevalence of major depressive disorder in patients with AN ranges from 65 to 81% [34], and the lifetime prevalence for an anxiety disorder is approximately 55% [35]. It is well established that depressed mood and anxiety symptoms are associated with a range of cognitive impairments including memory, inhibition, control, planning, attention, and flexibility [36–38]. It could thus be hypothesised that patients showing higher rates of psychological distress may also suffer cognitive impairments associated with inaccurate recall. These would be expected to impact the degree to which they could accurately report their PA on self-report measures.

In summary, there remains ambiguity in the literature regarding the accuracy of self-reported PA in patients with AN. It is not clear whether patients with AN will under or over-report their PA, and whether their accuracy is influenced by the intensity of activity. Furthermore, there is a paucity of research into the clinical features which may be associated with the accuracy of self-reported PA. Specifically, it has not yet been tested whether level of inaccurate reporting is associated with features such as level of compulsive exercise, motivation to change, and level of psychological distress. Therefore, this study has two aims.

Aims

The first aim of the study was to explore the relationship between self-reported PA and accelerometer data in patients with AN. Given the previous research, it was expected that patients would under-report their PA, and may be more likely to under-report light PA such as walking.

The second aim of this study was to examine the clinical characteristics associated with inaccurate reporting of PA. Due to limited existing research in characteristics associated with under-reporting in AN, the following exploratory hypotheses were suggested. Firstly, it was hypothesised that there will be an association between higher levels of compulsive exercise and higher accuracy in their self-report. Secondly, that there would be an association between lower motivation to change and under-report their PA. Finally, that higher psychological distress may be associated with greater inaccuracy on self-report.

Method

Participants

This study was nested within a trial of "CompuLsive Exercise Activity TheraPy (LEAP): a new approach to compulsive exercise in anorexia nervosa" [39]. This study was a multi-site, randomised controlled trial (RCT) which aimed to test a novel cognitive behavioural therapy for outpatients with AN about what constitutes healthy exercise, and equip them with skills to participate in balanced exercise. Adults with AN ($n = 78$; 4 males) were recruited into the RCT. To be eligible for inclusion, participants had to be at least 18 years old, have a primary diagnosis of AN using the Eating Disorder Examination (EDE) [40] interview, have a Body Mass Index (BMI) between 14 and 18.5 kg/m^2, and have exercised within the last month as indicated on the Exercise Participation Screening Questionnaire (EPSQ) or on the EDE-Q (at least one occasion in the past 28 days). Participants were recruited through public advertising, or referral from an eating disorder service.

All three recruitment sites approved ethics applications for the RCT: The Western Sydney University Human Research Ethics Committee in Australia; the National Health Service Research Ethics Committee in the UK, as part of the Health Research Authority; and the Institutional Review Board at Columbia University in New York, USA. Participants of the current accelerometer study ($n = 36$) were recruited only from Australia and the UK, as the US site did not collect accelerometer data. Written informed consent was provided by the participants for the treatment trial and completion of research measures. The Western Sydney University Human Research Ethics Committee (HREC) approved ethics for the current nested study and the addition of Louise Bezzina as an investigator (HREC approval number: H7732; amendment approved 11th September 2017).

At baseline, participants completed questionnaires and were asked to wear the accelerometer (GT3X+ ActiGraph, Manufacturing Technology, Fort Walton Beach, FL) on an elastic belt around their waist for 4 days (but not when in bed, while showering or swimming). The ActiGraph is an accelerometer device which has been validated in adults [41] and has been used in previous studies with patients with AN [19]. The software program ActiLife 6.9 was used for data processing and analysis. Sequences of more than 60 mins of continuous zero counts (indicating the accelerometer was not in use) were excluded from the analysis, and participants were required to have worn the device for at least 10 h during waking time for each day to be considered valid [42]. Freedson cut points [17] were used to convert the downloaded accelerometer counts per minute data into daily times (in minutes) participants spent in light, moderate, and vigorous intensity PA. Total minutes spent in PA per day were also calculated.

To meet inclusion for the current study, participants had to have worn the accelerometer for a minimum of 10 h per day for at least 2 days. Based on this criterion, 34 participants (32 female, 2 male) were included in the analysis of the current study. This comprised 24 participants from the Australian site, and 10 participants from the UK site. Analyses were completed on group differences between UK participants who wore the accelerometer and those who declined (50% of participants; at the UK site, accelerometer participation was optional), and no significant difference was found in eating disorder severity level as measured by the EDE global score. The average wear time was 14.4 h per day, for an average of 3.5 days. Demographic and clinical characteristics of the participants are found on Table 1.

Measures

Participants wore the accelerometer after their initial assessment with the research assistant. They also completed the following self-report questionnaires at baseline:

The Exercise Participation Screening Questionnaire (EPSQ) is a validated measure assessing common exercise types, with duration, frequency of sessions and intensity [43]. The EPSQ in its original form was administered as a respondent based interview over multiple time periods and we adapted this to a self-report format of current exercise. Thus, in this study it asked about exercise completed in the past four weeks, including the type of exercise, number of sessions per week, average duration per session, and self-rated intensity of each exercise. The types of exercise listed were walking, jogging, swimming, aerobics, weights, cycling, swimming,

Table 1 Demographic and clinical characteristics of the participants

Demographics / Clinical characteristics (*N* = 34)	M (SD)	Range (Min - Max)	95% CI
Age	26.3 (6.4)	18.3–29.1	24.1–28.5
Current BMI[a]	16.4 (1.2)	14.0–18.0	15.9–16.8
EDE[b] Global Score	3.4 (1.2)	0.7–5.4	2.9–3.8
"When do you think AN[c] started?" (age in years)	16.6 (4.8)	5–33	14.9–18.2
"When was AN diagnosed?" (age in years)	20.4 (6.6)	12–38	18.1–22.7
Years between diagnosis and enrolment in LEAP[d]	5.7 (6)	1.8–23.6	3.6–7.8
	N (%)		
Gender	Female: 32 (94.1%) Male: 2 (5.9%)		
AN Subtype (*n* = 32)	▪ AN-Restrictive subtype: 19 (59.4%) ▪ AN-Binge/Purge subtype[e]: 13 (40.6%) - Regular objective bulimic episodes: 7 (21.9%) - Self-induced vomiting: 3 (9.4%) - Laxative/diuretic use: 9 (28.1%)		
Country of birth	Australia: 21 (61.8%) United Kingdom: 9 (26.5%) Other: 4 (11.8%)		

[a]Body Mass Index, [b]Eating Disorder Examination, [c]Anorexia Nervosa, [d] CompuLsive Exercise Activity TheraPy (LEAP), [e] At least one behaviour, 4 or more episodes per month, over last 3 months

tennis and other. Participants frequently indicated pilates, yoga, resistance exercises (e.g., sit-ups, push-ups, lunges), and cardio machines as other. Participants self-rated the activity's intensity level (low, medium, or high) and the duration of each activity in a typical session (in minutes). These intensity levels were used to compare to the accelerometer activity counts of light, moderate and vigorous respectively. A daily average of minutes/day was calculated for each level of intensity of exercise.

The Eating Disorder Examination (EDE) [40] is a semi-structured interview administered by the research assistant to assess the psychopathology associated with the diagnosis of an eating disorder. It is comprised of four subscales (eating concern, weight concern, shape concern, and dietary restraint), one global score, and ratings of eating disorder behaviours to assess severity of symptoms. The EDE has been demonstrated to have robust psychometric properties [44]. The Cronbach's α was .89 in the current study.

The Anorexia Nervosa Stages of Change Questionnaire (ANSOCQ) [45] is a measure of motivation to change which has been validated in adult patients with AN. It consists of 20 questions, assessing three factors: weight change including motivation to reach a minimum healthy weight (weight gain), motivation to alter the relative importance of shape and weight compared to other aspects of life including accomplishments and fulfilment (eating, shape, and weight concerns), and motivation to improve relational and emotional concerns associated with AN (ego-alien aspects). Each question has 5 responses representing the various stages of change (pre-contemplation; contemplation; preparation; action; and maintenance) and the participant can select more than one statement per question, according to the answer/s which best represent their current beliefs. Example items include: *"There is no way I would be prepared to gain weight on these body parts"* (weight gain: pre-contemplation response); *"I have decided that I need to do something about the fear I have of becoming fat because it is controlling me"* (eating, shape and weight concerns: contemplation response); and *"My emotional problems have improved and I am trying to keep it this way"* (ego-alien aspects: maintenance response). Higher scores represent more motivation to change. A mean stage of change score is calculated: < 1.5 = pre-contemplation; 1.5–2.4 = contemplation; 2.5–3.4 = preparation; 3.5–4.4 = action; > 4.5 = maintenance. In the current study, the total score was used, and it's Cronbach's α was .91.

Kessler-10 item distress scale (K^{-10}) [46] is a 10-item measure of psychological distress including both anxiety and depression symptoms. The questionnaire includes questions such as *"Over the past four weeks (28 days), how often have you felt hopeless?"*. Higher scores indicate greater psychological distress, and the maximum score was 50. It has been shown to be valid and reliable in eating disorders research [47]. In the current study, the total score was used, and Cronbach's α was .89.

The Compulsive Exercise Test (CET) [23] is a 24-item measure designed to assess the core features of compulsive exercise in eating disorders. It has 5 subscales: Avoidance and rule driven behaviour, reflecting exercise governed by rules and consequences (e.g., *"If I cannot exercise I feel low or depressed");* Weight control exercise, reflecting exercise focused on shape and weight (e.g., *"I exercise to improve my appearance");* Mood improvement, regarding the positively reinforcing effects of exercise on mood (e.g., *"I feel less anxious after I exercise"*); Lack of exercise enjoyment, meaning performing exercise in an obligatory way, despite not gaining enjoyment from it (e.g., *"I find exercise a chore"*); and Exercise rigidity, assessing the pattern of inflexibility associated with exercise routines (e.g., *"My weekly pattern of exercise is repetitive"*). The CET uses a 6-point Likert scale from 0 (never true) to 5 (always true). Means for the five subscales are summed for the CET-Total, with higher scores indicating a greater level of compulsive exercise. The CET has demonstrated strong reliability, validity, and clinical utility in adult patients with AN [12]. The total score was used in the current study, and it's Cronbach's α was .93.

Statistical analysis

To address the first aim (i.e., explore the relationship between self-reported PA and accelerometer data in patients with AN), the discrepancy between self-reported PA and accelerometer data was calculated by subtracting the average time spent in PA based on accelerometer data from the self-reported PA (i.e. EPSQ - accelerometer = discrepancy). Negative values would therefore indicate under-reporting on the self-report measure (EPSQ). A paired-samples *t*-test (within-subjects) was then conducted to compare the total PA (averaged across intensity level) reported on the EPSQ and recorded on the accelerometer device. This analysis was then repeated as a paired samples *t*-test when PA was stratified by level of intensity (i.e. light, moderate and vigorous).

To address the second aim (i.e. examine the clinical characteristics associated with inaccurate reporting of PA), correlational analyses were used to examine the association between inaccurate reporting and clinical variables. The Shapiro-Wilk test was first used to test the distribution of the data due to the small sample size. Some measures (e.g., CET, and the discrepancy between overall self-report of exercise and accelerometer data) were non-normally distributed. As all analyses involved correlations with at least one non-normally distributed variable, non-parametric tests (Spearman's rho) were used in analyses. Based on the hypotheses, 2-tailed tests were used and correlational analyses were all within subjects. Results were considered significant when $p < 0.05$ and all statistical analyses were carried out using SPSS version 21.0.

Results

Accuracy of self-report (EPSQ) vs accelerometer data

The first aim of the study was to examine whether patients with AN accurately reported their total PA on the EPSQ compared to accelerometer data.

Results demonstrated that participants significantly under-reported their total minutes per day of PA on the EPSQ ($M = 91.8$, $SD = 96.0$) compared to accelerometer data ($M = 325.6$, $SD = 109.1$); $t\ (33) = -13.2$, $p < 0.001$. This indicated that when averaged across level of intensity, patients were significantly under-reporting their PA on the EPSQ compared to accelerometer data. We investigated factors which may have been associated with accuracy of reporting. There was no significant difference in accuracy of reporting between restricting and binge/purge subtype $t\ (30) = -1.1$, $p = 0.3$. Overall total PA accuracy was not correlated with eating disorder symptomatology (EDE global score), $r\ (32) = .21$, $p = 0.23$.

A Bland-Altman Plot (Fig. 1) was used to further explore the level of agreement between self-report and accelerometer measures by deriving the discrepancy in total PA and the 95% limits of agreement [48]. The discrepancy was − 233.9 min / day and the limits of agreement were 2.7 and − 470.4 min / day. This large difference indicates a poor agreement between the EPSQ and accelerometer data in measuring total daily PA.

The discrepancy between EPSQ and accelerometer data was then calculated for light, moderate, and vigorous PA to determine whether patients were differentially under-reporting for different intensity levels of PA. The mean minutes per day in each level of intensity of PA (as recorded by the accelerometer and EPSQ) are summarised in Table 2.

When stratified by intensity of exercise, it appeared that the discrepancy for total PA could be related to under-reporting of light PA. A paired-samples *t*-test was conducted to compare light PA recorded on the EPSQ and accelerometer device. There was a significant difference in reporting light PA on the EPSQ ($M = 17.8$, $SD = 53.0$) compared to the accelerometer ($M = 258.9$, $SD = 88.6$); $t\ (33) = -11.3$, $p < 0.001$. Results showed that participants were not significantly under reporting their moderate or vigorous PA ($p > 0.05$).

These results indicate that the under-reporting of light PA on the EPSQ explained the significant under-reporting of total PA.

Links between inaccurate reporting and clinical features

Spearman's correlational analyses were used to examine the relationship between under-reporting of exercise (total PA) and compulsive exercise, motivation to change, and psychological distress. The results of the correlations are summarised in Table 3.

The mean total compulsive exercise score was 15.6 ($SD = 4.6$). More accurate reporting of total PA on the EPSQ compared to accelerometer data was weakly, however significantly correlated with compulsive exercise, *r*

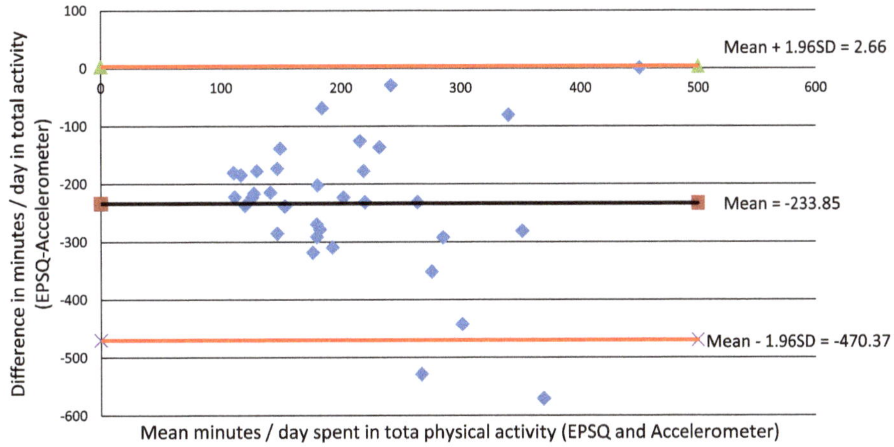

Fig. 1 Bland-Altman plot showing difference versus average values of self-reported (EPSQ) and objectively measured (Accelerometer) total physical activity. The plots show discrepancy with 95% limits of agreement in patients ($n = 34$). Negative values indicate under-reporting of PA on the self-report measure (EPSQ)

(32) = .36, $p = 0.04$. This is represented in Fig. 2. This suggested that a higher level of compulsive exercise was associated with increased accuracy on self-report measures compared to accelerometer data. When PA was stratified by level of intensity, there were no significant correlations found between under reporting light, moderate, or vigorous PA and compulsive exercise.

The mean total score for stage of change was 46.4 ($SD = 11.6$). Under-reporting of total PA on the EPSQ compared to accelerometer data was not significantly correlated with stage of change ($p > 0.05$), as shown in Fig. 3. However, when PA was stratified by level of intensity, there was a significant correlation between under-reporting of moderate PA and motivation to change, such that those who were more motivated to change were more likely to under-report their PA, r (32) = −.39, $p = 0.02$.

The mean score for psychological distress was 31.0 ($SD = 8.8$). Under-reporting of total PA on the EPSQ compared to accelerometer data was not significantly correlated with psychological distress ($p > 0.05$), as shown in Fig. 4. However, when PA was stratified by level of intensity, this trend appeared to be driven by the significant relationship between the discrepancy of self-reported light PA and distress, r (32) = .36, $p = 0.04$.

Discussion

The current study aimed to examine how accurately patients with AN self-reported their PA on the EPSQ compared to accelerometer data. Results indicated that patients with AN significantly under-reported their overall PA on the EPSQ compared to accelerometer data. It is difficult to compare these results to previous research outcomes given the different methods of self-reported and accelerometer PA assessment, length of time PA was monitored, and sample size. However, results were consistent with three previous studies which compared self-report measures to accelerometer data [16, 19, 20]. In contrast, this finding is inconsistent with the results of Keyes et al. [21], which found that patients with AN showed higher self-reported PA compared to healthy controls, while accelerometer-measured PA levels for patients with AN and controls were not significantly different. One possible explanation for this difference could be that their study did not include comparisons between the self-report and accelerometer data for each individual [21]. As such, individual differences in the accuracy of reporting may not have been captured. Further, several patients who had missing data on accelerometer devices were excluded from analyses, potentially underestimating accelerometer PA results.

Table 2 Mean minutes per day of physical activity recorded on accelerometers and EPSQ, and the discrepancy between these means

PA intensity	Accelerometer (mins/day)	EPSQ[a] (mins/day)	Discrepancy	p
Light	258.9	17.8	− 241.1	< 0.001
Moderate	55.6	53.7	−1.9	0.80
Vigorous	11.2	20.3	9.1	0.28
Total	325.6	91.8	−233.9	< 0.001

[a]Exercise Participation Screening Questionnaire

Table 3 Spearman's correlations between under-reporting on EPSQ (self-report vs accelerometer discrepancy) and compulsive exercise, motivation to change, and distress

Level of exercise discrepancy (EPSQ[a] vs Accelerometer)	Compulsive exercise (CET[b] total)	Motivation to change (ANSOCQ[c] total)	Distress (Kessler-10)
Light	0.03	0.05	0.36* ($p = 0.04$)
Moderate	0.24	−0.39* ($p = 0.02$)	−0.01
Vigorous	0.12	−0.03	0.08
Total	0.36* ($p = 0.04$)	−0.06	0.29

[a] Exercise Participation Screening Questionnaire, [b] Compulsive Exercise Test, [c] Anorexia Nervosa Stages of Change Questionnaire; *$p<.05$

A novel finding from the current study was that patients were more likely to under report their light PA compared to moderate and vigorous PA. Previous studies have not examined differential under-reporting as a function of intensity of exercise. This result is consistent with the qualitative data collected by Kolnes [26] and Bratland-Sanda et al. [19] which found that patients with AN tended to under-report their light PA in discussion with the researchers. However, it is notable that this finding contrasts with data showing that non-clinical samples are more accurate when reporting lighter intensity PA [18]. One possible explanation could be that patients with AN hold a different definition of 'light activity' to other groups. However, this hypothesis warrants further investigation. Future studies could reduce the potential for differential definitions to affect data by providing detailed instructions and examples to help clarify what kinds of activity would be categorised as 'light' in intensity.

Results indicated a positive association between higher levels of compulsive exercise (CET score) and higher accuracy on overall PA. This finding is consistent with previous research, which suggests that patients who engage in exercise of this quality are more likely to be rigid in their exercise regime and more likely to keep records [24, 26]. It may be the case that patients with compulsive exercise are more self-aware of their participation in PA and thus are better able to accurately report this on self-report measures.

Motivation to change (ANSOCQ stage of change score) was not related to accuracy on the self-report measure of total PA. However, there was a weak significant relationship between increased accuracy and lower motivation to change, and this effect was particularly strong for moderate intensity PA. This is inconsistent with previous research by Kolnes [26] and Bratland-Sanda et al. [19] who both hypothesised that participants may be more inaccurate in their self-report when they are less motivated to change and comply with treatment. Further, the finding that patients who were more motivated to change were more likely to under-report moderate intensity PA is counter-intuitive, and it is not clear why this effect would be limited to only moderate intensity exercise. One factor which may explain this finding is the limited variation in the data- all patients in the sample rated themselves as being between the contemplation and action stage of change. However, no participants were on the extreme ends of the scale (pre-contemplation and maintenance stage). This lack of

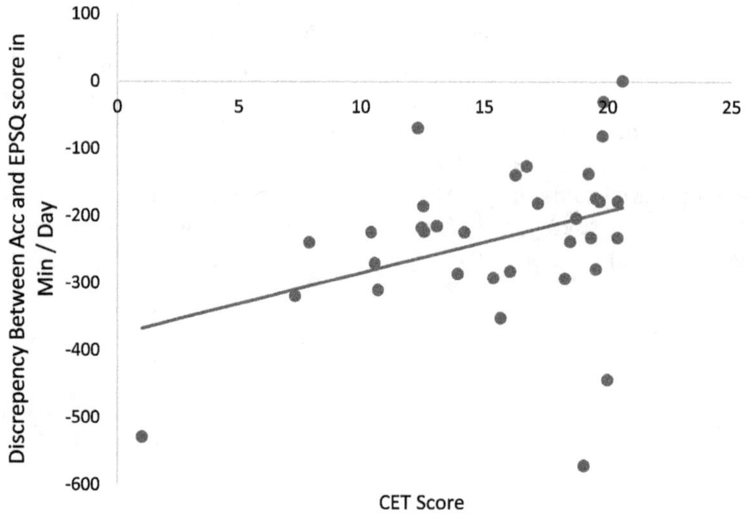

Fig. 2 Correlation between the discrepancy of accelerometer data and EPSQ score, and compulsive exercise (CET score) ($n = 34$). Negative values indicate under-reporting of PA on the self-report measure (EPSQ)

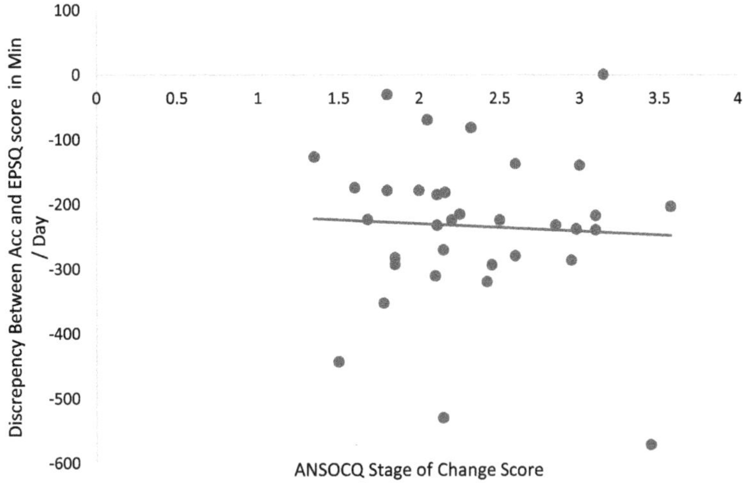

Fig. 3 Correlation between the discrepancy between accelerometer rand EPSQ score and motivation to change (ANSOCQ score) ($n = 34$). Negative values indicate under-reporting of PA on the self-report measure (EPSQ)

variation may have meant that any effect of motivation to change was not captured. Another possible factor that could influence motivation to change is level of ED symptomatology, however in this study we did not find a significant association between ED symptomatology and accuracy of reporting. Future research could replicate these analyses with a sample of patients in different stages of motivation to change to investigate this further.

Level of psychological distress (anxiety and mood symptoms on the K^{-10}) was not found to be related to under-reporting of total PA on self-report measures (i.e. the level of under-reporting was similar for those with high and low levels of distress). Interestingly, there was a slight, but non-significant trend towards higher distress being associated with more accurate reporting. Results indicated that this trend was driven by a significant relationship between higher distress and more accurate reporting of light PA. This result was inconsistent with the literature reporting that depression and anxiety symptoms may be associated with cognitive deficits in memory, which would be expected to lead to inaccurate reporting. Furthermore, it is not clear why the correlation between increased accuracy and increased distress was only significant for light intensity PA. One possible explanation for this could be that those who accurately reported their light PA had higher levels of self-focused attention and thus were more aware of the quantity of light PA they were engaging in, and may not deem it to be ‘good enough’ as it was not high intensity. It could be the case that this judgement could result in higher levels of psychological distress if the aim of exercise was to expend as much energy as possible. Self-focused

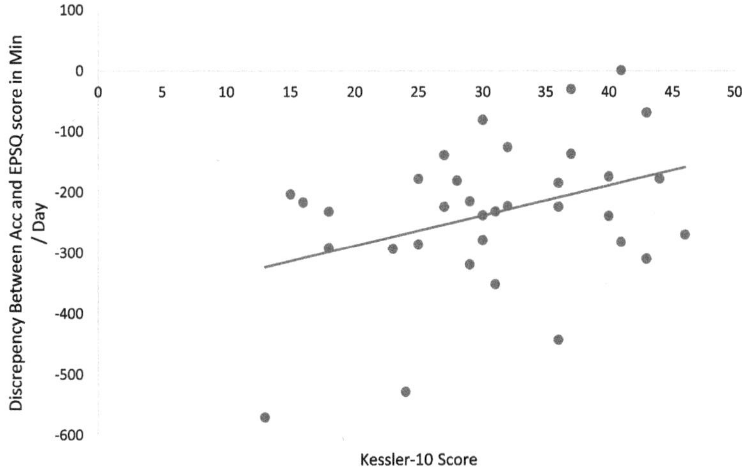

Fig. 4 Correlation between the discrepancy between accelerometer rand EPSQ score and psychological distress (Kessler-10 score) ($n = 34$). Negative values indicate under-reporting of PA on the self-report measure (EPSQ)

attention has been associated with negative affect [49], which provides further support for this idea. However, this finding warrants further investigation.

The current study had several strengths. It was novel as it was the first study to evaluate the EPSQ compared to an objective measure of PA in a sample of outpatients with AN. It was also the first study to measure the association between clinical characteristics and inaccurate reporting of PA. Another strength of the study was the use of accelerometer devices as an objective measure of PA. Accelerometer devices are considered the most reliable measure of PA to be used in a clinical setting for this population [15]. Furthermore, participants adhered to the study protocol – average wear time for the accelerometer was 14.4 h a day for an average of 3.5 days. Given PA was not a primary outcome of the larger RCT, this was a relatively long wear-time. Wear time was similar to other studies in the area, which have ranged from 3 days (16) to 7 days [19–21]. Furthermore, Trost, McIver, and Pate [50] reported that 3–5 consecutive days of wear time reliably estimated habitual PA. However, it is recognised that while accelerometer devices are relatively practical and valid in comparison to other direct or objective measures, accelerometry is also reliant on the patient's compliance with wearing the device [15]. Future research could consider applying stricter thresholds for time and days wearing the device to increase the accuracy of data. Furthermore, it may be more reliable to use a waterproof accelerometer device in future studies so that water-based activities, such as swimming, could be recorded.

The present research has several important clinical implications in the assessment and treatment of patients with AN. Firstly, the data suggest that clinicians should be aware that patients with AN may vary in the accuracy of their self-reported PA depending on the intensity of exercise (i.e. light, moderate, or vigorous), such that they may be more likely to under-report light PA compared to moderate or vigorous PA.

Secondly, there is preliminary evidence to suggest that the EPSQ may be an accurate measure of patients' moderate and vigorous PA. This is clinically relevant as the EPSQ appears to be an easy to administer, efficient, and inexpensive tool that can be used in a clinical context. However, the EPSQ may not be useful in determining overall PA due to the patients' tendency to under-report light PA on this measure, leading to a significant under-reporting of overall PA. Given the significant under-reporting of light PA on the EPSQ, it may be necessary to use another measure for capturing PA, particularly if the clinician suspects the patient may be engaging in excessive light PA. Results from the study demonstrated that accelerometers can more accurately measure light PA, although they can be time and cost-intensive to administer and interpret, as well as potentially intrusive for patients [18]. =Alternatively, a self-report measure which is more sensitive to light PA could be developed as part of future research.

Thirdly, findings suggest that patients whose exercise could be considered compulsive in quality, as measured by the CET scores, are more likely to accurately report their exercise than those whose exercise is less compulsive. Given the time and economic resources required when using accelerometer devices, it may be more important to prioritise their use to monitor patients whose PA is not classified as compulsive. Finally, the results provide preliminary evidence that clinicians should not assume that clinical characteristics such as psychological distress and motivation to change affect the accuracy of self-report PA.

The limitations of the current data are first that self-report PA data involved asking participants to reflect on their exercise over the previous month, then averaged to calculate a daily exercise average. As such, it relied heavily on participants' recall and was not administered in respondent based interview format as in its original use. This could in part explain the significant under-reporting of light PA (as opposed to moderate and vigorous PA) as it could be argued that light PA may be more easily forgotten as it is less strenuous and possibly more likely to be incidental. Further, the days represented in the patients' self-report were not the same days that the accelerometer was worn, and self-reported data reflected patient's recall of PA over the previous month while the accelerometer data was over an average of four days, meaning the length of time represented also differed. Researchers asked participants to complete a written diary style record of their activity whilst wearing the accelerometer, however there was not an adequate amount of written data suitable for inclusion in the study. Future studies could consider administering a modified version of the EPSQ measure daily, and asking the participant to reflect the same days that the accelerometer device was worn. This could also assist in future studies as a way of measuring participant's perception of how reflective the accelerometer data would be of their self-reported PA. Further, the sample was limited as it included 34 participants (with only two males) and analyses were only conducted on patients who agreed to wear an accelerometer device and complied with wear-time instructions. It is likely that this is a unique sample, and that those who did not agree to wear an accelerometer device could differ in the accuracy of their self-reported PA. An important consideration is that there were no consequences of patients reporting high or low PA, or engaging in more or less PA than usual. This is because only the researchers reviewed the accelerometer and self-report data, and data was collected at baseline limiting treatment interference.

However, we do acknowledge there may be a small motivation/compliance factor, as therapists collected the accelerometers and questionnaires from the patients. It is not clear how the current data would generalise to situations where the patient's clinician reviewed the self-report data, or if there were prescribed consequences for increased PA (e.g. increased caloric intake) in a therapy context. Future research could therefore consider testing the accuracy of the EPSQ in different settings (i.e. inpatient vs outpatient) and with patients at different stages of illness. Finally, given the small sample size included in the current study, there are limitations to the conclusions which can be drawn from the correlational analyses presented. Future studies could consider repeating the analysis with a larger sample to increase the strength of conclusions which can be drawn from correlational trends.

Conclusion

The present study has furthered our understanding of the relationship between self-reported PA and accelerometer data in outpatients with AN. Overall, results confirm previous research findings that patients with AN underestimate their PA on self-report measures. Results also showed that patients accurately self-reported moderate and vigorous PA, but significantly under-reported light PA on the EPSQ. Furthermore, higher levels of compulsive exercise were significantly associated with more accurate reporting of total PA. Clinical features, such as motivation to change and distress were less clearly associated with the accuracy of total self-report PA, but results suggest they may be associated with inaccurate reporting at different levels of intensity of PA. Associations between clinical features and the accuracy of self-report in the current study were weak and based on a relatively small sample size, and therefore further investigation is warranted before strong conclusions can be drawn. The results have clinical implications in understanding the utility, and potential shortcomings, of self-reported PA measures, and when accelerometer devices may be more appropriate. Results may also guide future research in understanding why patients under-report PA, which could help inform the development of self-report measures and treatment programs for patients with AN.

Abbreviations

AN: Anorexia Nervosa; ANSOCQ: Anorexia Nervosa Stages of Change Questionnaire; BMI: Body Mass Index; CET: Compulsive Exercise Test; EDE: Eating Disorder Examination; EPSQ: Exercise Participation Screening Questionnaire; IPAQ: International Physical Activity Questionnaire; LEAP: CompuLsive Exercise Activity TheraPy Programme.; PA: Physical Activity; RCT: Randomised Controlled Trial

Acknowledgements

We would like to acknowledge the following therapists and research officers involved in the LEAP trial.

Therapists: Tara Cousins, Lisa Dawson, Diane Kancijanic, Melissa Klein, Christopher Langham, Deborah Mitchison, Caitlin Shepherd, and Alex Withers.

Therapy Supervisor: Michelle La Puma.

Research Officers: Lauren Belak, Andreea Heriseanu, Jessica Lerman, Jacqui Wales, and Sarah Young.

Authors' contributions

This study was nested within the RCT "Taking a LEAP forward in the treatment of anorexia nervosa". PH, ST, CM, JA, SM, KP and EA were chief investigators of this trial. SC processed the accelerometer data and with SY conducted preliminary analysis. NF was involved in data collection. LB developed the study idea with SY, PH and ST. LB analysed the data and prepared the manuscript. All authors contributed to and approved the final manuscript.

Competing interests

ST and PH receive royalties from Routledge, Hogrefe, and Huber and McGraw-Hill publishers for printed contributions on eating disorders. SM received, and PH and ST receive honoraria from Shire Pharmaceuticals. PH received royalties from Oxford University Press and receives sessional fees and lecture fees from the Australian Medical Council, Therapeutic Guidelines publication, and New South Wales Institute of Psychiatry. PH and ST are Editors-in-Chief of this journal, and CM, JA, SM, KP, and SY are on the editorial board.

All authors have other published papers cited in this manuscript.

Author details

[1]University of Sydney, Sydney, Australia. [2]School of Medicine, Western Sydney University, Sydney, Australia. [3]Loughborough University, Loughborough, UK. [4]University of Warwick, Coventry, UK. [5]University of Nottingham, Nottingham, UK. [6]Columbia University, New York, USA. [7]Translational Health Research Institute, School of Medicine, Western Sydney University, Locked Bag 1797, Penrith, South NSW 2715, Australia.

References

1. American Psychiatric Association. Diagnostic and statistical manual of mental disorders : DSM-5: American Psychiatric Association. Arlington: DSM; 2013.
2. Gull WW. Anorexia nervosa (apepsia hysterica, anorexia hysterica). 1868. Obes Res. 1997;5(5):498–502.
3. Favaro A, Caregaro L, Burlina AB, Santonastaso P. Tryptophan levels, excessive exercise, and nutritional status anorexia nervosa. Psychosom Med. 2000;62(4):535–8.
4. Kron L, Katz JL, Gorzynski G, Weiner H. Hyperactivity in anorexia nervosa: a fundamental clinical feature. Compr Psychiatry. 1978;19(5):433–40.
5. Davis C, Katzman DK, Kaptein S, Kirsh C, Brewer H, Kalmbach K, et al. The prevalence of high-level exercise in the eating disorders: etiological implications. Compr Psychiatry. 1997;38(6):321–6.
6. Young S, Touyz S, Meyer C, Arcelus J, Rhodes P, Madden S, et al. Relationships between compulsive exercise, quality of life, psychological distress and motivation to change in adults with anorexia nervosa. J Eat Disord. 2018;6(1).
7. Haddad FS. Displaced stress fracture of the femoral neck in an active amenorrhoeic adolescent. Br J Sports Med. 1997;31(1):70–2.
8. Mond J, Myers TC, Crosby R, Hay P, Mitchell J. 'Excessive exercise'and eating-disordered behaviour in young adult women: further evidence from a primary care sample. Eur Eat Disord. 2008;16(3):215–21.
9. Cook BJ, Hausenblas HA. The role of exercise dependence for the relationship between exercise behavior and eating pathology: mediator or moderator? J Health Psychol. 2008;13(4):495–502.
10. Touyz S, Hay P, Noetel M. Is the neglect of exercise in anorexia nervosa research a case of "running out" of ideas or do we need to take a "LEAP" of faith into the future? J Eat Disord. 2017;5(1):35 Available from: http://jeatdisord.biomedcentral.com/articles/10.1186/s40337-017-0157-z.
11. Halmi KA, Goldberg SC, Casper RC, Eckert ED, Davis JM. Pretreatment predictors of outcome in anorexia nervosa. Br J Psychiatry. 1979;134(1):71–8.
12. Young S, Touyz S, Meyer C, Arcelus J, Rhodes P, Madden S, et al. Validity of exercise measures in adults with anorexia nervosa: the EDE, compulsive exercise test and other self-report scales. Int J Eat Disord. 2017;50(5):533–41.
13. Davies S, Parekh K, Etelapaa K, Wood D, Jaffa T. The inpatient management of physical activity in young people with anorexia nervosa. Eur Eat Disord Rev. 2008;16(5):334–40.
14. Pirke KM, Trimborn P, Platte P, Fichter M. Average total energy expenditure in anorexia nervosa, bulimia nervosa, and healthy young women. Biol Psychiatry. 1991;30(7):711–8.

15. Gümmer R, Giel KE, Schag K, Resmark G, Junne FP, Becker S, et al. High Levels of Physical Activity in Anorexia Nervosa: A Systematic Review. Eur Eat Disord Rev. 2015;23:333–44.
16. Van Elburg AA, Hoek HW, Kas MJH, Van Engeland H. Nurse evaluation of hyperactivity in anorexia nervosa: a comparative study. Eur Eat Disord Rev. 2007;15(6):425–9.
17. Freedson PS, Melanson E, Sirard J. Calibration of the Computer Science and Applications, Inc. accelerometer. Med Sci Sports Exerc. 1998;30(5):777–81.
18. Li H, Zhao Y, Wang Y, Kang J. Spectrophotometric determination of azithromycin based on the charge transfer reaction between azithromycin and alizarin. Fenxi Huaxue. 2004;32(5):598–600.
19. Bratland-Sanda S, Sundgot-Borgen J, Øyvind R, Rosenvinge JH, Hoffart A, Martinsen EW. "I'm not physically active - I only go for walks": physical activity in patients with longstanding eating disorders. Int J Eat Disord. 2010;43(1):88–92.
20. Alberti M, Galvani C, El Ghoch M, Capelli C, Lanza M, Calugi S, et al. Assessment of physical activity in anorexia nervosa and treatment outcome. Med Sci Sports Exerc. 2013;45(9):1643–8.
21. Keyes A, Woerwag-Mehta S, Bartholdy S, Koskina A, Middleton B, Connan F, et al. Physical activity and the drive to exercise in anorexia nervosa. Int J Eat Disord. 2015;48(1):46–54.
22. Adkins EC, Keel PK. Does "excessive" or "compulsive" best describe exercise as a symptom of bulimia nervosa? Int J Eat Disord. 2005;38(1):24–9.
23. Taranis L, Touyz S, Meyer C. Disordered eating and exercise: development and preliminary validation of the compulsive exercise test (CET). Eur Eat Disord Rev. 2011;19(3):256–68.
24. Meyer C, Taranis L, Goodwin H, Haycraft E. Compulsive exercise and eating disorders. Eur Eat Disord Rev. 2011;19(3):174–89.
25. Wyatt LM. Obsessive-compulsiveness and disordered eating in obligatory and non-obligatory exercisers [Internet]. ProQuest Dissertations and Theses. 1997. Available from: http://search.proquest.com/docview/304376256?accountid=14182%5Cn. Accessed 7 Aug 2019.
26. Kolnes LJ. "Feelings stronger than reason": Conflicting experiences of exercise in women with anorexia nervosa. J Eat Disord. 2016;4(1).
27. Guarda AS. Treatment of anorexia nervosa: insights and obstacles. Physiol Behav. 2008;94(1):113–20.
28. Geller J, Cassin SE, Brown KE, Srikameswaran S. Factors associated with improvements in readiness for change: low vs. normal BMI eating disorders. Int J Eat Disord. 2009;42(1):40–6.
29. Schebendach J, Mayer LES, Devlin MJ, Attia E, Walsh BT. Dietary energy density and diet variety as risk factors for relapse in anorexia nervosa: a replication. Int J Eat Disord. 2012;45(1):79–84.
30. Muñoz P, Quintana JM, Las Hayas C, Padierna A, Aguirre U, González-Torres MA. Quality of life and motivation to change in eating disorders. Perception patient-psychiatrist. Eat Behav. 2012;13(2):131–4.
31. Prochaska JO, Diclemente CC, Norcross JC. In search of how people change: applications to addictive behaviors. J Addict Nurs. 1993;5(1):2–16.
32. Godart NT, Flament MF, Perdereau F, Jeammet P. Comorbidity between eating disorders and anxiety disorders: A review. Int J Eat Disord. 2002;32:253–70.
33. Godart NT, Perdereau F, Rein Z, Berthoz S, Wallier J, Jeammet P, et al. Comorbidity studies of eating disorders and mood disorders. Critical review of the literature. J Affect Disord. 2007;97:37–49.
34. Fernandez-Aranda F, Pinheiro AP, Tozzi F, La Via M, Thornton L, Plotnicov K, et al. Symptom profile of major depressive disorder in women with eating disorders. Aust N Z J Psychiatry. 2007;41(1):24–31.
35. Kaye WH, Bulik CM, Thornton L, Barbarich N, Masters K. Comorbidity of anxiety disorders with anorexia and bulimia nervosa. Am J Psychiatry. 2004.
36. Ajilchi B, Nejati V. Executive functions in students with depression, anxiety, and stress symptoms. Basic Clin Neurosci. 2017;8(3):223–32.
37. Billingsley-Marshall RL, Basso MR, Lund BC, Hernandez ER, Johnson CL, Drevets WC, et al. Executive function in eating disorders: the role of state anxiety. Int J Eat Disord. 2013;46(4):316–21.
38. Rock PL, Roiser JP, Riedel WJ, Blackwell AD. Cognitive impairment in depression: a systematic review and meta-analysis. Psychol Med. 2014; 44(10):2029–40.
39. Hay P, Touyz S, Arcelus J, Pike K, Attia E, Crosby RD, Madden S, Wales J, La Puma M, Heriseanu AI, Young S. A randomized controlled trial of the compuLsive exercise activity TheraPy (LEAP): a new approach to compulsive exercise in anorexia nervosa. Int J Eat Disord. 2018;51(8):999–1004.
40. Fairburn C, Cooper Z, O'Connor M. Eating Disorder Examination. Edition 17. 0D. In: Cognitive behavior therapy and eating disorders [Internet]; 2014. p. 1–30. Available from: http://www.credo-oxford.com/pdfs/EDE_17.0D.pdf
41. Matthews CE. Calibration of Accelerometer Output for Adults. Med Sci Sport Exerc. 2005;37(Supplement):S512–22 Available from: https://insights.ovid.com/crossref?an=00005768-200511001-00004.
42. Matthews CE, Ainsworth BE, Thompson RW, Bassett DR. Sources of variance in daily physical activity levels as measured by an accelerometer. Med Sci Sports Exerc. 2002;34(8):1376–81.
43. Davis C, Kennedy SH, Ravelski E, Dionne M. The role of physical activity in the development and maintenance of eating disorders. Psychol Med. 1994;24(4):957–67.
44. Berg KC, Peterson CB, Frazier P, Crow SJ. Psychometric evaluation of the eating disorder examination and eating disorder examination-questionnaire: a systematic review of the literature. Int J Eat Disord. 2012;45(3):428–38.
45. Rieger E, Touyz S, Schotte D, Beumont P, Russell J, Clarke S, et al. Development of an instrument to assess readiness to recover in anorexia nervosa. Int J Eat Disord. 2000;28(4):387–96.
46. Kessler RC, Andrews G, Colpe LJ, Hiripi E, Mroczek DK, Normand SLT, et al. Short screening scales to monitor population prevalences and trends in non-specific psychological distress. Psychol Med. 2002;32(6):959–76.
47. Mond JM, Hay PJ, Rodgers B, Owen C, Beumont PJV. Assessing quality of life in eating disorder patients. Qual Life Res. 2005;14(1):171–8.
48. Martin Bland J, Altman DG. Statistical methods for assessing agreement between two methods of clinical measurement. Lancet. 1986;327(8476):307–10.
49. Nilly M, Winquist J. Self-focused attention and negative affect: a meta-analysis. Psychol Bull. 2002;128(4):638–62.
50. Trost SG, Mciver KL, Pate RR. Conducting accelerometer-based activity assessments in field-based research. In: Medicine and Science in Sports and Exercise; 2005.

4

"We don't really know what else we can do": Parent experiences when adolescent distress persists after the Maudsley and family-based therapies for anorexia nervosa

Ella Wufong*, Paul Rhodes and Janet Conti*

Abstract

Background: Maudsley Family Therapy (MFT), and its manualised version, Family-Based Therapy (FBT), are the only well-established treatment interventions for adolescent anorexia nervosa (AN), with treatment efficacy primarily measured by improvements in eating behaviours and weight restoration. A crucial component of this therapy is an intensive home-based refeeding intervention that requires a substantial commitment from parents for up to one year. While this treatment works to restore weight in a proportion of adolescents, very little is known about its impacts on family distress, relationships and identity, including in the 40% of families where the adolescent experiences ongoing eating disorder (ED) symptomatology and/or psychological distress during and post-treatment. Specifically, few studies have investigated the impacts of MFT/FBT treatment on family functioning or on how parents negotiate their identities, or who they understand themselves to be, in the context of this treatment intervention. This is a significant omission, given the substantive role assigned to parents to take responsibility for their child's eating restoration in the first treatment phase. This study seeks to address this gap through a qualitative exploration of parents' experiences of MFT/FBT, in cases where treatment was discontinued and/or their child continued to experience psychological distress post-treatment.

Methods: 13 parents participated in in-depth semi-structured interviews that scaffolded between their experiences and ways they negotiated and sustained their identities as parents within the context of MFT/FBT for their child. Interview data was analysed through a framework of critical discursive analysis to generate themes centred on these parents' experiences and identity negotiation.

Results: Key findings are that MFT/FBT: (1) provided a map for therapy that initially relieved parents' anxieties for their child and facilitated improvements in family functioning; (2) inadequately addressed parental guilt and blame with a form of externalisation of the illness; (3) perpetuated parental guilt by raising anxiety about AN and allocating responsibility for refeeding their child in phase 1 of the treatment; and (4) when ceased, left these parents struggling with an uncertain future, and fears for the wellbeing of their children.

(Continued on next page)

* Correspondence: e.wufong@westernsydney.edu.au;
j.conti@westernsydney.edu.au
Western Sydney University, Locked Bag 1797, Penrith 2751, Australia

(Continued from previous page)

Conclusions: The structure of MFT/FBT provided initial relief with some improvements in family communication patterns, however, when the adolescent experienced protracted ED symptoms and/or ongoing psychological distress post-treatment, these parents were left with uncertainty as to how to navigate their shifting roles and their child's ongoing struggles. This research highlights the need for treatments for adolescent AN that more comprehensively address both the adolescent and parents' psychological distress and also (re)build their senses of identity that have been challenged by AN and its effects.

Keywords: Adolescent anorexia nervosa, Maudsley family therapy, Family-based therapy, Parent experiences, Identity, Qualitative, Discourse

Plain English summary

The Maudsley model of family therapy for anorexia nervosa is a well-established intensive approach to the treatment of children and teens. It requires a substantial commitment from parents who must engage in intensive home-based refeeding and therapy for up to one year. Parents are encouraged to dedicate much of their lives to this process, with siblings also providing emotional support to the adolescent. While this treatment works for many very little is known about the effects it has on family distress, relationships and identity. Little is also known about these effects for families who it does not work for. In this project we interviewed thirteen families to find out more. Many described how the treatment did provide them with a road map that helped make them feel less anxious and restore family relationships for a while. In the long term, however, some described how the treatment could make them feel more guilty when it didn't work as well as had been promised and make them anxious about the future for their child.

Background

Maudsley Family Therapy (MFT), and its manualisation into Family-Based Treatment (FBT) are the most frequently researched treatment interventions for adolescent anorexia nervosa (AN), with reported long-term improvements in adolescent eating behaviour and weight restoration. This has led to these interventions meeting the American Psychological Society's (APS) "well established treatment" (level 1) criteria [1] and inclusion in the NICE treatment guidelines [2]. In the growing body of research on MFT and FBT, including treatment augmentations, there is a paucity of in-depth analysis of the experiences of parents whose adolescents and family are treated with MFT/FBT for adolescent AN. In particular there is an absence of the voice of the 40% of parents whose adolescents experience ongoing psychological distress and/or ED symptomatology post-treatment, despite weight restoration [3].

MFT was developed by clinicians and researchers at the Maudsley Hospital in London [4, 5] and later manualised by Lock and Le Grange [6, 7] into FBT [7]. MFT/FBT[1] is a pragmatic synthesis of a number of other family therapy approaches that have been used to treat AN [7]. The intervention borrows the "family meal" and allocating responsibility to the parents for their child's nutritional restoration from Minuchin's structural family therapy approach [8], the agnostic view of etiology from strategic family therapy [9, 10], therapist neutrality in relation to the family system from Milan systems therapy [11, 12], and the externalisation of the illness from Narrative Therapy (NT) [13]. A key feature of the approach is that it seeks to harness the parents (and siblings) as the fundamental resources in the "fight" against "the anorexia" ([7], p. 80). The first phase of treatment is focused exclusively on supporting the parents to assume control over their child's food intake, which continues until the adolescent has reached at least 90% of their expected body weight ([7], p. 179). The second phase of treatment focuses on transitioning control of eating back to the adolescent, and the final phase focuses on the adolescent's developmental needs.

With the measure of remission from AN as ≥95% Ideal Body Weight (IBW), less than half of adolescents who undergo FBT recover [14, 15], and a randomized controlled trial (RCT) of long-term outcomes of adolescents treated with FBT reported that although 89% of adolescents achieved weight gain to 90% IBW, around 40% of these adolescents had significant ongoing psychological distress at follow-up, as reported by them or their parents [3]. Furthermore, drop-out rates of approximately 20% have been reported for MFT/FBT interventions [16, 17]. Although argued by some to be the "gold-standard" treatment for AN [18] the effectiveness of this intervention is uncertain for a notable proportion of adolescents, outside the outcome measure of weight restoration.

Since its development, there has been a number of research studies that have augmented components of the MFT and FBT interventions. Variations on the delivery of these interventions have included treatment of the adolescent separated from the parents (parent-focused therapy), systemic family therapy and multi-family group interventions. These variations have been rated by the APS criteria as "possibly efficacious" (level 3) [1]. Further augmentations to the manualised FBT approach [19] have proliferated and include the addition of individual Cognitive Behaviour Therapy to target perfectionism [20], incorporation of the principles of exposure therapy [21], and Dialectical Behaviour Therapy [22]. A recent systematic review [23] has reported that while some of these augmentations focus on the young person's psychological issues, the majority increase the intensity of parent-driven behavioural intervention through multi-family therapy [24, 25], separated family therapy [26, 27], parent-focused therapy (PFT) [15], intensive family coaching [28] and day hospital permutations [29]. As high levels of expressed emotion (EE) and parental criticism have been hypothesised as possible impediments in the standard conjoint FBT model [30, 31], PFT avoids this issue by separating the adolescent from the parent in therapy and has been found to have improved treatment outcomes in families reporting high expressed emotion [26]. Notably evident in the majority of innovations in family interventions for adolescent AN is a reluctance to question the core principles of the original Maudsley model [32], or to include therapeutic practices that are seen as corrupting those principles.

Despite a focus on MFT/FBT augmentations, evidence for their benefit is not robust [1]. Most importantly there is no strong evidence to suggest how the manualised FBT model might be augmented to make it more responsive to the specific needs of a family struggling with MFT/FBT. A more responsive model has been developed by researchers and clinicians associated with the Maudsley Hospital in London—the "New Maudsley Approach" [33] aims to provide improved collaborative support and skills training for parents and incorporates elements of Motivational Interviewing [34] into its collaborative skills training program to address the treatment ambivalence that is often a feature of anorexia presentations [35]. The New Maudsley Approach is grounded in the belief that parents of children with AN are already experiencing high levels of stress and distress, and therefore interventions that intentionally raise anxiety levels—such as the orchestration of the "intense scene" in the first session of FBT ([7], p. 59) may ultimately prove unhelpful.

In the evidence base for the outcomes of MFT/FBT there is a notable omission of parental measures [36] and a paucity of in-depth research into parents' experiences and ways they negotiate the structure and components of the intervention. A metasynthesis of adolescents, parents, and clinicians who treat adolescent AN [37] has highlighted a dissonance between treatment "targets"; for example, the priority for clinicians was found to be AN and its eradication through focusing on weight gain and behaviour change, whereas adolescents were consistently found to be concerned with psychological and social functioning [38]. Parents also expected treatment targets to extend beyond a somatic focus and the authors argued that treatment that is overly focused on weight and behaviour change risks creating "pseudorecovery" ([37], p. 14) that is, physical recovery in the absence of psychological recovery, with a high risk of relapse. The issue of treatment targets has been echoed in several studies where adolescents expressed the view that an overemphasis on physical attributes rather than psychological factors was unhelpful and dehumanising [39–41]. From a parental perspective in another qualitative study, two fathers also expressed frustration at the emphasis on weight gain [42]. Likewise, a follow-up study of parents and adolescents at one-year follow-up after an FBT intervention found that a significant minority of participants reported an overemphasis on eating behaviours, and insufficient attention paid to causative factors and psychological issues [43].

This current study is an in-depth analysis of the experiences of 13 Australian parents who experienced MFT/FBT for AN treatment for their child and either dropped-out from this treatment or reported that their child continued to experience psychological distress and/or ED symptomatology, despite partial or full weight restoration. The aims of this research were, firstly, to build a more comprehensive understanding of how these parents ascribed meaning to their experiences and negotiated their identities in the context of MFT/FBT, which is important given the central role parents are assigned in this intervention to facilitate their child's weight and eating recovery. Secondly, this study sought to establish a platform to inform the development of future treatment interventions for adolescents who experience AN and their families.

Methods

Participants

Thirteen parents (nine mothers and four fathers) of 11 female adolescents were interviewed about their experiences of MFT/FBT intervention after their daughter's diagnosis of AN (see Table 1 for details). Although eight of the 11 adolescents had returned to within a normal weight range with MFT/FBT, one had lapsed into low body weight, and all the adolescents experienced ongoing psychological distress (reported by the parent and/or adolescent). Twelve of the 13 parents were living with the other birth parent of their children. Eleven of the parents participated in this study between 1 and 6 years post-MFT/FBT, and two parents reported MFT for their daughter being 15 years prior. All three adolescents who discontinued MBT/FBT before weight restoration continued to engage in individual therapy, with one subsequently reaching restoration to a normal weight. Three

Table 1 MFT/FBT treatment and reported adolescent outcome

Parent Pseudonyms	Family structure	Child age at interview	Child diagnosis age	MFT/ FBT age	MFT/ FBT mths	Individual therapy during MFT/FBT	Phase completed	Adolescent symptoms after MFT/FBT
Kristin & Nathan	Parents +3C	28	13	13	12	No	3	WR, ED, D (P, A)
Alice	Parents +2C	14	12	12	10	Yes. OCD	2 (current)	WR, ED, D (P)
Emily	Parents +2C	18	16	16	19	Yes. Depression & anxiety	2	WR, ED, D (P)
Jane	Parents +3C (NZ)	20	16	16	6	No	3	WR, ED, D (P, A)
Janice	Parents +2C	20	14	14	24	Yes. CBT, mindfulness, psychiatrist	3	WR, ED, D (P, A)
Kiera	Parents +3C	20	14	14	30	No	3	WR, ED (lapse after 3 years) & D (P)
Paul	Parents +4C	19	16	16	24	Yes. Depression & anxiety	3	WR, ED, D (recent hospitalisation) (P, A)
Terry	Parents +2C	18	14	14	6	No. Psychologists & psychiatrists before & after	2	WR, lapse into ED (low weight), D (P, A)
Margaret & Jack	Parents +2C	14	11	11	24	No. Until end of MFT/FBT	1 (DC)	Not WR, ED, D (gained weight with other ED treatment) (P, A)
Merrum	Parents separated +3C	18	17	17	3–4	No	1 (DC)	Not WR, ED, D (P, A)
Susan	Parents +2C	21	15	15	12–24	No. Psychologist when inpatient	1 (DC)	Not WR, ED, D (P, A)

Abbreviations: *C* child, *DC* discontinued, *WR* weight restored, *ED* eating disorder, *D* psychological distress, *P* parent report, *A* adolescent report

of the 11 adolescents were permitted to engage in individual therapy during MFT/FBT (see Table 2 for details of participants' AN treatments).

Procedure and materials

This study was approved by the Western Sydney University Human Research Ethics Committee (approval number: H11303). Participants responded to advertisements distributed through health professional networks, which invited them to participate in a research study with the question: "How can we improve Maudsley Family Therapy for Adolescent Anorexia?"

Semi-structured interviews were conducted in person, or via telephone. Three interviews were carried out by author (EW) in 2017, and the remainder by author (JC) and an additional researcher in 2016. The semi-structured interview schedule (Appendix A) allowed for unstructured questions that were guided by participant's responses in vivo [44] and drew from the paradigm of NT [45] to scaffold between the parent's experiences of the MFT/FBT intervention and ways that they negotiated their identities within this context. Analysis of these parent experiences, identity negotiations and dilemmas provided a foundation for ways MFT/FBT could be improved. The interviews were audio-recorded, and transcribed with the method of light transcription [46], where repetitive words, phrases and pauses (unless lengthy) that disrupt the flow and coherence of the accounts are removed, thereby enabling the analysis to track shifts in positioning and discursive resources used, rather than focusing on the more conversational elements of speaking. All names in the transcripts were replaced with participant-chosen pseudonyms, and participants were given a copy of the interview transcript to change and/or remove information that they considered potentially identifying. Participants were also given a copy of this paper to member-check the analysis of their transcripts as a form of validity (see Appendix B for parent review and feedback).

Analysis

To address the research questions and develop a richer understanding of these parents' experiences, patterns of identity negotiation, and dilemmas associated with key components of MFT/FBT, a critical discursive analysis framework [47, 48] was drawn upon to analyse the interview data. Analysis by the researchers (see Appendix C for researcher positioning statements) traced some of the discursive materials these parents used to piece together narratives of their experiences of MFT/FBT, including their active negotiation of dilemmas, ways they were positioned by and positioned themselves in relation to dominant discourses [49], and from these positions authored a unique sense of identity as parents. Initial coding of the interview data as relevant to the research questions was collapsed into a set of themes that were refined in a recursive process. Interview extracts that most richly represented the final set of themes and subthemes were then extracted and analysed in greater depth.

Results

Analysis traced these parents' experiences of key dimensions of the MFT/FBT interventions and concludes with the uncertainty faced by parents after ceasing treatment (see thematic map, Fig. 1).

Theme 1—A map for therapy

Although the 13 parents experienced initial relief through the MFT/FBT map, 11 were also troubled by the extent of the focus on their child's eating restoration—frequently at the exclusion of addressing their child's psychological distress—especially in the early phases of treatment.

"I felt helpless": Structure and standing together

Nine parents talked about a sense of relief on finding professionals who specialised in AN treatment and the structured MFT/FBT interventions.

> *Extracts 1*
>
> *Emily: I think I was extremely grateful to the Maudsley team, [...] the first people who actually talked to us, right, to explain things to us, who gave us a guideline.*
>
> *Janice: I felt helpless. I felt totally out of control. I had lots of people saying to me "Just—just make her eat. It's no big deal." Particularly [...] that generation who don't always get that this is a genuine mental illness. So, having a plan just made me feel like I had something secure to—to work on, to work with, to trust in. And I trusted the psychiatrist we were seeing emphatically.*
>
> *Jack: [...] the 95% Maudsley track record or whatever it was that rolled out gave me a high level of confidence 'will this work?' So follow it, follow them, follow ah it consistently, don't deviate because we haven't got any of that expertise or experience they do.*

These narratives exemplify the extent of these parents' pain and helplessness in the context of their child's AN experience. Being given a "guideline" by the Maudsley treatment team was experienced as a relief by Emily after a paucity of explanations in previous treatments. Diagnosis for Janice legitimated her daughter's experience as a "genuine mental illness"—and confirmed her insider knowledge of the complexity of her daughter's experience—that was not simply attributable to parental

Table 2 Adolescent treatments for ED and other psychological problems

Parent	Other eating disorder treatments	Eating disorder behaviours	Treatment for other problems
Kristin & Nathan	Psychiatrist, BN-Day program, DBT group (all C)	Current binge eating started 2 years after MFT/FBT	Psychiatrist and DBT group (C) for depression, self-harm
Alice	Inpatient (P)	Restriction, over-exercise	Psychiatrist (C) and inpatient (P), OCD (diagnosed at 11 years old), depression, self-harm, possible ASD
Emily	Inpatient (including nasogastric tube), dietician (P)	Restriction, over-exercise	Psychologist from age 14 for anxiety, depression, self-harm
Jane	Inpatient, (P) group, (C), psychologists (C & P)	Restriction, over-exercise, purging, binging	Depression, sub-clinical ASD symptoms (diagnosed at 10–12 years)
Janice	Psychologist (CBT & mindfulness), ED support group (C & P), psychiatrist (C)	Restriction, over-exercise, vomited once	Psychiatrist (C), OCD/depression currently on lithium and recently ceased escitalopram
Kiera	Nil. Thinking of seeing a psychologist	Restriction and over-exercise	Psychiatrist, Psychologists (P), anti-depressants (subsequent to anorexia diagnosis), self-harm
Paul	3 inpatient admissions (P), about to recommence hospital treatment	Restriction, over-exercise, purging and binge eating	Psychiatrists/psychologists/school counsellor (P) for depression, anxiety (included anti-depressants)
Terry	Inpatient then MFT/FBT (P), outpatient, multi-family therapy (P)	Restriction, over-exercise, purging	Psychiatrist/psychologist (C), self-harm, Conversion Disorder, depression, psychosis: medication including quetiapine
Margaret & Jack	Psychologist (NT) (C), inpatient admission (P)	Restriction, over-exercise	Psychologist (C), anxiety
Merrum	Psychologist (NT), dietitian, psychiatrist (C)	Restriction, over-exercise	Psychologist and Psychiatrist (C), anxiety, family counselling before ED (P)
Susan	Psychologist and psychiatrist (C), inpatient admissions (P)	Restriction, over-exercise, purging	Psychologist and psychiatrists for depression, OCD (C)

Abbreviations: *C* current, *P* past

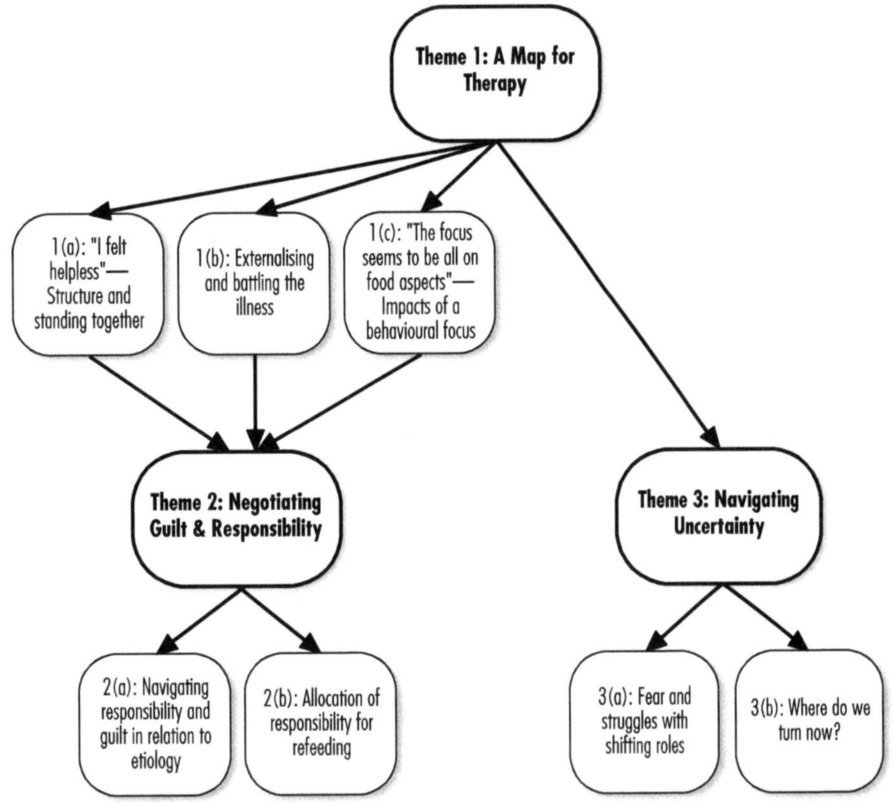

Fig. 1 Thematic Map of Parents' Experiences of MFT/FBT

incompetence in not being able to "just make her eat". The high evidence of success of MFT/FBT cited to Jack contributed to an initial confidence in handing over of "expertise" of their daughter's care, as AN had undermined his own expertise as her father.

The structure of MFT/FBT therapy also had the potential to assist in the restructuring of family relationships as outlined in nine of the parents' narratives.

Extracts 2

Emily: [...] they actually kind of guided us through some of the very, very hard conversations. Hard as in about feelings, about guilt, about perceptions, and about the effects it had on us [...] I think as a family we've grown a lot closer [...] in a way that we can respect each other.

Nathan: [...] the kids could complain about us, we could complain about them. So it, it developed an openness that hadn't been there previously.

Kiera: [...] we were a joint force. I think if you can work together really quickly it helps because an eating disorder can get around one of you, but if it knows that dad's there backing up everything that mum says and vice-versa, I think that helps.

Jane: [...] she announced that she appreciates what we did for her [...] She knows we're quite committed to it as best as we can.

These extracts highlight the scope for MFT/FBT in cultivating a sense of closeness in relationship between family members. For Emily, MFT/FBT provided a scaffold for her family to engage in "very hard conversations" that navigated questions about "guilt" and "perceptions". For other parents, these interventions provided a context for "openness" and for their child to have a voice (Nathan) and, through the structural family intervention, a unified voice to the parents (Kiera). MFT/FBT also provided opportunity for these parents to experience themselves as contributing positively and meaningfully to their children's lives through their commitment to their child's recovery.

Externalising and battling the illness

Nine parents talked specifically about their experiences of externalisation of the illness, including the process of separating their child's identity from the illness identity, and fighting the illness, rather than their child.

Extracts 3

Kiera: There was Sally and there was the eating disorder and once you separate them you realise that she is still there and we're fighting the eating disorder and she is too. [...] And it made it easier, that it wasn't just her doing this to herself.

Emily: I always said, you know, "You're my daughter, I love you, but anorexia, I can kick as often as I like. If I do something which obviously you don't like, I do it because it's against anorexia. It's not against you, but it is against the illness."

Margaret: I accept that when she was very sick, you know, we talk in these beautiful terms of "it was the eating disorder and not Hayley in the room" and all those euphemisms but effectively Hayley was still in the room but she was treated as though she wasn't. [...] that was probably the most unnerving thing that the person who I believe has been the key to recovery, i.e. herself (emotional tone), was deliberately excluded from the process and talked about as though she wasn't even in the room.

Kristin: [...] anorexia never leaves that person. They fight with it every day. [...] that disease is so strong!

Externalisation of the eating disorder enabled Kiera to resist minimising her daughter's experience to something she was "just doing" to herself and opened the path to position their responses and actions as "fighting the eating disorder". Externalisation of the illness also enabled these parents to focus their frustration and other negative emotions upon an anorexic entity, rather than their child. For example, externalisation with a battle metaphor enabled Emily to legitimise her strong emotional responses to her daughter's behaviours—"I love you, but anorexia I can kick as often as I like". Margaret positioned the practice of externalisation as euphemistic with the effect of Hayley herself also being externalized from the therapy ("deliberately excluded from the process").

The medical construction of AN as "disease" or "illness" set up an adversarial scenario [50] for these parents where they found themselves engaged in a "fight" to vanquish AN from their daughter's life. For some of the parents this became a protracted "fight" with the "disease", for example that led Kristin—after a decade of her daughter struggling with an eating disorder—to conclude that "anorexia never leaves that person". Michael White [50] has argued that the therapeutic practice of externalisation, when confined to an illness—or other adversarial—metaphor, risks the person (and their family) experiencing a sense of exhaustion, reduced personal agency and increased distancing from others when this does not occur. This was evident in Kristin's conclusion, "that disease is so strong!" and for Margaret in the inadvertent distancing of her daughter in the externalisation process where she argued that her daughter "was deliberately excluded from the process and talked about though she wasn't in the room".

"The focus seems to be on all the food aspects": Impacts of a behavioural focus

The parents' relief at the MFT/FBT map was followed by a number of their concerns with the narrowing of focus of the MFT/FBT script to their child's eating behaviour and weight restoration, particularly in the early phases. Although these parents understood the rationale for this symptom focus, they also expressed concerns including the implicit neglect of therapeutic focus on the broader contexts of their child's distress and the substantive impacts of being allocated the primary role of refeeding their child.

EXTRACT 4a

Kristin: What we've realised now is that, because it is a mental disease, so the anorexia, the Maudsley treats the eating part of it. On top of all of that, the big umbrella that's on top of that is the mental disease that continues for the rest of their days.

EXTRACTS 4b

Merrum: [...] when I said, "we're at the point now where we need to move on. When's the psychology part of this come in?" Cause I knew it was going to come. And "oh not yet. We're not ready for that yet" and I'm saying, but Kate is and I think Kate needs to speak.

Susan: Well I think that's when – I think they were supposed to be but – but it ended up being kind of like problem solving from one week to the next of how to get her to eat. You know you've only got an hour and [...] her OCD got completely out of control.

Margaret: I feel sad that, that she had to, on top of the disease that she is fighting, had to be treated in a way that denied her intelligence, that denied her innate ability to, to fight this herself and of course no parent is going to um, say "oh we'll just see whether she wants dinner tonight" and not be around.

These parents expressed concern that MFT/FBT too narrowly treated their daughter's AN symptoms. Within the narratives of the parents who reported that their child's weight was restored through MFT/FBT, there was a parallel process between their daughter's ongoing psychological distress and their own distress and worry that their child might bear the legacy of AN for "the rest of their days" (for example, extract 4a). In the narratives of parents whose child/family discontinued MFT/FBT before weight recovery (extracts 4b), there was significant concern expressed about the exclusion of focus on their child's broader distress, which parents witnessed through impacts such as their child losing their voice (Merrum) and their child's unaddressed symptoms of distress (Susan). Implicit in Margaret's rhetorical positioning was the assumption that parents will do what it takes to get their child well, however, the focus on parents should not exclude the adolescent's active involvement in their own recovery during any stage of treatment.

Extracts 5

Paul: Though, the focus seems to be all on the food aspects. But from my point of view, like as a parent, the food is the, it's the end product of the whole problem, what's going on underneath, what's causing all this?

Terry: [...] something causes it in the first instance and not being able to treat what causes it, as well as the anorexia itself, um, trying to separate the two is a problem. And I come back to the need for a more holistic approach [...] Something that recognises all the complementary parts and doesn't try and treat one in isolation of the other.

In drawing on a problem-solving discourse, Paul argued that there are underlying triggers for his daughter's experiences—that the eating behaviours are the effect, rather than the cause. Terry's argument for a "holistic approach" to treatment underscored the fragmented approach to therapy that can occur when mental illness is diagnosed and treated using a nosological framework. The biomedical discourse introduces a tendency to conceive of different expressions of problematic experiences as distinct and separate comorbidities, rather than interrelated parts of a whole. These fathers expressed misgivings about the MFT/FBT scripts, which were increasingly at odds with their own intuitions regarding their daughter's ongoing needs and struggles.

All of the parents recounted experiences of systemic family distress as they took up the responsibility for their child's eating restoration.

Extracts 6

Alice: [...] they talked to us a lot about the re-feeding and it sounds easy in principle, in theory, but when you actually do it at home it's not that easy when a teenager's screaming at the top of her lungs and you're getting yoghurt thrown at you. I found it really distressing when she didn't want to eat [...] Because you can't really put someone's mouth in a vice and make them eat it, can you?

Susan: I would say that extreme conflict's not worth you know. [...] if the girl doesn't think there is any option then that—there's absolutely no way that you can get out of eating then you'll eat but you know it's such a cost.

Janice: The Maudsley Method seemed to me, when I was feeling really negative, [...]a cheap way out for the government to treat my child, tell us to deal with it. I understand that families are the best approach to deal with this; [...] Because you feel a little thrown to the wolves. [...] once you close the door of your family home that's it; you're on your own.

Kristin: You want a live child at the end of it? This is what you have to do. [...] but you can only do that with support.

These parent narratives highlight how the apparent simplicity of the MFT/FBT interventions ("sounds easy in principle") obscured the reality of how distressing "re-feeding" their adolescent child was for the majority of parents interviewed. This "cost" (Susan) was in navigating the inevitable conflict and dilemmas faced by parents when their child refused to eat. Central to Alice's rhetorical question, "you can't really ... make them eat it, can you?" is a dilemma related to whether the psychological risks of forcing a child to eat can be justified in the name of saving their life.

The costs of these interventions were also a private cost for parents, and were positioned by Janice as "a cheap way out for the government to treat my child". This statement exposes the broader institutional investments in MFT/FBT to treat adolescent AN that are obscured by the uptake of parental discourses that assume that a "good" parent will unquestionably assume the role of "re-feeding". Taking up this parental role unquestionably ("you want a live child at the end of it?"—Kristin) obscured both the burden on these parents and families and the institutional positioning of MFT/FBT as a cost-effective treatment for adolescent AN [51].

Theme 2—Negotiating guilt and responsibility

All of the parents struggled to negotiate guilt related to their daughter's experience of AN and its treatment. The practice of allocation of responsibility for the "refeeding" of their child also held the potential to induce further guilt, particularly in contexts where anticipated weight gains were not achieved or maintained.

Navigating responsibility and guilt in relation to etiology

All the parents engaged in processes of negotiating the question of guilt related to the etiology of AN, taking up a diverse range of positions within a parent-blaming discourse.

Extracts 7

Terry: [...] we'd failed as parents. It's simple, you know? Parents are supposed to look after their kids and particularly in, in the traditional sense fathers are supposed to look after their families. [...] I felt that I'd failed in that.

Jack: [...] my role as provider, protector and nurturer it felt very, very fundamental that um, you know the basics of parenthood I failed.

Janice: I felt that we didn't deserve it. I felt that we'd been—this is going to sound terribly, um, ah, I can't think of the right terminology—I felt this happened to other people that weren't as good parents as we were. [...] I was knocked off my ivory tower. So I was very, very angry. [...] At the time I just, yeah, I thought I'd really failed as a parent to—to have sort of allowed this to happen, or not noticed this had happened. But it wasn't until the psychiatrist we first saw and he said the same to me, was that genetics loads the gun and the environment fires it. [...] that this wasn't my fault at all.

Emily: [...] you feel like well, what have I done? Well, for me as a mother it felt like, well as a parent, what have we done wrong. How (pauses) how did it go off the rails? Did we not pay enough attention? [...] But she still says, "Mum, you will not let me put on that much weight again." We have a good relationship and, you know, she doesn't say it to hurt me, but for me, that then triggers again, oh it was my fault.

Although eight parents talked about how the MFT/FBT therapists had explicitly absolved them of guilt, the majority of the parents' narratives continued to be positioned by parent-blaming discourses. This ranged from guilt about the cause, not noticing their child's symptoms and intervening sooner, and a sense of somehow having failed their child. In taking up a father-as-protector discourse, Terry and Jack assumed their child's AN experience to be a neglect of their responsibilities ("supposed to look after their families"). Janice simultaneously took up and rejected the parent-blaming discourse with her anger being understood as an identity violation and in defense of herself and her husband as "good parents". Despite seeking to free herself from this discourse, she nevertheless remained entangled in the assumption that AN arises from faulty parenting. Emily was caught in a position where she felt responsible and guilty for not discerning AN earlier, responsible for the "refeeding" process, and her daughter's weight gain-related distress. These extracts highlight that the guilt experienced by parents was complex and multifaceted, and not readily amenable to straightforward anti-blame rhetoric.

Allocation of responsibility for refeeding

All of the parents expressed how they struggled with self-blame in the context of being allocated responsibility for their adolescent's eating restoration.

Extracts 8

Alice: Yeah, and when things aren't going well you do kind of blame yourself. Like I really blame myself for her going backwards at Christmas. I should have been more watchful about what had happened ...

Emily: My daughter said, "That dietician saved me from dying because she made me eat." [...] She accepts people with knowledge, and so she goes like right, this lady is a specialist, she is a very no nonsense specialist, and my daughter accepted that that's the way she is, and she goes, "Okay. I will do what that lady tells me."

Alice experienced guilt when her daughter's weight dropped and blamed herself for not continuing the hypervigilance around her daughter's eating. Here it is evident that although the MFT/FBT script maintains that parents are not responsible for AN, being allocated responsibility for refeeding places parents in a position where they are directly responsible for weight recovery, and therefore recruited into further guilt when this is not achieved or maintained. By insisting on the inclusion of a dietician in the treating team, Emily was able to free herself from the position of being solely responsible for her daughter's eating, which reduced conflict within her family. For Margaret and Jack, whose daughter was unable to gain weight with the MFT/FBT intervention, the protracted struggles experienced by their daughter to gain weight resulted in the purportedly non-blaming intervention having a paradoxical effect (extracts 9).

Extracts 9

Margaret: [...] because it was ground hog day. [...] it turned into this sort of circular um, blaming is probably going too far, but a sort of circular evaluation of, of where we'd gone wrong, because the framework clearly works so if we've not succeeded, ***we've*** *gone wrong. [...] (Interviewer: How did that affect how you saw yourself as a mother?) Oh my goodness I was, I have never been so challenged in my life as a mother. I felt wretched. It's such a, a fundamental thing to feed and protect your child and anorexia has already challenged that in its essence and then to, on a weekly basis, be in a context (emotional tone to voice) where you're failings are on show and also on show to your children.*

Jack: Well no in our case we were on trial. I'd be shocked if Margaret didn't even use that expression. [...] I felt like she was on trial in those sessions towards the end and Hayley's failure to put on weight was Margaret's failure to feed her enough ultimately. And I didn't come to her defense, either in the room or afterwards, you know, well enough or consistently enough.

The experience of "groundhog day" with MFT/FBT built on the already established sense of falling short of the "fundamental thing to feed and protect your child" for Margaret. The ongoing allocation of responsibility for Hayley's eating restoration to Margaret and Jack and the search for ways to get Hayley to eat created a context for the allocation of blame—"**we'd** gone wrong". For Margaret, this contributed to an erosion of her sense of identity as a mother ("I felt wretched"). Jack also expressed concern about how this non-blaming approach, when protracted, also become mother blaming.

Theme 3—Navigating uncertainty

For these parents, the reallocation of responsibility to their daughters for eating and self-care, and their transition to autonomy in the later phases of MFT/FBT, were troubling to negotiate, especially in the context of their child's ongoing psychological distress and/or ED symptomology.

Fear and struggles with shifting roles

Around half the parents expressed fear that their child's struggles might continue for the rest of their lives.

Extracts 10

Jane: [...] she's always, gets upset easy and could get depressed easily, you think there's so many more years to go, you know. How's her life going to go? Is she going to constantly live with being a bit depressed, or not?

Kristin: Yeah, and it will never go and I think, for me, that bothers me [emotional voice] because she's my daughter, you know?

Paul: I think it's the not knowing that is the hardest of it. I mean, if you have a flu or a cold, you know you're going to get over it. [...] That it's got a set a time for you to recover from it ...

Terry: I think we're all realistic enough to know that once you've suffered anorexia, it's probably something that will be there in the background for the rest of your life...

These parents questioned whether their child's psychological distress is an experience they will "constantly live with" (Jane) and "will never go" (Kristin), as these parents sought to renegotiate their relationship with hope for their child's future. Paul's struggle with uncertainty about his daughter's recovery highlighted the limitations of applying a medical discourse to AN [52], as recovery from AN is not as simple or certain as recovery from a "flu or a cold". For Terry, the diagnosis of AN entailed suffering "that will be there in the background for the rest of your life". His use of "your" signifies that the suffering was not only for his daughter but also for his family, because for parents there is also the prospect of lifelong distress as they seek to support their child.

Six parents' narratives highlighted their struggles in re-allocating responsibility to their child for their eating in light of their ongoing fears.

Extracts 11

Emily: I actually have difficulty then again letting go, because it was then, okay I have to be in charge to be really the boss against this illness. [...] Kelly said to me, "Mum, don't talk about it anymore. I don't want to be that person with anorexia all the time. We have to let it go." [...] it's hard to not identify then [as] the mother of a child with anorexia.

Jane: To some extent you just have to say, "Well look, what else can I do?" Just what will be will be, to a little extent. [...] it's the same as you can lead a horse to water but you can't make them drink and they're growing up and you have to let them go eventually.

Kiera: I think that's part of the Maudsley that when they're younger that you do the parenting thing and make the decisions and take over, which is what you do best, and last year when she was 19 that still needed to be the case because she wasn't able to do that for herself. [...] I told her when she was younger, I had to look into her eyes and tell her that dad and I would be her strength until she was able to be stronger for herself [sobs].

A turning point for Emily in rethinking her role as "the boss against this illness" and renegotiating her identity as "the mother of a child with anorexia" was when her daughter resisted totalisation of her identity as "that person with anorexia". Jane was also faced with knowing that she had done everything she could as a mother—which she depicted through metaphor ("lead a horse to water")—to mark out the limitations of the extent to which parents can make their child eat, particularly as they get older and to allow for uncertainty to "a little extent". Kiera talked about the necessity of taking responsibility for her daughter's eating when she lapsed at age 19 as she sought to continue to be strong for her daughter with the hope that one day she will have the "strength" to do this for herself. Shifting from an authoritarian stance in phase one of the intervention was troubling for these parents as they were faced with the fear of their daughter lapsing, greater uncertainty around their child's future, and renegotiating their roles and identities as parents.

Where do we turn now?

For the four parents whose daughters did not gain weight with MFT/FBT, there was a sense of helplessness and fear that the front-line, evidence-based treatment did not work for their child.

Extracts 12

Susan: One of them [treatment team] said basically they were running out of options, I mean they—we had kind of—they did come up with lots of options but we were kind of scraping the bottom of the barrel.

Margaret: I think it was a combination of um, of fear of, what else, if not this? We'd also had a period where we really did feel Hayley needed hospitalisation [...] and in spite of her statistics, they clearly weren't 'bad' enough to be hospitalised and we weren't prioritised enough. So I think I'd felt absolutely abandoned by the system.

Merrum: I'm not an expert but I could tell that my child was ready for the next part and they weren't listening. [...] But I just felt like her voice wasn't being heard and it was so important for her. As soon as kids verbalise things, they own it.

For Susan, not gaining weight after numerous hospitalizations and MFT/FBT created a parallel process of helplessness through the family system and her treatment team. Margaret and her husband Jack experienced a sense of "abandonment" as they fell through the cracks of a treatment system that was unable to be tailored to their daughter's unique situation. Merrum struggled to negotiate her identity as a mother with the sense of herself as "not an expert" in AN treatments. Nevertheless, her refusal to sideline her expertise to the treatment team led her to draw on her insider knowledge as a mother that prioritised her daughter's voice in her recovery.

All parents whose child's weight was restored with MFT/FBT expressed uncertainty and unease regarding the ongoing eating-related and psychological distress that their daughters were experiencing, and a sense of struggle about where to turn to next.

Extracts 13

Kiera: [...] we should have had her seeing a psychologist [post-treatment] just to cope with the stress of things. [...] because we just thought that she was cured. A bit naïve with all the stuff that we know now...

Paul: It's like a virus, changing to another—the treatment works for the initial virus but it doesn't work for the new virus now. [...] Whereas now we have more of an understanding but we still feel quite helpless in it, because we don't really know what to do. I mean, apart from helping our daughter get some more therapy, we don't really know what else we can do.

In the context of their child's ongoing difficulties, these parents sought to understand how it was that their child had not recovered. After discharge from treatment, Kiera reported being surprised to learn that it is not uncommon for AN to have a much longer course, leaving her with the retrospective understanding of herself as "naïve". Paul expanded upon the medical discourse through likening his daughter's ongoing struggles to a "virus" which mutates out of their control. A dualistic medical discourse of illness and cure failed to provide a trajectory beyond recovery or chronic illness, leaving these parents feeling "helpless" and struggling to know where to turn next.

These parents struggled to know where to turn to next, particularly as MFT/FBT had been positioned to many of them—through the certainty of scientific discourse—as the only "evidence-based" treatment for adolescent AN. They were positioned on the outside of this discourse, in a place of uncertainty about the next step and how to stand for their child in the face of ongoing ED symptoms and psychological distress.

Discussion

The structure and promise of MFT/FBT were initially experienced as ameliorating these parents' anxieties about their child's struggle with AN. Although the intervention went some way towards addressing their guilt through non-blaming rhetoric and the practice of externalisation of the illness, these parents' complex relationship with guilt—particularly when coupled with their child's ongoing ED symptoms and psychological distress—meant that this non-blaming approach paradoxically became experienced as parent-blaming. Being allocated responsibility for their child's eating in the early phases of treatment was also troubling for these parents. In particular, they expressed frustrations with the focus on weight gain and eating behaviours at the expense of psychological processes and, in some instances, their child's loss of voice. When they completed or discontinued MFT/FBT they were faced with an uncertain future in relation to their child and were unsure where to turn in the face of their child's ongoing ED symptomatology and/or psychological distress.

Behavioural focus of MFT/FBT

Most parents in this study expressed concerns with the extent of the behavioural focus and emphasis on weight and eating restoration, particularly in the early phases of MFT/FBT. This was particularly distressing for parents whose child did not gain weight, with the concomitant increased systemic interpersonal conflict and heightened self-blame. These parents' experiences are echoed by a parent interviewed in an Australian Broadcasting Commission report on AN treatments, where one mother whose child later ended her own life said: "One psychiatrist was giving us advice about what we should do and I said I didn't know if I could do this, hold Tess down and put food in her mouth without hurting her," she said. "He said I needed to go into therapy so I could find out why it was that I couldn't save my daughter's life." (see news article at the following link: https://www.abc.net.au/news/2017-05-04/australian-health-system-failing-patients-with-eating-disorders/8485300\).

All parents whose child initially regained weight were also troubled by their child's recurrent psychological distress post-treatment, particularly depression and ED symptoms, leaving these parents without a map to navigate their responsibilities for their child's recovery. Although there is evidence that early weight gain is a predictor of improved psychological outcomes [53], AN is commonly associated with a range of other mental health problems [54, 55]. Additionally, it is notable that from the parents' perspectives, their daughter's concerns about body weight and shape were not ameliorated by MFT/FBT—despite weight gain—which is consistent with the findings of other research [56]. Given the difficulty of treating AN—and the great distress of the families involved—it is understandable that clinicians need to prioritise the adolescent's medical safety. However, these parents expressed clear concern about the apparent limitations of MFT/FBT in addressing their child's comorbid psychological issues—whether pre-existing or concomitant with AN. Early treatment focus on nutritional restoration with the assumption that this will also reduce an adolescent's distress is problematic, as an absence of comprehensive intervention for adolescent and parent systemic distress in the early phases of treatment means that these issues are effectively relegated until the later phases of therapy. As argued by Greg Dring, "if the therapist spends the first sixteen sessions of the work discouraging the discussion of feelings, relationship issues and developmental difficulties in a personal way, then it may be very difficult to revive such discussion at a later stage when, in any case, the work is about to be concluded." ([57], p. 66).

Parental guilt and the etiological stance of MFT/FBT

The agnostic etiological stance of MFT/FBT and the explicit absolving of guilt and blame was experienced as helpful by most parents in this study. However, since the treatment involves a focus on modifying parenting practices, it remains an open question as to what role parenting styles and family dynamics play in the development or maintenance of AN, noting also that a recent study has found that parent-focused treatment was more effective than FBT [15]. Most of these parents harboured lingering guilt and regret about their roles in potentially influencing and/or struggling to discern the onset or relapse of AN. Parents also sought to understand the causal factors associated with their child's experience of AN through the uptake of the dominant medico-scientific discourse, in which deterministic causation is a fundamental feature.

Despite the agnostic etiological stance of MFT/FBT, these parents took up a wide range of etiological positions, which underscored the uniqueness of each family's experiences and understandings of AN. This included: an innate, organic, disease model; a genetics and environment model; a sociocultural model; an emotional coping model; a controlling mothers model; a confluence of factors model; and a self-confidence and control model. MFT/FBT attempts to pragmatically sidestep these considerations with its agnostic stance, however this also created significant frustration in parents who argued that underlying or associated psychological difficulties were sidelined by the intervention.

In the context of having a child with significant health issues, feelings of guilt and responsibility are inevitable within the prevailing dominant parenting discourses.

Despite the anti-blame rhetoric of MFT/FBT, these parents continued to be both positioned and troubled by parenthood discourses that hold parents responsible for their child's distress and difficulties. The experiences of persistent and residual guilt expressed by these parents support the view that MFT/FBT does not adequately address guilt and responsibility in a family-systemic manner [57]. Instead, parents were left to understand and interpret their child's experiences and actions, and therapeutic opportunities were therefore lost to re-ascribe meaning to guilt, including the possibility of (re)authoring their identity narratives [45] through what might be absent but implicit in guilt [58], such as a valuing of their responsibility in the parental role.

Externalisation

Externalisation is a feature of NT [13], and it has been adopted by MFT/FBT to externalise the illness [7], with the intention of therapeutically shifting parental blame and criticism to an externalised entity. When externalisation is confined to a dualistic biomedical discourse, an adolescent's experience is constructed as an illness/disease that is totalised as bad, with recovery—as the antithesis of illness/disease—constructed as entirely good [59, 60]. Michael White [50] has argued that dualistic conceptions of AN set up the task of therapy as adversarial and risk leading to a sense of exhaustion when this does not eventuate. Instead relational, rather than dualistic, externalisation [52] has been proposed in which the adolescent's voice is at the centre of a therapeutic conversation that maps the real effects of AN on their life and identity, fostering the generation of their own experience-near metaphors [45] to richly depict both their AN experience and fuel the building of counter-narratives that depict their processes of re-covering their life and identity [52] from AN.

Beyond MFT/FBT

When MFT/FBT is positioned to parents as an effective, gold-standard treatment within a biomedical discourse, parents are recruited into an understanding that there is a likelihood that their children will be "cured" of their "disease". This risks a sense of hopelessness and helplessness when the treatment does not lead to the elimination of AN. Parents in this study expressed fears for their child's futures as they negotiated the transition to independence and adulthood, in the presence of ongoing psychological distress. Even more concerning for these parents was the apparent understanding that once MFT/FBT failed, their daughter's life trajectory would inevitably be one filled with chronic mental health issues. What was evident in parental narratives was their commitment to their children, and some of the ways that they sought to preserve their identities as parents, within a therapeutic context where there was limited opportunity for them to re-author durable and sustaining identities for themselves and their child.

Clinical implications

This study has questioned the core tenets of MFT/FBT, including the practices of allocating responsibility to parents for re-feeding and weight restoration and the deferring of addressing in detail an adolescent's distress until the final phase of treatment. Additionally, the practice of externalisation of the illness is limited in its effectiveness at reducing blame and responsibility to parents, particularly in contexts where the child does not progress on to recovery. The central metaphor of illness in externalisation also risks excluding the adolescent, who may not conceptualise their experiences in the terms of this discourse [52]. It also constructs the task of therapy within an adversarial framework, resulting in a sense of exhaustion if recovery does not eventuate [50].

This study highlights the need for further research into the development of more comprehensive treatments for AN. It also highlights the importance of therapists tailoring treatments to a person and family's needs and preferences, which is a critical—and sometimes neglected—facet of evidence-based practice [61]. In particular, it is clear that parents want and need treatments that address the range of issues related to their child's difficulties from the outset of treatment—treatments that are not rigidly focused upon eating behaviours and weight gain at the exclusion of addressing other psychological problems within the broader context of their lives.

Research scope

This study was interested in exploring the experiences of a group of parents who were concerned to improve the first-line treatment for adolescent AN, including those who were currently experiencing or had discontinued this therapy. The children of these parents continued to experience psychological distress during and post-treatment; with some continuing to experience ED symptomatology. More research is needed into the diverse experience of parents who experience MFT/FBT along with their adolescent child and siblings, and this research represents one facet of the complex array of possible experiences. Although the themes that were constructed from the data were present across the parent narratives, future research with larger sample sizes might consider variables such as time post-MFT/FBT intervention, the age and gender of the adolescent, parental separation, the extent of sibling involvement in treatment, and the inter-relationships between parent, adolescent and sibling experiences of MFT/FBT.

Conclusions

Parent's experiences of their child's struggles with AN are complex. MFT/FBT interventions respond to this complexity through an early focus on eating and weight restoration. The substantive risk of this approach, particularly when applied as a first-line treatment for all adolescents who experience AN, is the potential to inadequately address the psychological distress of adolescents and their families, particularly in the early phases of treatment. Since MFT/FBT interventions are family-based, and harness parents as the primary treatment providers, it is crucial that parents' experiences and voices are heard and inform the development of improved treatments for AN. These parents have highlighted the need for therapeutic interventions to be mindful of the unintended effects of allocating responsibility to parents for re-feeding their adolescent, and to more comprehensively address their child's distress (particularly in the earlier phases), as well as parental guilt, blame, and exhaustion from efforts to fight and vanquish AN. The findings of this study invite practitioners and researchers to consider therapeutic interventions that move beyond a behavioural focus on AN symptoms, including in the earlier phases of treatment—interventions that more holistically address the impacts of AN on the life and identity of the adolescent and their family and that provide a space for parents to re-author their stories as stories of standing for their child in hope, and as stories of survival.

Abbreviations

AN: Anorexia nervosa; APS: American Psychological Society; ED: Eating disorder; FBT: Family-based therapy; IBW: Ideal body weight; MFT: Maudsley family therapy; NT: Narrative Therapy; PFT: Parent-focused therapy

Acknowledgements

The authors would like to acknowledge the collaborative work of the following researchers who contributed to the paper by Conti et al. (2017) that formed a foundation for the analysis of this paper: Dr. Daphne Hewson (formerly Macquarie University), Professor Tanya Meade (Western Sydney University), Dr. Jamie Calder (Australian Catholic University) and Sara Cibralic (formerly Western Sydney University).
The authors would like to acknowledge Emma Sheens (University of Sydney), Sara Cibralic (formerly WSU), Jamie Calder (ACU), Daphne Hewson (formerly Macquarie University) and Tanya Meade (WSU) in their support of this research. This research has been supported by a Women's Research Fellowship Grant from Western Sydney University.

Authors' contributions

Each of the authors have made substantive contributions to this paper. EW interviewed participants, coded and analysed the data and wrote the first draft of this manuscript. JC conceived this research, interviewed participants, analysed the data and edited the manuscript. PR conceived this research, and edited the final manuscripts. All authors read and approved the final manuscript.

Authors' information

EW has a Master of Clinical Psychology degree from Western Sydney University, JC is a senior lecturer in Clinical Psychology at Western Sydney University and PR is an Associate Professor in Clinical Psychology at Sydney University.

Competing interests

The authors declare that they have no competing interests.

References

1. Lock J. Family therapy for eating disorders in youth: current confusions, advances, and new directions. Current opinion in psychiatry. 2018;31:431–5.
2. NICE. National Institute for Clinical Excellence (NICE). Eating disorders: core interventions in the treatment of anorexia nervosa, bulimia nervosa and related eating disorders [Internet]. nice.org.uk. 2017. Available from: https://www.nice.org.uk/guidance/ng69. [cited 12 June 2017].
3. Lock J, Couturier J, Agras WS. Comparison of long-term outcomes in adolescents with anorexia nervosa treated with family therapy. J Am Acad Child Adolesc Psychiatry. 2006;45:666–72.
4. Dare C, Eisler I. Family therapy for anorexia nervosa. Handbook of treatment for eating disorders. New York: Guilford Press; 1997.
5. Dare C, Eisler I, Russell GFM, Szmukler GI. The clinical and theoretical impact of a controlled trial of family therapy in anorexia nervosa. J Marital Fam Ther. 1990;16:39–57.
6. Lock J, Le Grange D, Agras S, Dare C. Treatment manual for anorexia nervosa : a family-based approach. New York: Guilford Press; 2001.
7. Lock J, Le Grange D. Treatment manual for anorexia nervosa : a family-based approach. Second Edition. New York: Guilford Press; 2013.
8. Minuchin S, Rosman BL, Baker L. Psychosomatic families. Cambridge, MA and London, England: Harvard University Press; 1978.
9. Haley J. Uncommon therapy: the psychiatric approach of Milton H. Erickson, MD. New York: W.W. Norton and Company; 1973.
10. Madanes C. Strategic family therapy. San Francisco: Jossey-Bass; 1991.
11. Palazzoli MS, Boscolo L, Cecchin G, Prata G. Paradox and Counter paradox. Lanham: Jason Aronson; 1978.
12. Palazzoli MS. Self-starvation: from the intraphysique to the transpersonal approach. London: Chaucer; 1978.
13. White M, Epston D. Narrative means to therapeutic ends. New York: W. W. Norton & Company; 1990.
14. Agras WS, Lock J, Brandt H, Bryson SW, Dodge E, Halmi KA, et al. Comparison of 2 family therapies for adolescent anorexia nervosa. JAMA Psychiatry. 2014;71:1279.
15. Le Grange D, Hughes EK, Court A, Yeo M, Crosby RD, Sawyer SM. Randomized clinical trial of parent-focused treatment and family-based treatment for adolescent anorexia nervosa. J Am Acad Child Adolesc Psychiatry. 2016;55:683–92.
16. Dejong H, Broadbent H, Schmidt U. A systematic review of dropout from treatment in outpatients with anorexia nervosa. Int J eat Disord. Wiley subscription services, Inc., A Wiley Company; 2012;45:635–647.
17. Lock J, Le Grange D, Agras WS, Moye A, Bryson SW, Jo B. Randomized clinical trial comparing family-based treatment with adolescent-focused individual therapy for adolescents with anorexia nervosa. Arch Gen Psychiatry. 2010;67:1025–32.
18. Murray SB, Thornton C, Wallis A. A thorn in the side of evidence-based treatment for adolescent anorexia nervosa. Aust N Z J Psychiatry. Sage UK: London, England; 2012;46:1026–1028.
19. Loeb KL, Le Grange D, Lock J. In: Loeb KL, Le Grange D, Lock J, editors. Family Therapy for Adolescent Eating and Weight Disorders. New York: Routledge; 2015. p. 1–453.
20. Hurst K, Zimmer-Gembeck M. Focus on perfectionism in female adolescent anorexia nervosa. Int J Eat Disord. 2015;48:936–41.
21. Hildebrandt T, Bacow T, Greif R, Flores A. Exposure-based family therapy (FBT-E): an open case series of a new treatment for anorexia nervosa. Cogn Behav Pract. 2014;21:470–84.
22. Johnston JAY, O'Gara JSX, Koman SL, Baker CW, Anderson DA. A pilot study of Maudsley family therapy with group dialectical behavior therapy skills training in an intensive outpatient program for adolescent eating disorders. J Clin Psychol. 2015;71:527–43.
23. Richards IL, Subar A, Touyz S, Rhodes P. Augmentative approaches in family-based treatment for adolescents with restrictive eating disorders: a systematic review. Eur Eat Disord Rev. 2018;26:92–111.
24. Gelin Z, Fuso S, Hendrick S, Cook-Darzens S, Simon Y. The effects of a multiple family therapy on adolescents with eating disorders: an outcome study. Fam Process. 2015;54:160–72.
25. Gelin Z, Hendrick S, Simon Y. Multiple family therapy for adolescents with anorexia nervosa: a one-year follow-up. European Psychiatry. 2015;30:643.
26. Eisler I, Dare C, Hodes M, Russell G, Dodge E, Le Grange D. Family therapy for adolescent anorexia nervosa: the results of a controlled comparison of two family interventions. J Child Psychol Psychiatry. 2000;41:727–36.
27. Eisler I, Simic M, Russell GFM, Dare C. A randomised controlled treatment trial of two forms of family therapy in adolescent anorexia nervosa: a five-year follow-up. J child Psychol psychiatry. Blackwell Publishing Ltd. 2007;48:552–60.
28. Lock J, Le Grange D, Agras WS, Fitzpatrick KK, Jo B, Accurso E, et al. Can adaptive treatment improve outcomes in family-based therapy for

adolescents with anorexia nervosa? Feasibility and treatment effects of a multi-site treatment study. Behav Res Ther. 2015;73:90–5.
29. Henderson K, Buchholz A, Obeid N, Mossiere A, Maras D, Norris M, et al. A Family-Based Eating Disorder Day Treatment Program for Youth: Examining the Clinical and Statistical Significance of Short-Term Treatment Outcomes. Eating Disorders. 2013;22:1–18 Routledge 2nd ed.
30. Le Grange D, Hoste RR, Lock J, Bryson SW. Parental expressed emotion of adolescents with anorexia nervosa: outcome in family-based treatment. Int J eat Disord. 2011;44:731–4 Wiley subscription services, Inc., A Wiley Company.
31. Schwarte R, Timmesfeld N, Dempfle A, Krei M, Egberts K, Jaite C, et al. Expressed Emotions and Depressive Symptoms in Caregivers of Adolescents with First-Onset Anorexia Nervosa-A Long-Term Investigation over 2.5 Years. Eur Eat Disord Rev. 2017;25:44–51.
32. Rhodes P, Gosbee M, Madden S, Brown J. "Communities of concern" in the family-based treatment of anorexia nervosa: towards a consensus in the Maudsley model. Eur Eat Disord Rev. 2005;13:392–8.
33. Treasure J, Smith G, Crane A. Skills-based caring for a loved one with an eating disorder. 2nd ed. New York: Routledge; 2016.
34. Miller WR, Rollnick S. Motivational interviewing, third edition. 3rd ed. New York: Guilford Press; 2012.
35. Macdonald P, Hibbs R, Corfield F, Treasure J. The use of motivational interviewing in eating disorders: a systematic review. Psychiatry Res. 2012; 200:1–11.
36. Fisher CA, Skocic S, Rutherford KA, Hetrick SE. Family therapy approaches for anorexia nervosa. Cochrane Database of Syst Rev. 2018, Issue 10. Art. No.: CD004780. https://doi.org/10.1002/14651858.CD004780.pub3.
37. Sibeoni J, Orri M, Valentin M, Podlipski M-A, Colin S, Pradère J, et al. Metasynthesis of the Views about Treatment of Anorexia Nervosa in Adolescents: Perspectives of Adolescents, Parents, and Professionals. Jiménez-Murcia S, edn.. PLoS ONE. 2017;12:e0169493.
38. Sibeoni J, Orri M, Colin S, Valentin M, Pradère J, Revah-Levy A. The lived experience of anorexia nervosa in adolescence, comparison of the points of view of adolescents, parents, and professionals: a metasynthesis. Int J Nurs Stud. 2017;65:25–34.
39. Bezance J, Holliday J. Adolescents with anorexia nervosa have their say: a review of qualitative studies on treatment and recovery from anorexia nervosa. Eur Eat Disord Rev. 2013;21:352–60.
40. Colton A, Pistrang N. Adolescents' experiences of inpatient treatment for anorexia nervosa. Eur Eat Disord Rev. 2004;12:307–16.
41. Offord A, Turner H, Cooper M. Adolescent inpatient treatment for anorexia nervosa: a qualitative study exploring young adults' retrospective views of treatment and discharge. Eur Eat Disord Rev. 2006;14:377–87.
42. Tierney S. The Treatment of Adolescent Anorexia Nervosa: A Qualitative Study of the Views of Parents. Eating Disorders. 2006;13:369–79 2nd ed.
43. Le Grange D, Gelman T. Patients' perspective of treatment in eating disorders: a preliminary study. South African journal of psychology, vol. 28. London, England: Sage UK; 1998. p. 182–6.
44. Miles J, Gilbert P. A handbook of research methods for clinical and health psychology. New York: New York: Oxford University Press; 2005.
45. White M. Maps of narrative practice. New York: W. W. Norton & Company; 2007.
46. Edley N. Analysing masculinity: interpretative repertoires, ideological dilemmas and subject positions. Discourse as data. SAGE: Los Angeles; 2001.
47. Wetherell M, Taylor S, Yates SJ. Discourse as data. SAGE: Thousand Oaks; 2001.
48. Burr V. Social constructionism. London: Routledge; 2003.
49. Harré R, Gillett G. The discursive mind. London: Sage; 1994.
50. White M. On anorexia. Narrative practice. New York: W. W. Norton & Co; 2011.
51. Lock J, Couturier J, Agras WS. Costs of remission and recovery using family therapy for adolescent anorexia nervosa: a descriptive report. Eat Disord. 2008;16:322–30.
52. Conti JE. Recovering identity from anorexia nervosa: Women's constructions of their experiences of recovery from anorexia nervosa over 10 years. Journal of Constructivist Psychology Routledge. 2016;17:1–23.
53. Garner DM, Rockert W, Olmsted MP, Johnson C, Coscina DV. Psychoeducational principles in the treatment of bulimia and anorexia nervosa. In: Garner DM, Garfinkel PE, editors. Handbook of psychotherapy for anorexia nervosa and bulimia. New York: Guilford Press; 1985.
54. Swanson SA. Prevalence and correlates of eating disorders in adolescents. Arch Gen Psychiatry. 2011;68:714.
55. Bühren K, Schwarte R, Fluck F, Timmesfeld N, Krei M, Egberts K, et al. Comorbid Psychiatric Disorders in Female Adolescents with First-Onset Anorexia Nervosa. European Eating Disorders Review. 2013;22:39–44 4 ed.
56. Accurso EC, Ciao AC, Fitzsimmons-Craft EE, Lock JD, Le Grange D. Is weight gain really a catalyst for broader recovery?: the impact of weight gain on psychological symptoms in the treatment of adolescent anorexia nervosa. Behav Res Ther. 2014;56:1–6.
57. Dring G. Finding a voice. London: Karnac Books; 2015.
58. White M. Reflections on narrative practice: Dulwich Centre Publications; 2000.
59. Conti JE. "I Don't think anorexia is the way out": reconstruction of meaning in Women's narratives of anorexia nervosa over 10 years. J Constr Psychol. 2015;29:165–83.
60. Conti J, Rhodes P, Adams H. Listening in the dark: why we need stories of people living with severe and enduring anorexia nervosa. J Eat Disord. 2016;4:79.
61. Sackett DL, Rosenberg WMC, Gray JAM, Haynes RB, Richardson WS. Evidence based medicine: what it is and what it isn't. BMJ. 1996;312:71–2.

5

Physical restraint during inpatient treatment of adolescent anorexia nervosa: frequency, clinical correlates and associations with outcome at five-year follow-up

Thomas Blikshavn[1,2], Inger Halvorsen[1*] and Øyvind Rø[1,3]

Abstract

Background: Studies of the use and effects of physical restraint in anorexia nervosa (AN) treatment are lacking. The purpose of this study was to describe the frequency of physical restraint in a specialized program for adolescents with AN, and to examine if meal-related physical restraint (forced nasogastric tube-feeding) was related to 5-year outcome.

Method: Thirty-eight (66% of 58) patients with AN (mean age 15.9, SD = 1.9) admitted to a regional, specialized adolescent eating disorders (ED) inpatient unit. Patient data, including restraint episodes, were obtained from hospital records, and outcome was assessed at a 5-year follow-up.

Results: A total of 201 restraint episodes occurred over 5513 days of inpatient treatment, including 109 meal-related episodes and 56 episodes to avoid self-harm. Twelve (32%) patients experienced at least one restraint episode during the admission, of which eight (21%) experienced meal-related restraint. Four patients represented 91% of all restraint episodes, experiencing 10 or more episodes during admission. Meal-related restraint was significantly associated with a higher rate of persisting ED diagnosis, but not with weight gain during admission, EDE-Q global score or BMI at follow-up.

Conclusions: Restraint episodes occurred rather infrequently. A small number of patients ($n = 4$) accounted for a high proportion of episodes (91%). More knowledge is important to reduce the need for restraint in treatment for AN.

Keywords: Physical restraint, Forced nasogastric tube feeding, Anorexia nervosa, Eating disorders, Adolescent

Plain English summary

It is an important goal for health services to provide treatment voluntarily and without the use of coercion. However, in severe anorexia nervosa it is sometimes necessary to use physical restraint, that is, the patient is physically held by the staff, to provide nutrition by tube feeding. Previous studies on the use of physical restraint in anorexia nervosa are lacking, and more knowledge is important to reduce the need to use restraint in treatment.

This study describes the frequency of physical restraint in a specialized program for adolescents with anorexia nervosa, and investigates if the use of physical restraint was related to 5-year outcome. About two thirds of the patients did not experience any restraint episodes, neither to provide tube feeding, nor to avoid harm. However, a small number of patients experienced a large number of restraint episodes, i.e., four of the 38 participants (11%)

* Correspondence: inger.halvorsen@uus.no
[1]Regional Department for Eating Disorders, Division of Mental Health and Addiction, Oslo University Hospital, P.O. Box 4956 Nydalen, N-0424 Oslo, Norway
Full list of author information is available at the end of the article

accounted for 91% of all physical restraint episodes. Thus, more knowledge on patients with many restraint episodes is important to avoid escalation of resistance to treatment and further use of restraint. Patients who had experienced restraint episodes for tube feeding had a higher rate of persisting eating disorders at 5-year follow-up compared to those without restraint episodes.

Introduction

Involuntary treatment for eating disorders (ED) is utilized as a last resort in cases where there is considerable risk to the patient that cannot be managed in a less restrictive way [1–3]. The restoration of normal body weight, which depends upon meals being administered several times daily, represents a uniquely challenging cornerstone of treatment [4]. To our knowledge, no quantitative studies until the present have examined the extent to which weight restoration is facilitated by the use of physical restraint, that is, the use of physical force to restrict or control the patient. In the literature, the general view is that interventions involving physical restraint have no inherent therapeutic effects in the treatment of children and adolescents [5] and may be associated with negative psychological outcomes [6, 7]. However, the literature has largely concerned itself with physical restraint to manage patient aggression [8, 9], and therefore may not generalize to physical restraint utilized to administer nutrition in ED.

One qualitative study specifically examined the experiences of both caregivers and patients who had previously received nasogastric tube feeding (NGT) during inpatient treatment for ED in adolescence, where more than half of the patients had been restrained due to resistance to the procedure [10]. Briefly summarized, it was found that NGT was experienced negatively at the time, but was retrospectively perceived as helpful. The majority of participants did not believe there had been any viable alternatives to NGT feeding. Neither physical resistance nor reported negative reactions to the treatment had any obvious relationship to outcome.

Studies of involuntarily-treated adolescents with anorexia nervosa (AN) suggest that some patients are subject to physical restraint for treatment purposes, but the type and frequency of restraint episodes are seldom reported. For example, a large study of all specialist inpatient ED units in Scotland between 2009 and 2011 reported that 17 of 89 adolescent patients had been formally detained, and 10 had received NGT feeding [11]. Yet the extent to which NGT was administered against the patients' will, and/or with physical restraint was not reported. The only study to date that compared outcome for adolescent AN between involuntarily admitted patients versus those admitted with parental consent found that NGT was used in 68.8% versus 11.7% of groups, respectively, although the rate of using physical restraint to administer NGT was not mentioned [12]. A Danish register-based study of involuntary measures in the treatment of AN reported that 18% of patients had experienced at least one involuntary measure, with 2% of these patients experiencing more than 100 recorded involuntary measures [13]. Involuntary NGT feeding was the most frequent involuntary measure employed, and was most prevalent in the age group 15–17 years. However, no data were available on how many meals were delivered via NGT and/or if physical restraint had been used to administer nutrition.

A large study of restraint utilized in acute general adolescent mental health units in Norway found that a small number of patients with AN were exposed to exceptionally high levels of physical restraint [14]. Specifically, 1896 of a total of 4173 restraint episodes were related to compulsory feeding. These episodes occurred in 21 patients with AN (i.e., an average of 90 episodes per patient), from a total of 4099 registered patients. Thus, nearly half (45%) of the restraint episodes registered at Norwegian acute mental health inpatient units for adolescents were related to compulsory feeding for a small number of patients with AN.

Two recent systematic reviews on compulsory treatment in AN are supportive of a beneficial outcome of compulsory treatment [15, 16]. Only one previous study has investigated outcome in adolescents with AN that had received compulsory treatment [12], and findings also concur with the more general notion of therapeutic benefit. However, the scant research evidence on compulsory treatment in adolescents with AN may not generalize to treatment delivered via physical restraint. Research is lacking on the type, frequency and effects of use of physical restraint in treatment of AN. Thus, we do not know the extent to which physical restraint is utilized, the characteristics of patients and the treatment institutions involved, and if such events influence the course and outcome of the ED.

Aims of the study

This study aimed to describe the use of physical restraint in a specialized inpatient ED unit for adolescents, and to investigate whether the frequency and occurrence of restraint were associated with weight gain during admission and five-year outcome. Specifically, we investigated whether patients subjected to meal-related physical restraint during the index admission would have less weight gain during the admission and poorer outcome at follow-up in terms of readmissions during the follow-up period, and/or persistence of ED diagnosis, lower BMI and higher EDE-Q global score at follow-up.

Methods

Setting and participants

The Regional Department for Eating Disorders (RASP) at Oslo University Hospital is a tertiary, specialized ED treatment center, with a catchment area of approximately 2.9 million people. Patients are referred from their local specialized mental health services and have received prior treatment without remission. Most adolescents have received both outpatient family-based treatment (FBT) and prior inpatient treatment. Since 2008, a family-based inpatient treatment model has been offered at RASP for adolescents, based upon the evidence for outpatient FBT as well as Norwegian policies allowing parents/guardians to accompany patients under the age of 18 years during the inpatient stay. The child and adolescent inpatient unit admits patients up to 18 years old, and has beds for a maximum of five patients and their families. Details regarding the adaptation of FBT to an inpatient treatment setting have been described elsewhere [17, 18].

The current quantitative study is part of a five-year follow-up of patients who had received family-based inpatient treatment between May 2008 and June 2014. All former patients ($n = 58$) were successfully contacted and invited to participate. No exclusion criteria were applied. Of 58 patients invited, consent was obtained from 38 (66%) of the patients. If multiple hospital admissions had occurred during the follow-up period, only data from the first admission were used. At admission, all patients had a DSM-5 diagnosis of AN. Average age at admission was 15.9 years (SD = 1.9), and mean duration of inpatient treatment was 20.3 (SD = 13.7) weeks. Four of the participants were male. When comparing the 38 participants with the 20 non-participants, we found no significant differences for the following demographic and clinical characteristics at baseline: compulsory treatment status, admission BMI percentile, duration of admission, weight gain during the admission, and age at the time of the follow-up. Furthermore, no significant differences were found regarding having an entry in the restraint protocol, or having been exposed to meal-related physical restraint.

Treatment was carried out in close collaboration with the parents with the aim to support the parents' competency and confidence in their own ability to help their child to eat sufficiently. The ED unit emphasized avoiding the use of coercion in treatment. Coercion was only used when deemed absolutely necessary to ensure adequate nutrition and vigorous efforts to achieve patient co-operation had failed. A weekly weight gain of about one kg was recommended during the admission. The unit provided a structured regime to achieve this, i.e. by providing meal plans, prescribing supplemental nutritional drinks, or NGT feeding if the patient did not finish her/his meal, and recommending how much activity and rest the child needed. The program's meal protocol stated that the patients had to finish every meal in 30 min, followed by another 15 min to drink supplemental nutritional drinks if required. If the meal was not completed, either with regular food or nutritional drinks, NGT feeding of the remaining nutrients was prescribed. The tube was inserted after the non-completed meal and removed following replacement of the missing nutrients, based on an assumption that the patient would manage adequate oral food-intake at the next meal. Most patients completed all their meals with regular food, or supplemental nutritional drinks, with support from their parents and nursing staff. In cases of NGT feeding, the staff strongly encouraged and emphasized efforts to enlist the patient's collaboration. However, if the patient physically resisted prescribed NGT feeding despite these efforts, a psychiatrist or clinical psychologist with the approved competence to make decisions according to the Mental Health act could, under certain circumstances, recommend that staff use physical restraint by holding the patient to administer forced NGT feeding. Parental consent was required to administer NGT feeding for patients below the age of 16, and for those above 16 years, compulsory admission and a legally valid decision on compulsory nutrition was required. The unit did not use pharmacological restraint/sedation, or mechanical restraint.

Procedure

Information about this study, and a consent form with a decline option, were mailed to former patients and their families. Non-respondents were contacted by telephone. Patients that agreed to participate received questionnaires by mail prior to the follow-up interview. The follow-up interview was conducted at the hospital for 27 participants, at the patients' home ($n = 7$), by telephone ($n = 3$), and elsewhere ($n = 1$). Average age at follow-up was 20.2 years (SD = 2.6), and median time to follow-up was 5.2 years (95% CI 3.8–5.5). The interviews were conducted between May 2015 and January 2016 by five experienced clinicians. All were employed at the ED department, and four had been involved in the treatment in the unit during the study period. All interviews were recorded, and any uncertainties about diagnoses were discussed by interviewers before diagnoses were coded.

Measures

Data from the treatment phase

Clinical data from the treatment phase were obtained from hospital records, including weight and height at admission and discharge. BMI percentiles for age and sex were calculated using a Norwegian version of a weight-for-height ratio calculator based on reference data from Child Growth Foundation, UK [19].

Data regarding physical restraint during the treatment phase In Norway, the use of coercive measures in mental health care is regulated by the Norwegian Mental Health Act, section 4–8. The types of coercive measures regulated by the law are physical holding, mechanical restraint, seclusion and medication to avoid harm. Justifications for the use of coercive measures in section 4–8 are exclusively limited to averting serious harm to the patient, others, or property. Coercion for treatment purposes (meal-related restraint) was also recorded as a coercive measure under section 4–8. The law requires that each unit has a restraint protocol where every episode with use of restraint is entered, and that this protocol be checked by independent, official, control commissions. Data on the use of restraint for nutritional treatment were therefore available. In addition to the restraint protocol, the patient records were also examined by the first author for any described episodes of physical restraint. For each episode, it was noted on which shift in the unit it occurred, justification, duration, and number of staff involved.

Follow-up assessment

Treatment received for eating disorders during the follow-up period Information regarding inpatient and outpatient treatment was obtained from patients during the follow-up interview. If re-admitted to our study unit, readmission data were also available from the patient records. Fourteen (39%) of the participants had received additional inpatient treatment, and 34 (89%) outpatient treatment for an ED during the follow-up period.

Eating disorder diagnoses at follow-up DSM-5 ED diagnoses at follow-up were assessed by the Eating Disorder Examination 16.0 (EDE) [20]. Only the diagnostic items in the EDE were used for the present study.

Eating disorder symptoms The Eating Disorder Examination Questionnaire 6.0 (EDE-Q) [21, 22] was used to measure ED symptoms during the previous 28 days. The mean of the four subscales, dietary restraint, eating concern, weight concern, and shape concern, was calculated to obtain a global EDE-Q score.

Body weight, height, and body mass index (BMI) Weight and height was measured during the follow-up examinations conducted at the hospital ($n = 17$). Self-reported body weight and height from the EDE interview were used if the participant did not want to be weighed ($n = 10$) or if the interview was conducted elsewhere ($n = 11$). Body mass index (BMI; kg/m^2) was calculated from the obtained values. Mean BMI in the group with measured weighed/height (19.9, SD = 3.3) did not differ from the group with self-reported weight/height (19.9, SD = 2.9, n.s.).

Categorization by legal status during the treatment phase

By Norwegian law, involuntary treatment status is formally only applicable to persons at the age of consent, which is 16 years old for health-related matters. Below the age of 16, the legal basis of treatment is consent by parents/caregivers. The patients were therefore categorized into three groups based on legal status during the index admission: 1) Parental consent (< 16 years, $n = 19$), 2) Voluntary treatment (≥ 16 years, $n = 15$), and 3) Involuntary treatment (≥ 16 years, $n = 4$)).

Statistical analyses

All analyses were done using SPSS for Windows, version 23.0. Categorical variables were analyzed using the chi-squared test, or, for expected cell numbers below 1, the Fischer's exact test. Group comparisons for normally distributed continuous variables were made using Independent Samples T-test, and where normality could not be assumed, Mann-Whitney U-test was used. Reported p-values are two-tailed. Effect size estimates are Cohen's d for normally distributed variables. For the Mann-Whitney U test, effect sizes are estimated by r, as proposed by Cohen [23], and for chi-square test results by the phi coefficient (ϕ). By convention, for Cohen's d, an effect size of 0.2, 0.5, and 0.8 were considered a small, medium and large effect size, respectively, and likewise, for the effect size estimates r and ϕ, the numbers 0.1, 0.3, and 0.5 represent a small, medium, and large effect size [24].

The study was approved by the Regional Medical Ethics Committee.

Results

During the study period, the only type of coercive measure utilized on the unit was physical holding (physical restraint), while other coercive measures regulated by the law, such as mechanical restraint, seclusion and medication to avoid harm, were not used.

Number of patients subject to meal-related and non-meal related physical restraint

Twelve (31%) of the 38 patients had at least one recorded episode of physical restraint, of whom eight (21%) were subject to meal-related restraint (see Fig. 1). Males and females had similar occurrence of restraint episodes. Six patients had five or more events, all of whom had at least five meal-related events, accounting for 96% of the total number of recorded restraint events. These six patients had similar clinical characteristics at admission as the other 32 patients in terms of duration of illness, age at onset, age at admission and previous

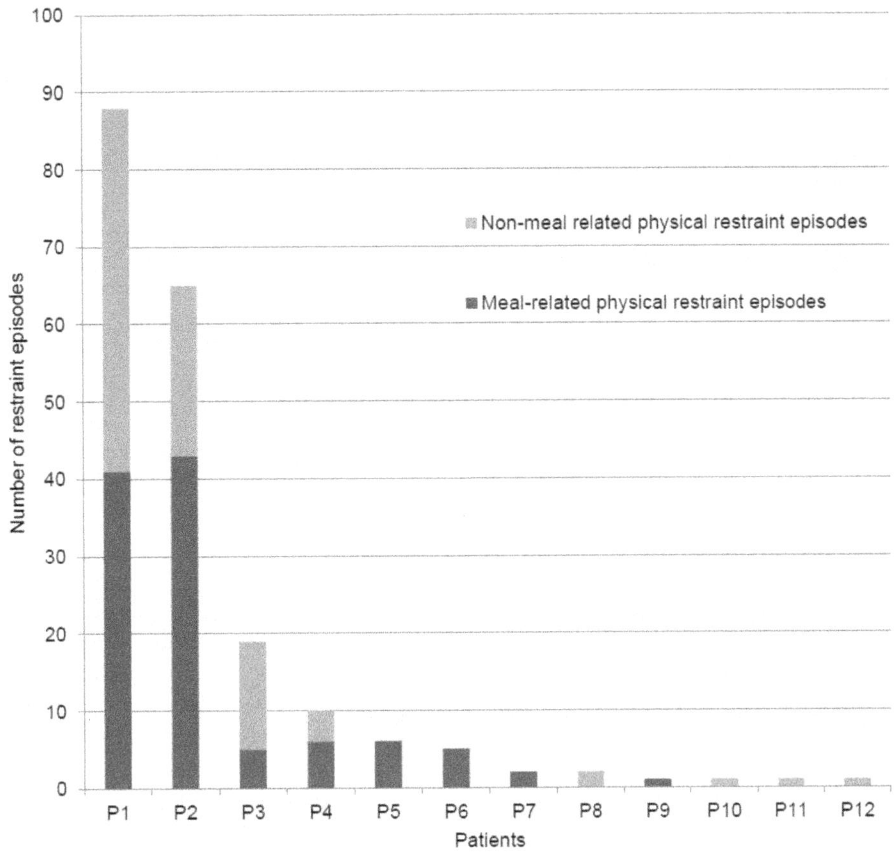

Fig. 1 Number of physical restraint episodes among participants. Distribution of number of restraint episodes among individual patients with ≥1 restraint episode, sorted in descending order

inpatient treatment. Further, four of these six patients had at least 10 events, accounting for 91% of all recorded restraint events (see Fig. 1).

Among patients admitted with parental consent (n = 19, < 16 years), eight patients (42%) had at least one restraint episode, including five (26%) with meal-related restraint. Among the voluntarily admitted patients (n = 15, ≥ 16 years), there was only one single event of restraint, which was related to self-harm. Three of the four patients in the involuntary group (≥ 16 years) had physical restraint episodes, and all these three patients had more than ten restraint episodes, including both meal-related restraint and non-meal related restraint episodes. These three involuntarily admitted patients accounted for the majority (79%) of all recorded restraint episodes.

Recorded events of physical restraint on the unit

A total of 201 occurrences of physical restraint were recorded over a total of 5513 days of inpatient treatment (treatment-days) for the 38 patients. Of the restraint episodes with a known cause (n = 170, see Table 1), restraint to administer nutritional treatment (54%, n = 109) or restraint employed to avoid serious self-harm (28%, n = 56) accounted together for 97% (n = 165) of the episodes. Across the 5513 inpatient treatment days, there was an average of 27.4 treatment-days per restraint episode for any reason, and an average of 50.6 treatment-days per meal-related restraint episode. Of the 201 recorded events, 24% of the events (n = 48) had missing data on at least one of the following parameters: the number of staff involved: n = 38 (19%), the reason for physical restraint: n = 31 (15%), the duration of physical restraint: n = 10 (5%), and the time of the day: n = 1. No episode of physical restraint occurred during the night shift, while 125 (63%) events occurred during day shift and 74 (37%) during the evening shift. The majority (n = 69, 63%) of the 109 meal-related restraint episodes took place during the first 8 weeks of the admission. However, three patients with multiple episodes during the first 8 weeks also had a large number of meal-related restraint episodes (n = 40) after the first 8 weeks of the admission.

Duration of physical restraint and number of staff involved

Meal-related events (n = 100) had a mean duration of 19.4 min (SD = 9.2 min), while self-harm related events

Table 1 Numbers of physical restraint episodes in the unit, categorized by legal status of the patient and justification[a]

	Meal-related	Self-harm related	Preventing harm to others	Preventing damage to property	Unknown justification	SUM (%)
Events during admission on parental consent (in 8 of the 19 patients on parental consent)	19	14	3	1	4	41 (21%)
Events during formal involuntary admission (in 3 of the 4 involuntary admitted patients)	90	41	1	0	27	159 (79%)
	109	55	4	1	31	200 (100%)

[a] One single event to avoid self-harm in a voluntarily admitted patient is omitted from table

($n = 56$) had a mean duration of 35.2 min (SD = 24.2 min). Of the episodes in which the number of staff involved in the event was known ($n = 163$), the mean number of staff was 3.5 (SD = 1.2) for both parental ($n = 35$) and involuntary ($n = 127$) admissions. Meal-related events ($n = 105$) had a mean number of 3.8 (SD = 1.1) staff members and self-harm related events ($n = 53$) had a mean number of 2.8 (SD = 1.0).

Body mass index at admission and discharge

Mean BMI was 15.2 (SD = 1.9) at admission and 18.3 (SD = 1.7) at discharge, while mean BMI percentile was 5.5 (SD = 14.2) at admission and 22.9 (SD = 19.6) at discharge. Mean weight gain during the admission was 7.4 (SD = 4.5) kg. No difference was found between the group of eight patients with meal-related restraint episodes and the 30 patients without any meal-related restraint episodes regarding mean BMI and BMI-percentile at admission, discharge, or weight gain during the admission.

Associations between meal-related physical restraint and outcome

At follow-up, sixteen (42%) of the former patients met criteria for a DSM-5 ED diagnosis (AN: $n = 8$, BN: $n = 2$, other/unspecified feeding or eating disorder: $n = 6$). The proportion with an ED diagnosis was significantly higher in the group who experienced meal-related physical restraint during admission, χ2 (1, $N = 38$) = 4.380, $p < 0.04$, $\phi = 0.34$ (see Table 2). All the six patients with the highest numbers of restraint episodes still had an ED diagnosis at follow-up. The number of readmissions to inpatient treatment during follow-up, EDE-Q global score, and BMI at follow-up, tended to be less favorable in the group with meal-related restraint, with small-medium effect sizes, but these differences were not statistically significant.

Discussion

Approximately two-thirds of adolescent patients admitted to an inpatient family-based treatment program for AN had no recorded episode of meal-related or non-meal related physical restraint across a six-year study period. One-third of patients experienced at least one episode of either forced NGT feeding and/or physical restraint to avoid harm. Interestingly, we found that a small number of patients accounted for almost all of the restraint episodes. Specifically, six patients who had five or more restraint episodes accounted for 97% of all restraint episodes that occurred on the unit. We found that patients subjected to meal-related physical restraint had a higher rate of persistent ED diagnosis at a 5-year follow-up compared to those without a history of meal-related restraint episodes. However, there were no significant differences in the number of readmissions, BMI or EDE-Q global score at follow-up between those with versus without a meal-related restraint episode, although findings did indicate a tendency toward a more favorable

Table 2 Eating disorder outcome at follow-up in patients with and without meal-related physical restraint episodes during the admission

	All patients $n = 38$	Meal-related physical restraint $n = 8$	No meal-related physical restraint $n = 30$	Test	*P*-value	Effect size[c]
Inpatient treatment during follow-up (number of patients)	14	5	9	χ^2 (1, N = 38) = 2.792	$p < 0.10$	$\varphi = 0.27$
Any DSM-5 ED diagnosis at follow-up (number of patients)	16	6	10	χ^2 (1, $N = 38$) = 4.380	$p < 0.04$	$\varphi = 0.34$
Follow-up EDE-Q global score (mean (SD))	2.15 (1.48)[a]	2.32 (1.52)	2.09 (1.50) [b]	t (32) = 0.380	$p < 0.71$	$d = 0.15$
Follow-up BMI (kg/m2) (median)	19.5 (95%CI: 18.2–20.6)	18.5 (95%CI: 15.6–20.8)	19.7 (95%CI: 19.0–20.7)	U = 75.500 Z = − 1.594	$p < 0.12$	$r = -0.26$

[a] $n = 34$, [b] $n = 26$, [c]by convention, for d, the values 0.2, 0.5 and 0.8 represent a small, medium, and large effect size, respectively, and likewise for r and φ by the values 0.1, 0.3, and 0.5

outcome in patients without any meal-related restraint episodes.

To our knowledge, there are no prior studies describing the frequency of physical restraint used in the treatment of adolescent AN. Thus, it is difficult to estimate if the rate of physical restraint found in our study is lower or higher than expected. In the present study, the participants were a selected group of inpatients referred to a tertiary ED department following unsuccessful in- and outpatient treatment offered at local specialized mental health services. Their long and complex illness and treatment courses could have been associated with elevated rates of restraint episodes. Legal coercion for the treatment for AN has been found to be associated with factors such as previous admissions, complexity of the patients' condition, and elevated health risks/low BMI [25], which are indeed factors that characterize the patient group in our study. It is likely these illness and patient-related characteristics would be associated with increased use of restraint to carry out the treatment. On the other hand, however, the treatment we provided on a specialized ED unit might have contributed to reduced use of physical restraint to administer nutrition. Staff training and expertise in meal-support therapy have been associated with greatly decreased rates of NGT feeding in this population [26], which is likely to reduce the rates of meal-related physical restraint.

The observed number of restraint episodes among the involuntary patients was particularly high, as 79% of all restraint episodes in the unit were accounted for by three of these four patients. In contrast, only one restraint episode was recorded among the 15 voluntarily admitted patients (see Table 1). A main reason for involuntary admission to treatment was that extensive past attempts to achieve weight gain voluntarily had proven unsuccessful, and legal authority to make decisions on forced nutrition was therefore deemed necessary. Forced nutrition was not legally possible to administer among voluntarily treated patients over 16 years, and, thus, there were no meal-related restraint episodes in this group. A larger proportion of patients below 16 years had at least one meal-related restraint episode (42%) compared to patients above 16 years (21%). As feeding in the younger patients was based on parental consent, forced nutrition could therefore be conducted without meeting the legal requirements and procedures necessary to establish compulsory treatment. Also, the younger, less mature patients might have poorer impulse control and more acting out, for instance in response to distress related to the treatment.

The higher number of physical restraint episodes during the day shift, and no restraint episodes during the night shift, was attributable to the unit's procedure not to administer NGT feeding at night. Furthermore, during the process of data collection, it became evident that although the immediate behavior prevented by physical restraint was typically coded as self-harm, the behavior was often preceded by food- or meal-related events on the unit (e.g. receiving the message that calories would be increased, or having finished a meal). To the extent that food-related anxiety [27, 28] constitutes a common denominator, the relative absence of triggering food- or meal-related events at night would be relevant in explaining the observed temporal pattern.

The use of physical restraint in the treatment of AN involves complex ethical dilemmas for health authorities, institutions, as well as the staff that carries out the restraint. Physical restraint might also be extremely resource-intensive and demanding, both financially and with respect to the staff's expertise. We found that each restraint episode involved a large number of staff (mean 3.5, SD = 1.2) for a significant time period (mean 22.9 min, SD = 16.9). The meal-related restraint episodes were particularly demanding given the challenges involved in administering safe tube-feeding while patients physically resisted the procedure. Typically, most of the staff on the unit were involved in the restraint episodes to prevent harm, which could not be planned beforehand, and staff was often "borrowed" from another unit to carry out meal-related restraint. During admissions of patients with numerous physical restraint episodes, extra staff had to be engaged. Restraint episodes were also demanding for the specialists responsible for treatment, as each episode required assessment, decision-making, and documentation by a psychiatrist or clinical psychologist certified with the approved competence to make decisions based on the Mental Health Act. Additionally, the use of physical restraint, particularly to administer forced feeding, is demanding and distressing for the staff, the patient, her/his family, as well as other patients and families admitted to the unit. Thus, achieving the successful re-nourishment in AN inpatient treatment which minimizes the use of physical restraint, is important for ethical reasons, health service economy, staff resources and well-being, as well as for the adolescents affected by AN and their families.

The highly skewed distribution of physical restraint episodes across patients is in concert with prior research, including a study on the use of involuntary measures in AN [13], as well as studies from outside the ED field, such as general adolescent inpatient populations in Norway [29], single adolescent psychiatric facilities in the US [30, 31], and child and adolescent inpatient treatment settings [32, 33]. Moreover, similar findings are reported for adult patients [34–36].

Our findings entail several important implications for the use of physical restraint and management during inpatient treatment in adolescent AN. First, interventions delivered ubiquitously to all patients in order to reduce the probability of physical restraint may not be very effective in reducing overall numbers, as the majority of patients experience little or no physical restraint. Additional investigation of those with frequent physical restraint episodes may lead to a better understanding of how to reduce or eliminate restraint in this group. Second, and in line with the health authorities' focus on reduced use of involuntary treatment and coercive measures in mental health services, treatment units should aim to deliver treatment voluntarily as much as possible. However, the reduction of restraint episodes might be obtained by selective targeting, with treatment units achieving substantial reductions in restraint episodes by subtle changes in admission policy, transfer of selected patients to another unit, or early discharge, none of which would be of any apparent benefit to the patients in question [36]. Because of this, further studies on physical restraint in the treatment of EDs should ideally include multiple sites, and also account for the amount of physical restraint delivered in non-psychiatric settings, particularly in somatic units. Finally, countertransference reactions appear important in understanding the clinician-patient dynamics in adolescent AN [37]. Also, staff emotional reactions appear relevant in understanding the escalation and persistence of patient aggression [38], which might be relevant for restraint rates. In our opinion, the contribution of clinician emotional reactions and behaviors to the emergence of coercion in treatment settings in general, and particularly to escalation of forced NGT feeding episodes, deserves further investigation.

Emotion regulation difficulties may also contribute to the emergence of physical restraint in the treatment setting, but the present study is not able to elucidate this question. Emotion regulation difficulties may be unrelated to weight status, and appear to be insensitive to weight normalization, at least in the short term [39]. This may particularly inform our understanding of patients with recurrent physical restraint episodes. Qualitative data suggest that awareness and tolerance of negative emotions, both of which are central tasks in emotion regulation, are central to the recovery process, or, conversely, that lack thereof contribute to relapse after weight restoration [40]. It could be of clinical relevance to include measures related to emotion regulation difficulties in future research on physical restraint in AN treatment.

In the present study, patients with meal-related restraint did not differ significantly from those with no meal-related restraint in terms of clinical characteristics or weight status during admission. Further, differences in the number of readmissions and BMI and EDE-Q global score at follow-up did not reach statistical significance. However, the proportion of patients who had an ED diagnosis at 5-year follow-up was significantly higher in the group who experienced meal-related coercion during hospitalization, with a medium effect size ($\phi = 0.34$). Given the small number of patients exposed to meal-related restraint, however, both negative and positive findings should be interpreted with caution. Notably, all outcome measures at follow-up trended toward a poorer outcome for those who experienced meal-related coercion during admission, and, except for the EDE-Q global score, effect sizes were consistent with a medium effect. Also, it is noteworthy that all the six patients with highest numbers of restraint episodes still had an ED diagnosis at follow-up. In sum, we believe that the current study, being the first of its kind, suggests that a history of meal-related restraint may be of clinical importance to long-term outcome, justifying further investigation of this clinically challenging problem.

The main limitation of the current study is the small number of patients in the group of interest, leading to a high risk of type II errors. About 1/3 of those treated during the study period did not participate in this follow-up study, although the non-participants did not significantly differ from participants on a number of background variables, including formal involuntary status, registered restrained episodes, or the presence of meal-related physical restraint, which lends support to the representativeness of the results for our patient group. The focus of the study was on physical restraint, but, as the few involuntary patients accounted for the majority (79%) of the restraint episodes, we are not able to distinguish the effect of having experienced physical restraint episodes on outcome from the effect of having received involuntary treatment. Also, as the study population is from a tertiary treatment center, the participants are a highly selected group, and may not be representative of other inpatients settings for ED. Legislation and organization of health services for the most severely ill patients with AN differ between countries, which also constitutes a limitation in the generalizability of the results of this study.

Conclusion

The use of involuntary treatment and coercive measures in mental health services entails complex ethical dilemmas, especially for the treatment of AN, in which life and physical health might be at risk and patients often refuse medically necessary procedures to ensure weight gain. More knowledge of the use of physical restraint in the treatment of adolescent AN is important, and, if possible, a reduction in the use of such measures. On this tertiary inpatient unit for adolescents with severe AN, the occurrence of physical restraint was rather infrequent. Only a small number of patients accounted for the vast majority of physical restraint episodes. Physical restraint seemed to be related to poorer prognosis at a 5-year follow-up, as evidenced by the persistence of an ED diagnosis. Additional research with larger samples is necessary to better understand the use and effects of physical restraint in AN.

Abbreviations

ED: Eating disorder; NGT: Nasogastric tube feeding; AN: Anorexia nervosa; BMI: Body mass index (kg/m^2); FBT: Family-based treatment; EDE-Q: The eating disorder examination questionnaire

Acknowledgements

The authors thank senior researcher Deborah L. Reas, PhD, for proofreading the manuscript.

Authors' contribution

The first author has had the main responsibility for planning the study, data collection, data analyses and writing of the first draft of the paper. The second author is the project leader for the larger study of which this study is part of. She has given consultation on all parts of this study, and completed the writing of the paper. The third author has been a consultant on all parts of the study and has participated in the writing of the paper. The author(s) read and approved the final manuscript.

Competing interests

The authors have no competing interests.

Author details

[1]Regional Department for Eating Disorders, Division of Mental Health and Addiction, Oslo University Hospital, P.O. Box 4956 Nydalen, N-0424 Oslo, Norway. [2]Department of Child and Adolescent Mental Health, Akershus University Hospital, Lørenskog, Norway. [3]Division of Mental Health and Addiction, Institute of Clinical Medicine, University of Oslo, Oslo, Norway.

References

1. National Institute for Clinical Excellence (NICE). Eating disorders: recognition and treatment. nice.org.uk. 2017. Available from: https://www.nice.org.uk/guidance/ng69.
2. Herpertz-Dahlmann B, van Elburg A, Castro-Fornieles J, Schmidt U. ESCAP expert paper: new developments in the diagnosis and treatment of adolescent anorexia nervosa -a European perspective. Eur Child Adolesc Psychiatry. 2015;24(10):1153–67. https://doi.org/10.1007/s00787-015-0748-7.
3. Westmoreland P, Johnson C, Stafford M, Martinez R, Mehler PS. Involuntary treatment of patients with life-threatening anorexia nervosa. J Am Acad Psychiatry Law. 2017;45(4):419–25.
4. Lock J, Agras WS, le GD CJ, Safer D, Bryson SW. Do end of treatment assessments predict outcome at follow-up in eating disorders? IntJ Eat Disord. 2013;10. https://doi.org/10.1002/eat.22175.
5. Day DM. Examining the therapeutic utility of restraints and seclusion with children and youth: the role of theory and research in practice. Am J Orthop. 2002;72(2):266–78. https://doi.org/10.1037/0002-9432.72.2.266.
6. Mohr WK, Anderson JA. Faulty assumptions associated with the use of restraints with children. J Child Adolesc Psychiatr Nurs. 2001;14(3):141–51. https://doi.org/10.1111/j.1744-6171.2001.tb00305.x.
7. Valenkamp M, Delaney K, Verheij F. Reducing seclusion and restraint during child and adolescent inpatient treatment: still an underdeveloped area of research. J Child Adolesc Psychiatr Nurs. 2014;27(4):169–74. https://doi.org/10.1111/jcap.12084.
8. Delaney KR. Evidence base for practice: reduction of restraint and seclusion use during child and adolescent psychiatric inpatient treatment. Worldviews Evid-Based Nurs. 2006;3(1):19–30. https://doi.org/10.1111/j.1741-6787.2006.00043.x.
9. Masters KJ, Bellonci C, Bernet W, Arnold V, Beitchman J, Benson RS, Bukstein O, Kinlan J, McClellan J, Rue D, Shaw JA, Stock S, American Academy of C, Adolescent P. Practice parameter for the prevention and management of aggressive behavior in child and adolescent psychiatric institutions, with special reference to seclusion and restraint. J Am Acad Child Adolesc Psychiatry. 2002;41(2 Suppl):4S–25S. https://doi.org/10.1097/00004583-200202001-00002.
10. Neiderman M, Farley A, Richardson J, Lask B. Nasogastric feeding in children and adolescents with eating disorders: toward good practice. Int J Eating Disord. 2001;29(4):441–8. https://doi.org/10.1016/S0883-9417(98)80059-9.
11. Morris J, Simpson AV, Voy SJ. Length of stay of inpatients with eating disorders. Clin Psychol Psychother. 2015;22(1):45–53. https://doi.org/10.1002/cpp.1865.
12. Ayton A, Keen C, Lask B. Pros and cons of using the mental health act for severe eating disorders in adolescents. Eur Eat Disord Rev. 2009;17:14–23. https://doi.org/10.1002/erv.887.
13. Clausen L, Larsen JT, Bulik CM, Petersen L. A Danish register-based study on involuntary treatment in anorexia nervosa. Int J Eating Disord. 2018;51(11):1213–22. https://doi.org/10.1002/eat.22968.
14. Furre A, Sandvik L, Friis S, Knutzen M, Hanssen-Bauer K. A nationwide study of why and how acute adolescent psychiatric units use restraint. Psychiatry Res. 2016;237:60–6. https://doi.org/10.1016/j.psychres.2016.01.067.
15. Clausen L, Jones A. A systematic review of the frequency, duration, type and effect of involuntary treatment for people with anorexia nervosa, and an analysis of patient characteristics. J Eat Disord. 2014;2(1):29–0029. https://doi.org/10.1186/s40337-014-0029-8.
16. Elzakkers IF, Danner UN, Hoek HW, Schmidt U, van Elburg AA. Compulsory treatment in anorexia nervosa: a review. Int J Eat Disord. 2014. https://doi.org/10.1002/eat.22330.
17. Halvorsen I, Reas DL, Nilsen JV, Ro O. Naturalistic outcome of family-based inpatient treatment for adolescents with anorexia nervosa. Eur Eating Disord Rev. 2018;26(2):141–5. https://doi.org/10.1002/erv.2572.
18. Halvorsen I, Ro O. User satisfaction with family-based inpatient treatment for adolescent anorexia nervosa: retrospective views of patients and parents. J Eat Disord. 2019;7:12. https://doi.org/10.1186/s40337-019-0242-6.
19. Frampton I, Wilkinson A. Weight for height, Norwegian version. 4.23 edn. Early onset research team. London: St. George's Hospital Medical School; 2006.
20. Fairburn CG, Cooper Z, O'Connor M. The eating disorder examination (16. 0D). In: Fairburn CG, editor. Cognitive behavior therapy and eating disorders. New York: Guilford Press; 2008. ISBN: 1593857098.
21. Fairburn CG, Beglin SJ. Assessment of eating disorders: interview or self-report questionnaire? Int J Eat Dis. 1994;16(4):363–70. https://doi.org/10.1002/1098-108X(199412)16:4<363::AID-EAT2260160405>3.0.CO;2-#.
22. Ro O, Reas DL, Lask B. Norms for the eating disorder examination questionnaire among female university students in Norway. Nord J Psychiatry. 2010;64(6):428–32. https://doi.org/10.3109/08039481003797235.
23. Cohen J. Statistical power analysis for the behavioral sciences. 2nd ed. HillsdaleJ: L. Erlbaum Associates; 1988. ISBN: 0805802835.
24. Fritz CO, Morris PE, Richler JJ. Effect size estimates: current use, calculations, and interpretation. J Exp Psychol Gen. 2012;141(1):2–18. https://doi.org/10.1037/a0024338.
25. Carney T, Tait D, Touyz S. Coercion is coercion? Reflections on trends in the use of compulsion in treating anorexia nervosa. Australas Psychiatry. 2007;15(5):390–5. https://doi.org/10.1080/10398560701458202.
26. Couturier J, Mahmood A. Meal support therapy reduces the use of nasogastric feeding for adolescents hospitalized with anorexia nervosa. Eat Disord. 2009;17(4):327–32. https://doi.org/10.1080/10640260902991236.
27. Levinson CA, Byrne M. The fear of food measure: a novel measure for use in exposure therapy for eating disorders. Int J Eat Disord. 2015;48(3):271–83. https://doi.org/10.1002/eat.22344.
28. Steinglass JE, Sysko R, Glasofer D, Albano AM, Simpson HB, Walsh BT. Rationale for the application of exposure and response prevention to the treatment of anorexia nervosa. Int J Eating Disord. 2011;44(2):134–41. https://doi.org/10.1002/eat.20784.
29. Furre A, Falk RS, Sandvik L, Friis S, Knutzen M, Hanssen-Bauer K. Characteristics of adolescents frequently restrained in acute psychiatric units in Norway: a nationwide study. Child Adolesc Psychiatry Ment Health. 2017;11:3. https://doi.org/10.1186/s13034-016-0136-1.
30. Baeza I, Correll CU, Saito E, Amanbekova D, Ramani M, Kapoor S, Chekuri R, De Hert M, Carbon M. Frequency, characteristics and management of adolescent inpatient aggression. J Child Adolesc Psychopharmacol. 2013;23(4):271–81. https://doi.org/10.1089/cap.2012.0116.
31. Pogge DL, Pappalardo S, Buccolo M, Harvey PD. Prevalence and precursors of the use of restraint and seclusion in a private psychiatric hospital: comparison of child and adolescent patients. Admin Pol Ment Health. 2013;40(3):224–31. https://doi.org/10.1007/s10488-011-0396-2.
32. Delaney KR, Fogg L. Patient characteristics and setting variables related to use of restraint on four inpatient psychiatric units for youths. Psychiatr Serv. 2005;56(2):186–92. https://doi.org/10.1176/appi.ps.56.2.186.

33. Goren S, Singh NN, Best AM. The aggression-coercion cycle: use of seclusion and restraint in a child psychiatric hospital. J Child Fam Stud. 1993;2(1):61–73. https://doi.org/10.1007/bf01321301.
34. Hendryx M, Trusevich Y, Coyle F, Short R, Roll J. The distribution and frequency of seclusion and/or restraint among psychiatric inpatients. J Behav Health Serv Res. 2010;37(2):272–81. https://doi.org/10.1007/s11414-009-9191-1.
35. Knutzen M, Bjorkly S, Eidhammer G, Lorentzen S, Mjosund NH, Opjordsmoen S, Sandvik L, Friis S. Characteristics of patients frequently subjected to pharmacological and mechanical restraint--a register study in three Norwegian acute psychiatric wards. Psychiatry Res. 2014;215(1):127–33. https://doi.org/10.1016/j.psychres.2013.10.024.
36. Whitehead PD, Liljeros F. Heavy-tailed distribution of seclusion and restraint episodes in a state psychiatric hospital. J Am Acad Psychiatry Law. 2011; 39(1):93–9.
37. Satir DA, Thompson-Brenner H, Boisseau CL, Crisafulli MA. Countertransference reactions to adolescents with eating disorders: relationships to clinician and patient factors. Int J Eating Disord. 2009;42(6): 511–21. https://doi.org/10.1002/eat.20650.
38. Haugvaldstad MJ, Husum TL. Influence of staff's emotional reactions on the escalation of patient aggression in mental health care. Int J Law Psychiatry. 2016;49(Pt A):130–7. https://doi.org/10.1016/j.ijlp.2016.09.001.
39. Haynos AF, Roberto CA, Martinez MA, Attia E, Fruzzetti AE. Emotion regulation difficulties in anorexia nervosa before and after inpatient weight restoration. Int J Eating Disord. 2014;47(8):888–91. https://doi.org/10.1002/eat.22265.
40. Federici A, Kaplan AS. The patient's account of relapse and recovery in anorexia nervosa: a qualitative study. Eur Eat Disord Rev. 2008;16(1):1–10. https://doi.org/10.1002/erv.813.

6

Set-shifting, central coherence and decision-making in individuals recovered from anorexia nervosa

Tone Seim Fuglset

Abstract

Background: The aim of this study was to review the existing literature and evaluate whether deficits in set-shifting, central coherence and decision-making persist in individuals recovered from anorexia nervosa (AN-REC).

Method: A systematic review approach was used. Literature was identified via searches in PubMed, PsychInfo and Embase database. The main search resulted in 158 articles. After exclusion of 135 articles, 23 articles were included in the review.

Results: The majority of studies on set-shifting showed that set-shifting difficulties persist after recovery. Central coherence might also be trait related, however findings are inconsistent. Few studies have investigated decision-making in AN-REC, however those studies that do exist suggest that decision-making is not impaired in AN-REC.

Conclusions: Novel treatment strategies based on neuroscience research are emerging, focusing on targeting the underlying mechanisms of the illness, including neuropsychological functioning. Whether these functions are trait or state related could have implications for how they are targeted in treatment.

Keywords: Anorexia nervosa, Recovered, Executive functions, Systematic review

Plain English summary

Studies have consistently shown that patients with anorexia nervosa have altered neuropsychological functions in some cognitive domains. An important question is whether these difficulties persist after the patients have recovered from their illness. If they *do* persist, this could be related to traits and might be considered as predisposing factors of the illness. If these difficulties normalize with recovery, they are likely a consequence of the illness state. In this study, relevant scientific literature was gathered to investigate whether deficits in the neuropsychological functions i) set-shifting, ii) global processing and iii) decision-making still persists after recovery. In total, 23 studies were included in this review article. The majority of studies on set-shifting indicate that this function is impaired in individuals recovered from anorexia nervosa. Studies including global processing and decision-making are more unclear, as the results are inconsistent.

As anorexia nervosa is an illness that is difficult to treat, there is an urgent need for new and better treatment methods. There has been an increased interest in incorporating findings from neuroscientific research in developing new treatment strategies. These strategies are focusing on the underlying mechanisms of the illness, such as neuropsychological functioning. It would be beneficial to know whether neuropsychological deficits are related to predisposing traits or is a consequence of the illness state, as it might influence how we clinically approach the symptoms and behaviors that we see in anorexia nervosa.

Background

Anorexia nervosa (AN) is considered to be one of the most difficult psychiatric disorders to treat. There is a lack of efficient treatment approaches, especially for adult patients. The aetiology of AN is still unclear, however neuroscientific research has contributed to the

Correspondence: Tone.Seim.Fuglset@helse-mr.no
Division of Mental Health and Addiction, Møre and Romsdal Hospital Trust, Parkvegen 84, 6412 Molde, Norway

development of theoretical models of the illness, linking the core symptoms of AN such as restrictive eating to alterations in brain circuits [1–4].

It has been suggested that neuropsychological deficits mediate between underlying neurobiological functioning and the symptom and behaviors that we see in these patients [5]. Neuropsychological studies have repeatedly demonstrated significant deficits in executive functions such as set-shifting, central coherence and decision-making. Set-shifting refers to the ability to move back and forward between different tasks or mental sets, and is often used as a measure of cognitive flexibility. Patients with AN often have a rigid thinking style, which also involves eating and weight. These patients also often struggle with adapting to environmental changes. Studies have consistently shown that AN patients perform worse on set-shifting tasks compared to healthy controls [6]. Central coherence refers to a bias towards processing details (local processing) at the expense of paying attention to the bigger picture (global processing). A range of studies have demonstrated weak central coherence in patients with AN, suggesting that these patients have a local processing style, and show greater global integration difficulties [7]. Furthermore, decision-making is also likely impaired in patients with AN, as demonstrated repeatedly by several studies (rewieved in [8]). Clinical observations of patients often show that they struggle with making and trusting decisions. This could apply to decisions regarding food and what to eat, but also in other settings outside a meal situation.

A commonly raised question in this field is whether neuropsychological alterations such as deficits in set-shifting, central coherence and decision-making persist after recovery. If they *do* persist, they could be stable traits and not related to the state of the illness. Considering an increased interest in neuroscientific-based treatment methods that has emerged during recent years, it would be beneficial to determine whether such neuropsychological deficits are trait – or state related as it could have implications for how we approach these deficits clinically.

Aim of study

The aim of the present study is to systematically review the literature to evaluate whether deficits in set-shifting, central coherence and decision-making persist in individuals recovered from AN (AN-REC), and to discuss whether these neuropsychological functions are likely to be state or trait related.

Methods

Search strategy and selection of studies

Relevant literature was identified via searches in PubMed, PSychINFO and Embase databases using the search terms [anorexia nervosa] AND [recovered OR recovery OR mental health recovery] AND [set shifting OR central coherence OR decision making].

In total, the main search resulted in 158 articles. A supplemental search was performed by a manual search in Google Scholar, which resulted in five studies. After removal of duplicates, a total of 86 articles were assessed for eligibility. Studies were included if they met the following inclusion criteria:

1. Study included an AN-REC or an AN weight recovered (AN-WR) sample and comparison with a healthy control group/normative scores.
2. Manuscript written in English.
3. Study published in peer-reviewed journals.
4. Abstracts and titles were screened for relevance and eligibility, and 57 articles were excluded. The full texts of the remaining 29 articles were examined in more detail. Of these, six studies were excluded as they were not relevant for the current review (did not include recovered patients or did not include relevant neuropsychological tests). In all, 23 articles were included in the present study. Figure 1 illustrates a PRISMA flow chart of the search strategy.

Study characteristics

One study included both males and females in their sample [9], another study did not specify the gender of the participants [10], and the remaining studies included females only. Nineteen studies included an adult sample, (age ≥ 18 years), whereas only two studies included an adolescent sample (age < 18 years) [11, 12]. Two studies included both adolescents and adults [13, 14]. Definition of recovery varied across studies, see Table 1 for an overview of the different definitions of recovery.

Results

The studies included in this review were published between 2002 and 2017. The distribution across neuropsychological functions were as follows:

1) Set-shifting: 16
2) Central coherence: 8
3) Decision-making: 4

Set-shifting

A variety of tests was used to investigate set-shifting, including Fixed Set Task, Cognitive Shift Task, Trail Making Task (TMT), Brixton Test, CatBat Test, Uznadze Illusion Task, Verbal Fluency Test, Haptic Illusion Test, Wisconsin Card Sorting Test (WCST) and Berg's Card Sorting Test. The majority of studies found poorer set-shifting in AN-REC compared to healthy controls [9, 10, 14–16, 22, 24, 26, 28]. They demonstrate that set-shifting difficulties persist after recovery, and that AN-REC does not differ from

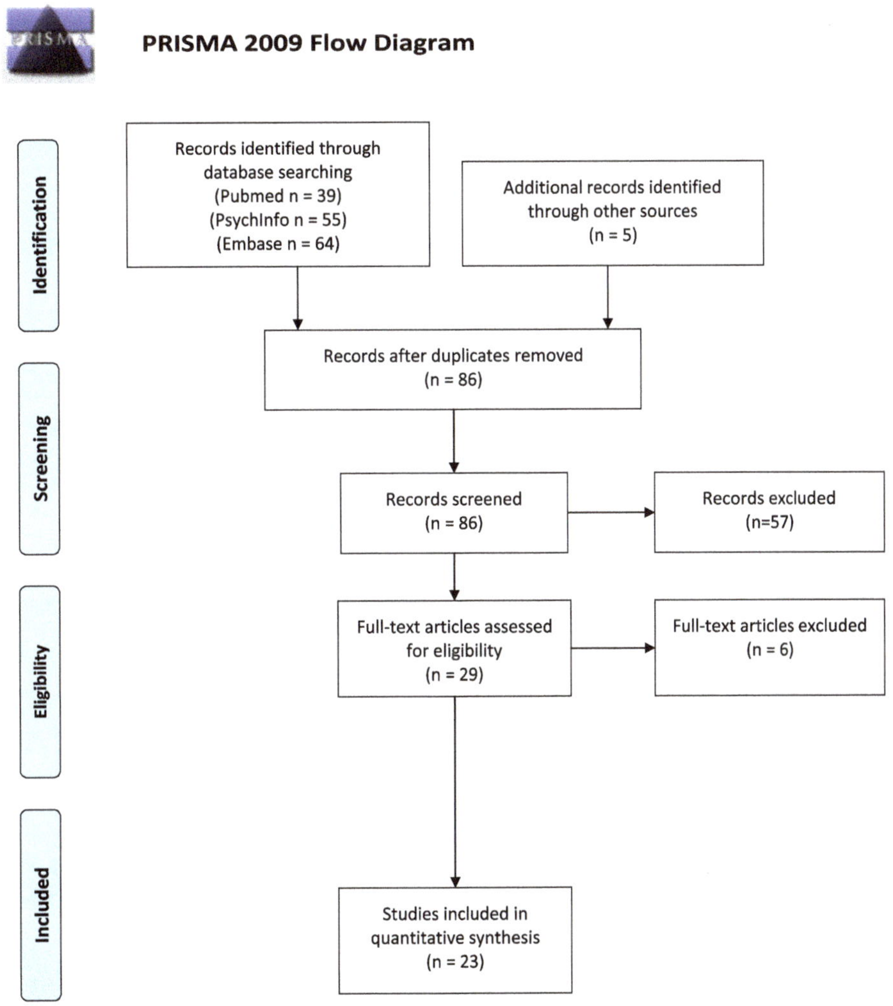

Fig. 1 PRISMA 2009 Flow Diagram

acute AN patients. Results from two of the studies showed a trend towards poorer set-shifting, but the findings were not significant [30, 31]. Similarly, one study found some evidence for poorer set-shifting in AN-REC [21]. Four studies reported no differences between AN-REC and healthy controls, suggesting that there are no set-shifting difficulties in recovered patients [11, 12, 18, 20].

Central coherence

Most studies used the Rey Complex Figure Test (RCFT) to investigate central coherence, but also the Embedded Figures Test, Sentence Completion Task, Homograph Reading Task, National Adult Reading Test and Fragmented Pictures Task were utilized. Four of eight studies found no differences between the AN-REC and the acute group, suggesting weak central coherence in the AN-REC group [13, 14, 19, 24]. One study found that AN-REC had no inefficiencies in global processing but a superior local processing [27]. Three studies found no significant differences in central coherence between the AN-REC group and healthy controls [9, 11, 22].

Decision-making

Only four studies have investigated decision-making in AN-REC. In a study using intertemporal choice task, no differences were observed between AN-REC and healthy controls (HC) [29]. Similar results were found in a study using the Iowa gambling task (IGT) [17]. Another study using the IGT actually reported better performance in the AN-REC group [25]. On the other hand, the same test resulted in poorer decision-making in AN-REC Table 2 [22].

Discussion

The aim of this review was to systematically examine the literature to evaluate whether deficits in set-shifting, central coherence and decision-making persist in individuals recovered from AN-REC, and to discuss whether

Table 1 Overview of criteria for recovery and duration of recovery. The articles are presented chronologically according to year of publication

Authors	Criteria	Duration of recovery
Tchanturia et al., 2002 [10]	Criteria for AN in the past	Minimum 1 year
	BMI 19–24	
	Regular menstruation	
	Normal eating patterns	
Tchanturia et al., 2004 [15]	Stable BMI	Minimum 1 year
	Regular periods	
	No psychotropic medication	
Holliday et al., 2005 [16]	Normal weight	At least 1 year
	Regular menses	
Tchanturia et al., 2007 [17]	BMI between 20 and 25	At least 1 year
	Regular menstruation	
Nakazato et al., 2009 [18]	History of AN diagnosis according to the DSM-IV	At least 1 year
	BMI between 18.5–24	
	Regular menstrual cycles	
	Binge and purge behavior absent	
	No prescribed psychotropic medication	
Lopez et al., 2009 [19]	BMI between 19 and 26	In the current year
	No binging, purging, food restriction or excessive exercise	
Nakazato et al., 2010 [20]	History of AN diagnosis according to the DSM-IV	At least 1 year
	BMI between 18.5–24	
	Regular menstrual cycles	
	Binge and purge behavior absent	
	No prescribed psychotropic medication	
Roberts et al., 2010 [21]	Healthy BMI (> 17.5)	1 year
	Regular periods	
	No AN or BN behaviors	
Tenconi et al., 2010 [14]	Normal weight	At least 3 years
	Regular menses	
	No ED symptoms and good social and interpersonal outcome	
Harrison et al., 2011 [13]	Restored regular menstruation	At least 1 year
	No scores above 4 on EDE-Q	
	BMI > 18.5	
Bühren et al., 2012 [12]	Patients were tested before and after weight rehabilitation	Mean duration of hospital treatment was 122 +/− 33 days, range: 57–193 days
Danner et al., 2012 [22]	BMI > 18.5 and recovered menstrual cycle	At least 12 consecutive months
	EDE-Q and BDI not different from HC	
Favaro et al., 2012 [23]	Asymptomatic	At least 3 months
Harrison et al., 2012 [24]	Restored regular menstruation	At least 1 year
	No scores above 4 on EDE-Q	
	BMI > 18.5	
Lindner et al., 2012 [25]	No DSM-IV criteria	At least 1 year
	BMI between 18.5 and 26	
	Regular menstrual cycles	

Table 1 Overview of criteria for recovery and duration of recovery. The articles are presented chronologically according to year of publication *(Continued)*

Authors	Criteria	Duration of recovery
	No ED specific cognitions	
Tchanturia et al., 2012 [26]	BMI > 18.5	At least 1 year
	Restored menstruation	
	Absence of ED behaviors	
Lindner et al., 2013 [27]	No DSM-IV criteria	At least 1 year
	BMI between 18.5 and 26	
	Regular menstrual cycles	
	No ED specific cognitions	
Lindner et al., 2014 [28]	No DSM-IV criteria	At least 1 year
	BMI between 18.5 and 26	
	Regular menstrual cycles	
	No ED specific cognitions	
Ritschel et al., 2015 [29]	If > 18 years old, BMI > 18.5	At least 6 months
	If < 18 years old, BMI > 10th BMI percentile	
	Menstruation	
	No binge, purge or restrictive eating pattern	
Talbot et al., 2015 [9]	BMI ≥ 18.5	Past 3 months (at minimum)
	No binging, purging, restricting and driven or compulsive exercise	
	Scores on all subscales of EDE-Q within 1 SD of population	
	norms	
Ely et al., 2016 [30]	Stable weight between 90 and 120% of ideal body weight	Prior 12 months
	Regular menstrual cycles	
Sultson et al., 2016 [31]	BMI > 18.5	At least 12 months
	Recovered menstrual cycle	
	No differences from HC on the EDE-Q	
Bentz et al., 2017 [11]	If > 16 years old, BMI > 18.5	At least 1 year
	If 14–15 years old, BMI-percentile corrected for age > 25th percentile	
	No present ED pathology	
	Global EDE-Q score within 1 SD of non-AN mean	
	MROAS ≥9	

AN anorexia nervosa, *BDI* Beck's depression inventory, *BMI* body mass index, *BN* bulimia nervosa; *DSM-IV* Diagnostic and Statistical Manual of Mental Disorders, 4th Edition, *ED* eating disorders, *EDE-Q* Eating disorders examination questionnaire *HC* healthy controls, *MROAS* Morgan Russel Outcome Assessment Schedule, *SD* standard deviation

these neuropsychological functions are likely to be state or trait related. The current review used 23 studies. The majority of studies in set-shifting suggest that this function is impaired in AN-REC. The evidence base for central coherence, on the other hand, is more unclear as findings are inconsistent. Few studies have investigated decision-making in AN-REC, however most studies so far suggest that this function is not different from healthy controls.

State or trait?

The majority of findings in this review suggest that set-shifting difficulties could be trait characteristics rather than a state marker. Tchanturia et al. suggest that impaired set-shifting could represent a vulnerability factor for AN [10] and that some aspects of set-shifting could be a trait rather than a state marker [15]. Likewise, in the study by Holliday et al. [16] there were no differences between acute AN and those who had fully recovered from AN. A

Table 2 Review of the literature of set-shifting, central coherence and decision-making in individuals recovered from anorexia nervosa. The articles are presented chronologically according to year of publication

Authors	Neuropsychological function	Tests	Aim of study	Sample	Age Mean (SD)	Main findings	Effect size (test)	Conclusion
Tchanturia et al., 2002 [10]	Set-shifting	Fixed set task Cognitive shift task	To examine perceptual and cognitive set-shifting	AN = 30 AN-REC = 16 HC = 23	AN = 25.2 (6.7) AN-REC = 30.0 (6.0) HC = 27.6 (6.4)	Significant differences between AN/AN-REC compared to HC	$d = 1.37$ (Fixed set task) $d = 0.72$ (Cognitive shift task, perseverations)	Impaired set-shifting could represent a vulnerability factor for AN
Tchanturia et al., 2004 [15]	Set-shifting	TMT Brixton test Picture set test Cat bat tests Uznadze illusion task	To investigate set-shifting in current and past AN patients	AN = 34 AN-REC = 18 HC = 36	AN = 27.2 (8.3) AN-REC = 28.4 (6.8) HC = 25.9 (4.8)	Set-shifting difficulties was observed in the AN group, and to a lesser degree in the AN-REC group	$d = 0.87$ (Picture set test) $d = 0.88$ (illusions)	Some aspects of set-shifting in AN appear to be a trait rather than state marker
Holliday et al., 2005 [16]	Set-shifting	Haptic illusion task Brixton Test TMT CatBat task	To investigate whether set-shifting difficulties are familial	47 pairs of sisters disconcordant for AN: AN-REC = 23 AN = 21 AN-WR = 3 HS = 47 HC = 47	AN (AN-REC + AN+ AN-WR) = 26.3 (10.2) HS = 27.6 (9.6) HC = 26.5 (6.1)	Set-shifting difficulties persists after recovery	N/A	Suggest that set-shifting difficulties are trait characteristics and may inform the search for the endophenotype of AN
Tchanturia et al., 2007 [17]	Decision making	IGT	To determine whether decision-making is impaired in AN-REC	AN = 29 HC = 29 AN-REC = 14	AN = 28.5 (9.17) HC = 26.3 (7.9) AN-REC = 28.9 (7.4)	No differences between AN-REC and HC. AN grop did poorer than AN-REC and HC	–	Impaired IGT performance could be a consequence of starvation
Lopez et al., 2009 [19]	Central coherence	Embedded figures test Unsegmented/ segmented block design RCFT SCT	To examine whether AN-REC women have weak central coherence	AN-REC = 42 HC = 42	AN-REC = 25 HC = 26	Weak central coherence in the AN-REC group	$d = 0.53$ (Rey order) $d = 0.73$ (Style) $d = 0.57$ (CC Index)	Suggest that weak central coherence is a stable trait and an endophenotype for AN

Table 2 Review of the literature of set-shifting, central coherence and decision-making in individuals recovered from anorexia nervosa. The articles are presented chronologically according to year of publication *(Continued)*

Authors	Neuropsychological function	Tests	Aim of study	Sample	Age Mean (SD)	Main findings	Effect size (test)	Conclusion
		Homograph reading task					*d* = 1.15 (SCT)	
Nakazato et al., 2009 [18]	Set-shifting	WCST	To establish whether set-shifting difficulties are present in AN and AN-REC	AN = 29 AN-REC = 18 HC = 28	AN = 28.3 (11.0) AN-REC = 32.2 (11.1) HC = 26.9 (5.8)	No significant differences between AN-REC and HC	–	Strongly suggest that impairment in set-shifting normalizes with recovery
Nakazato et al., 2010 [20]	Set-shifting	WCST TMT	Determine whether serum glutamine is associated with set-shifting ability	AN = 27 AN-REC = 18 HC = 28	AN = 27.7 (10.6) AN-REC = 32.2 (11.1) HC = 26.9 (5.8)	No differences between AN-REC and HC	–	Serum concentrations does not appear to be associated with executive functions
Roberts et al., 2010 [21]	Set-shifting	TMT WCST Brixton test Haptic illusion	To add clarity to set-shifting in EDs	AN-R = 35 AN-BP = 33 BN = 30 AN-REC = 30 AN sister = 30 BN sister =20 HC = 88	AN-R = 23.71 (6.39) AN-BP = 25.58 (7.64) BN = 26.43 (6.84) AN-REC = 32.13 (11.64) AN sister = 24.23 (6.44) BN sister = 27.60 (8.71) HC = 28.43 (8.47)	Some evidence for poorer set shifting in AN – REC	*d* = 0.64 (WCST)	It is likely a familial trait, and related to the maintenance of the illness
Tenconi et al., 2010	Set-shifting Central coherence	WCST	To explore suitability for endophenotypes in ED	AN = 60	AN = 26.2 (6.9)	No differences between AN and AN-REC	–	Impaired set-shifting and low central coherence might be an

Table 2 Review of the literature of set-shifting, central coherence and decision-making in individuals recovered from anorexia nervosa. The articles are presented chronologically according to year of publication *(Continued)*

Authors	Neuropsychological function	Tests	Aim of study	Sample	Age Mean (SD)	Main findings	Effect size (test)	Conclusion
[14]		TMT RCFT		AN-WR = 63 AN-REC = 30 HC = 120	HC = 27.4 (4.5)			endophenotype of AN
Harrison et al., 2011 [13]	Central coherence	RCFT GEFT FPT	To replicate findings of weak central coherence	AN = 50 BN = 48 AN-REC = 35 HC = 89	ED group = 27.13 (9.3) AN-REC = 29.00 (10.62) HC = 28.5 (9.93)	Superior detail processing skills was associated with having an ED and recovered from AN	*d* = 0.58 (RCFT) *d* = 0.31 (GEFT)	AN-REC are skilled at detailed processing. Weak central coherence may be a factor that perpetuates ED behaviors
Bühren et al., 2012 [12]	Set-shifting	Visual set-shifting task	To investigate set-shifting in AN before and after weight gain	AN = 28 HC = 27	AN = 15.6 (1.5) HC = 15.0 (1.7)	No deficits in set-shifting abilities.	–	Speculate that findings could be related to short duration of illness
Danner et al., 2012 [22]	Set-shifting Central coherence Decision making	BCST RCFT IGT	To examine set-shifting in women AN-REC	AN = 16 AN-REC = 15 HC = 15	AN = 25.63 (5.41) AN-REC = 24.33 (4.72) HC = 25.8 (4.69)	Poor set-shifting and decision making in AN-REC compared to HC. No differences between the groups in central coherence	*d* = 1.16 (BCST perseverative errors) *d* = 1.14 (BCST total errors *d* = 1.05 (BCST categories completed) *d* = 1.36 (Total IGT score)	Suggest that impaired decision-making and set-shifting is a stable trait in AN
Favaro et al., 2012	Central coherence	RCFT	To explore functional connectivity of networks involved in visuospatial and somatosensory processing	AN = 29 AN-REC = 16 HC = 26	AN = 25.8 (6.9) AN-REC = 23.8 (4.8) HC = 26.7 (6.7)	No differences between AN-REC and HC in central coherence	–	Results could be due to a milder form of the illness in the AN-REC group, measures by minimum BMI and duration of illness
Harrison et al., 2012 [24]	Set-shifting Central coherence	WCST Brixton task FPT RCFT	To explore cognitive and social emotional functioning	ED = 100 ED-REC = 35 HC = 90	N/A	ED-REC did not differ from the acute group.	–	Suggest that cognitive style is a trait.
Lindner et	Decision making	IGT	To examine decision-	AN-REC = 100	AN-REC =	AN-REC did better in decision-	*d* = 0.35 (IGT)	Findings are in contrast to previous

Table 2 Review of the literature of set-shifting, central coherence and decision-making in individuals recovered from anorexia nervosa. The articles are presented chronologically according to year of publication *(Continued)*

Authors	Neuropsychological function	Tests	Aim of study	Sample	Age Mean (SD)	Main findings	Effect size (test)	Conclusion
al., 2012 [25]			making and planning in AN-REC	HC = 100	34.49 (7.13) HC = 34.53 (7.26)	making		findings of impaired decision making in AN-REC
Tchanturia et al., 2012 [26]	Set-shifting	WCST	To explore WCST performance and other clinical outcomes	AN = 171 BN = 82 AN-REC = 90 HC = 199	AN = 25.4 (8.2) BN = 27.3 (8.3) AN-REC = 30.7 (11.1) HC = 27.7 (8.8)	AN-REC showed better performance than AN, but did more perseverative errors than HC	*d* = 0.50 (WCST perseverative errors)	This large dataset supports previous studies which indicate poor cognitive flexibility in people with EDs.
Lindner et al., 2013 [27]	Central coherence	RCFT	To examine central coherence as a possible endophenotype in AN	AN-REC = 100 HC = 100	AN-REC = 34.49 (7.13) HC = 34.53 (7.26)	AN-REC group showed better accuracy in the copy condition	*d* = 0.46 (RCFT copy condition)	No inefficiencies in global processing but a superior local processing
Lindner et al., 2014 [28]	Set-shifting	BCST	To explore whether set-shifting is inefficient after full recovery of AN	AN-REC = 100 HC = 100	AN-REC = 34.49 (7.13) HC = 34.53 (7.26)	AN-REC achieved fewer categories, more perseverations and spent less time for shifting set	*d* = 0.39 (BCST categories) *d* = 0.35 (BCST perseverations) *d* = 0.36 (BCST reaction time)	Suggest that set-shifting is inefficient after full recovery
Ritschel et al., 2015 [29]	Decision making	Intertemporal choice task	To investigate delay discounting in ill and recovered AN	AN = 34 AN-REC = 33 HC = 54	AN = 15.29 (2.7) AN-REC = 21.67 (3.1) HC = 18.75 (4.4)	No group differences in delay discounting	–	Suggest that delay discounting is not a trait marker for AN
Talbot et al., 2015 [9]	Set-shifting and central coherence	WCST Matching familiar figures test RCFT	To investigate whether impaired set-shifting and weak central coherence represent state or trait	AN = 24 AN-WR = 10 AN-REC = 15 HC = 43	AN = 21.0 (18-27)[a] AN-WR = 21.5 (19–25) [a]	Poorer set-shifting in AN –REC and AN-WR compared to HC.	*d* = 0.79 (WCST)	This study found no support that weak central coherence is an endophenotype for AN

Table 2 Review of the literature of set-shifting, central coherence and decision-making in individuals recovered from anorexia nervosa. The articles are presented chronologically according to year of publication *(Continued)*

Authors	Neuropsychological function	Tests	Aim of study	Sample	Age Mean (SD)	Main findings	Effect size (test)	Conclusion
					AN-REC = 24.0 (21–32) [a] HC = 19.0 (18–25) [a]	No differences between the groups on measures of local and global processing		
Ely et al., 2016 [30]	Set shifting	Color-Word interference test	To identify deficits specific to inhibition or task-switching	AN-REC = 47 HC = 24	AN-REC = 26.68 (1.83) HC = 25.08 (6.11)	Differences between the groups trended toward – but was not – significant	–	Suggest that cognitive control impairments in AN is related to anxiety, and not a neuropsychological deficit
Sultson et al., 2016 [31]	Set-shifting	BCST	To investigate whether activation in frontal and parietal regions is associated with set-shifting ability	AN = 16 AN-REC = 15 HC = 15	AN = 25.57 (5.8) AN-REC = 24.79 (4.5) HC = 25.80 (4.7)	No differences between AN-REC and HC, but a trend towards more perseverative errors and completing less categories than HC	–	Higher activation in frontal regions involved in self-referential processing and cognitive control is associated with poor set-shifting ability in AN-REC
Bentz et al., 2017 [11]	Set shifting and local processing	TMT GEFT	To investigate impairments of social functioning and potential associations with neurocognitive functions	AN = 43 AN-REC = 28 HC = 41	AN = 16.1 (1.5) AN-REC = 18.4 (1.6) HC = 17.7 (2.2)	No differences between the groups on neurocognitive functions	–	Young AN and AN-REC did not differ from HC

Effect sizes for significant differences between AN-REC and HC. Cohen's d effect size: small ($d = 0.2$), medium ($d = 0.5$) and large ($d = 0.8$)
AN anorexia nervosa, *AN – REC* anorexia nervosa recovered, *AN – WR* anorexia nervosa weight restored, *BN* bulimia nervosa, *BCST* Berg's Card Sorting Test, *ED's* eating disorders, *CC index* Central Coherence index, *ED-REC* eating disorders recovered, *FPT* Fragmented pictures task, *GEFT* Group Embedded Figures Test, *HC* healthy controls, *HS* Healthy sister, *IGT* Iowa Gambling Task, *N/A* Not applicable, *RCFT* Rey Complex Figure Test, *SCT* Sentence completion task, *TMT* Trail making test, *WCST* Wisconsin Card Sorting Test. The main findings represents significant differences in the experimental group (AN-REC) compared to a healthy control group
[a] Median values with upper and lower quartiles

common question is whether neuropsychological deficits in AN-REC represent scarring effects after many years of starvation and underweight. Due to methodological challenges, this is difficult to determine, and still debated. However, Holliday et al. [16] further suggest that reduced cognitive and perceptual flexibility could reflect a familial trait that is associated with a greater risk of developing AN, and not a scar due to the illness. Set-shifting difficulties as a trait is also supported by Harrison et al. [13] who reported a less adaptive cognitive style and social and emotional profile would be a trait that is associated with the eating disorder. They also suggest that this could be a maintaining factor, having the least adaptive cognitive style would be associated with a more chronic and severe form of the illness. Furthermore, they found that both individuals currently ill and recovered from AN have a fragmented perseverative cognitive style with social and emotional difficulties. A rigid cognitive style accompanied with social emotional difficulties was associated with a more persistent and severe form of illness. Danner et al. [22] also suggest that this is a stable impairment, as their results show that problems with set-shifting persist in AN-REC. Similar results was reported in the study by Talbot et al. [9], who found that individuals that have fully recovered from AN, still have impairments in set-shifting. They claim that full recovery from AN does not signify normal neuropsychological functioning. The results from Lindner et al. [28] showed that AN-REC showed inefficient set-shifting or flexibility, i.e. they stayed longer to the old rule instead of changing to the new rule. In summary, these studies suggest that difficulties with set-shifting could be trait-related.

On the other hand, some studies failed to detect any differences between AN-REC and HC on a set-shifting task. Bentz et al. [11] did not find any differences between the groups (AN, AN-REC and HC) in cognitive flexibility. Similarly, Bühren et al. [12] and Nakazato et al. [18] found no deficits in set-shifting in AN-REC. Ely et al. [30] failed to show any differences in cognitive inhibition and set-shifting in a remitted sample of AN patients and HC. They suggests that cognitive control impairments in AN is related to anxiety and does not reflect a neuropsychological deficit.

Results from studies on central coherence are more ambiguous. Based on the existing literature, it is difficult to determine whether deficits in central coherence is state or trait-related. Findings from some studies in this review show that AN-REC have persistent deficits in central coherence, while other studies indicate normal global processing in AN-REC. In the study by Danner et al. [22], those with poor set-shifting also showed weaknesses in central coherence. They suggest that these deficits could be specific to a subpopulation of individuals with AN, and that this could be linked to a rigid thinking style. Lopez et al. [19] found that AN-REC did "extremely well" on the EFT, which benefit from enhanced detailed function and suggest that weak central coherence could be a stable trait. Likewise, Harrison et al. [13] reported that AN-REC are skilled at detailed processing and that weak central coherence may be a factor that perpetuates eating disorder behavior. They also suggest that cognitive style could be a trait of the illness [24].

Lindner et al. [27] did not find any inefficiency in global processing in the recovered group. Similarly, Talbot et al. [9] did not find any differences in measures of local and global processing. Therefore, based on the existing literature, caution should be made when determining whether central coherence is related to state or trait of AN.

Decision-making is a complex construct, and few studies have investigated decision-making in AN-REC. However, according to the existing studies, it may seem like AN-REC does not have difficulties with decision-making tasks. In a study using the IGT, Tchanturia et al. [17] found that the AN-REC group performed just as well as the HC group, and they question whether poor decision-making is related to starvation. Another study using the IGT actually reported that AN-REC did better than HC [25]. One possible explanation could be that the AN-REC group have lower risk-taking behaviors. In a delay discounting task which included a monetary reward, Ritschel et al. [29] found no differences in delay discounting between AN-REC and HC. They suggest that altered self-control might be limited to disorder-relevant reinforcers, such as food. One study, using the IGT, reported that decision-making was impaired in AN-REC, and suggest that impaired decision-making is a stable trait in AN [22].

Neuropsychological endophenotypes in AN?

There has been an increased interest in determining possible endophenotypes for eating disorders. Endophenotypes can be defined as observable behavioral characteristics that underlie and contribute to disease vulnerabilities, but are not a part of the disease itself. There are three criteria of an endophenotype: i) the candidate trait is associated with the illness, ii) is state-independent, and iii) is present in unaffected family members [32]. The endophenotypes for AN are still unclear, however it has been argued that both set-shifting and central coherence could be potential endophenotypes for AN [9].

In the current review, persistent impairments in set-shifting is the most robust finding, as opposed to central coherence and decision-making. As an endophenotype needs to be trait-related and also present in family members, it is worth mentioning that two studies in this review also included unaffected family members. Holliday et al.

[16] found that set-shifting deficits in women with AN were shared with their healthy sisters. Both patients and their sisters took longer to set-shift on the CatBat cognitive set-shifting task and the Haptic Illusion task. They suggest that their study provides further support for the possibility that set-shifting may be a part of the endophenotype in AN. Similarly, Tenconi et al. [14] found that AN patients and their sisters share impairments in set-shifting. They also suggest that set-shifting is a cognitive endophenotype for AN. Poor set-shifting as an endophenotype could contribute to rigid and compulsive behaviors that are often seen in individuals with AN.

Further research with unaffected family members and AN-REC is needed to further investigate endophenotypes for AN, however, set-shifting difficulties could be a possible endophenotype for this illness.

Clinical implications

There has been an increased interest in incorporating findings from neuroscientific studies to the development of treatment strategies for AN. Cognitive Remediation Therapy (CRT) involves cognitive training which addresses difficulties with flexibility and global processing [33]. The aim of this treatment is to modify and improve these deficits, and apply new cognitive skills to eating-related tasks. A more recently developed treatment, Temperament-based treatment with support (TBT-S) [34] is also based on neuroscientific research. Here, the patients learn strategies to cope with their deficits, and learn how to use their personality traits in constructive ways. A complete understanding of the neuropsychological deficits in patients with AN, and whether they normalize with recovery, might influence how we develop such treatment strategies. An important issue is whether treatment should aim to alter these neuropsychological deficits, or whether the treatment should be adjusted to this specific neuropsychological thinking style.

Limitations

Some weaknesses in the literature included in this review are important to consider. First, there is a lack of consensus in the eating disorder field on a standard definition of recovery of AN. This could offer challenges when comparing results across studies. In the current review, the majority of studies include a BMI > 18.5 and the absence of eating disorder symptoms as criteria for recovery. Although the majority of studies require that the recovered state should have been at least 1 year, other studies require a duration of 6 months and 3 months.

Conflicting results across studies could also be due to variations in clinical measures, such as duration of illness, severity degree and AN subtype (restrictive and binge/purge). Severely affected patients with a long duration of illness might have larger scarring effects compared to individuals with shorter duration of illness and less symptom severity. However, determining these variables accurately is difficult. Most studies do not define the term duration of illness and how it is assessed. In addition, duration of illness can be measured in various ways, such as by diagnosis date, what time the symptoms emerged, or what time the patient was entered into treatment. When it comes to severity degree, McGuire et al. [35] have proposed a theoretical model for the definition and conceptualization of severity of AN. According to this model, there should be a staging system, which is based on symptom severity. The main purpose of this system is to make appropriate treatment options, however it would also be beneficial for scientific purposes.

Few studies have separated patients into different subtypes. Neuropsychological difficulties could vary within the AN group, and by not separating individuals into subgroups, important findings could be overlooked. However, which group of patients that have neuropsychological difficulties is yet to be established, as studies are few and the findings are inconsistent. Lindner et al. [28] divided the AN-REC group by subtypes and found that the restricting group performed worse on a set-shifting task than HC. At the same time, Danner et al. [22] suggest that neuropsychological impairments are not a general problem for AN, but these are specific for a subpopulation within both ill and recovered patients. Therefore, there could be subgroups of patients that have problems with set-shifting which could be independent from AN diagnostic subtype, a topic in need of further investigation.

Other differences in study design, such as sample size, might also affect the results. Lack of power calculations estimating the sample size necessary to detect significant differences between groups, could contribute to conflicting findings. In the current review, studies within the central coherence domain showed various findings. One study that failed to find significant results had a sample size of fifteen in the AN-REC group. In addition, conflicting findings could also be reflected by the large variety of tests that have been used within the same cognitive domain.

An important area of research is focused upon which factors that distinguish adolescent patients from adults. Adolescents seem to have a better prognosis than adults [36]. Studies have consistently shown that adults with AN have altered executive functioning, and some of these functions might be trait related. However, when do state difficulties occur? Moreover, are they related to the maintenance of the illness? Future studies should compare neuropsychological performance in adolescents versus adults with AN. Future studies should also focus on differentiating predisposing factors and perpetuating factors. Predisposing factors include inherent characteristic, such as genetics and personality traits, while perpetuating factors are conditions that maintain the symptoms of the illness. Predisposing and perpetuating factors are not necessarily the same, and determining these could contribute to the development of better treatment strategies.

Conclusion

The majority of studies in this review suggest that deficits in set-shifting persist after recovery, and could be trait related. Set-shifting difficulties could also be an endophenotype for AN as it is present in unaffected family members. Central coherence might also be trait related, however findings are inconsistent. Few studies have investigated decision-making in AN-REC, however existing studies suggest that decision-making is not impaired in AN-REC.

There is an urgent need for better treatment approaches for individuals with AN, and especially for adult patients. Novel treatment strategies based on neuroscience research are emerging, focusing on targeting the underlying mechanisms of the illness, including neuropsychological functioning. These new treatments include elements such as practicing and improving specific cognitive skills and teaching effective tools and strategies to manage eating disorder symptoms in a collaborative manner. The factors that sustain the illness are most likely different from the factors that contribute to the onset of the illness. It would therefore be beneficial to determining these factors so they could be correctly targeted in treatment.

Abbreviations

AN: Anorexia nervosa; AN-REC: Anorexia nervosa recovered; BN: Bulimia nervosa; CRT: Cognitive remediation therapy; HC: Healthy controls; IGT: Iowa gambling task; RCFT: Rey complex figure test; TBT-S: Temperament-based treatment with support; TMT: Trail making test.; WCST: Wisconsin Card Sorting Test; WR-AN: Weight-recovered anorexia nervosa

Acknowledgements

The author would like to thank Dr. Bente Talseth-Palmer for valuable comments and for proof-reading the manuscript.

Authors' contributions

TSF conducted the literature search, analyzed the data and wrote the paper. All authors read and approved the final manuscript.

Authors' information

TSF has a PhD in Psychology from the University of Oslo and has previously worked at the Regional Department for Eating Disorders at Oslo University Hospital. She is currently in a postdoctoral position in Møre and Romsdal Hospital Trust located in Molde, Norway.

Competing interests

The author declares that she has no competing interests.

References

1. Godier LR, Park RJ. Compulsivity in anorexia nervosa: a transdiagnostic concept. Front Psychol. 2014;5:778.
2. Kaye WH, Fudge JL, et al. New insights into symptoms and neurocircuit function of anorexia nervosa. Nat Rev Neurosci. 2009;10(8):573–84.
3. O'Hara CB, Campbell IC, et al. A reward-centred model of anorexia nervosa: a focussed narrative review of the neurological and psychophysiological literature. Neurosci Biobehav Rev. 2015;52:131–52.
4. Steinglass J, Walsh BT. Habit learning and anorexia nervosa: a cognitive neuroscience hypothesis. Int J Eat Disord. 2006;39(4):267–75.
5. Frampton I, Rose M. Eating disorders and the brain. In: Lask B, Bryant-Waugh R, editors. Eating disorders in children and adolescents. 4th ed. Hove: Routledge; 2013.
6. Wu M, Brockmeyer T, et al. Set-shifting ability across the spectrum of eating disorders and in overweight and obesity: a systematic review and meta-analysis. Psychol Med. 2014;44(16):3365–85.
7. Lang K, Lopez C, et al. Central coherence in eating disorders: an updated systematic review and meta-analysis. World J Biol Psychiatry. 2014;15(8):586–98.
8. Wu M, Brockmeyer T, et al. Reward-related decision making in eating and weight disorders: a systematic review and meta-analysis of the evidence from neuropsychological studies. Neurosci Biobehav Rev. 2016;61:177–96.
9. Talbot A, Hay P, et al. Cognitive deficits as an endophenotype for anorexia nervosa: an accepted fact or a need for re-examination? Int J Eat Disord. 2015;48(1):15–25.
10. Tchanturia K, Morris RG, et al. An examination of perceptual and cognitive set shifting tasks in acute anorexia nervosa and following recovery. Eat Weight Disord. 2002;7(4):312–5.
11. Bentz M, Jepsen JRM, et al. Neurocognitive functions and social functioning in young females with recent-onset anorexia nervosa and recovered individuals. J Eat Disord. 2017;5:5.
12. Buhren K, Mainz V, et al. Cognitive flexibility in juvenile anorexia nervosa patients before and after weight recovery. J Neural Transm (Vienna). 2012; 119(9):1047–57.
13. Harrison A, Tchanturia K, et al. Measuring state trait properties of detail processing and global integration ability in eating disorders. World J Biol Psychiatry. 2011;12(6):462–72.
14. Tenconi E, Santonastaso P, et al. Set-shifting abilities, central coherence, and handedness in anorexia nervosa patients, their unaffected siblings and healthy controls: exploring putative endophenotypes. World J Biol Psychiatry. 2010;11(6):813–23.
15. Tchanturia K, Morris RG, et al. Set shifting in anorexia nervosa: an examination before and after weight gain, in full recovery and relationship to childhood and adult OCPD traits. J Psychiatr Res. 2004;38(5):545–52.
16. Holliday J, Tchanturia K, et al. Is impaired set-shifting an endophenotype of anorexia nervosa? Am J Psychiatry. 2005;162(12):2269–75.
17. Tchanturia K, Liao PC, et al. An investigation of decision making in anorexia nervosa using the Iowa gambling task and skin conductance measurements. J Int Neuropsychol Soc. 2007;13(4):635–41.
18. Nakazato M, Tchanturia K, et al. Brain-derived neurotrophic factor (BDNF) and set-shifting in currently ill and recovered anorexia nervosa (AN) patients. Psychol Med. 2009;39(6):1029–35.
19. Lopez C, Tchanturia K, et al. Weak central coherence in eating disorders: a step towards looking for an endophenotype of eating disorders. J Clin Exp Neuropsychol. 2009;31(1):117–25.
20. Nakazato M, Hashimoto K, et al. Serum glutamine, set-shifting ability and anorexia nervosa. Ann General Psychiatry. 2010;9:29.
21. Roberts ME, Tchanturia K, et al. Exploring the neurocognitive signature of poor set-shifting in anorexia and bulimia nervosa. J Psychiatr Res. 2010; 44(14):964–70.
22. Danner UN, Sanders N, et al. Neuropsychological weaknesses in anorexia nervosa: set-shifting, central coherence, and decision making in currently ill and recovered women. Int J Eat Disord. 2012;45(5):685–94.
23. Angela Favaro, Paolo Santonastaso, Renzo Manara, Romina Bosello, Giulia Bommarito, Elena Tenconi, and Francesco Di Salle (2012). Disruption of Visuospatial and Somatosensory Functional Connectivity in Anorexia Nervosa, Biological Psychiatry, 72:864–870.
24. Harrison A, Tchanturia K, et al. Social emotional functioning and cognitive styles in eating disorders. Br J Clin Psychol. 2012;51(3):261–79.
25. Lindner SE, Fichter MM, et al. Decision-making and planning in full recovery of anorexia nervosa. Int J Eat Disord. 2012;45(7):866–75.
26. Tchanturia K. Poor cognitive flexibility in eating disorders: examining the evidence using the Wisconsin card sorting task, vol. 7; 2012. p. 1.
27. Lindner SE, Fichter MM, et al. Central coherence in full recovery of anorexia nervosa. Eur Eat Disord Rev. 2013;21(2):115–20.
28. Lindner SE, Fichter MM, et al. Set-shifting and its relation to clinical and personality variables in full recovery of anorexia nervosa. Eur Eat Disord Rev. 2014;22(4):252–9.

29. Ritschel F, King JA, et al. Temporal delay discounting in acutely ill and weight-recovered patients with anorexia nervosa. Psychol Med. 2015; 45(6):1229–39.
30. Ely AV, Wierenga CE, et al. Anxiety impacts cognitive inhibition in remitted anorexia nervosa. Eur Eat Disord Rev. 2016;24(4):347–51.
31. Sultson H, van Meer F, et al. Associations between neural correlates of visual stimulus processing and set-shifting in ill and recovered women with anorexia nervosa. Psychiatry Res Neuroimaging. 2016;255:35–42.
32. Gottesman II, Gould TD. The endophenotype concept in psychiatry: etymology and strategic intentions. Am J Psychiatry. 2003;160(4):636–45.
33. Leppanen J, Adamson J, et al. Impact of cognitive remediation therapy on neurocognitive processing in anorexia nervosa. Frontiers Psych. 2018;9:96.
34. Wierenga CE, Hill L, et al. The acceptability, feasibility, and possible benefits of a neurobiologically-informed 5-day multifamily treatment for adults with anorexia nervosa. Int J Eat Disord. 2018;51(8):863–9.
35. Maguire S, Le Grange D, et al. Staging anorexia nervosa: conceptualizing illness severity. Early Interv Psychiatry. 2008;2(1):3–10.
36. Fisher M. The course and outcome of eating disorders in adults and in adolescents: a review. Adolesc Med. 2003;14(1):149–58.

7

Extreme anorexia nervosa: medical findings, outcomes and inferences from a retrospective cohort

Dennis Gibson[1,2], Ashlie Watters[1,2], Jeana Cost[1,3], Margherita Mascolo[2] and Philip S. Mehler[1,2,3*]

Abstract

Background: Extreme anorexia nervosa (AN) is defined as a BMI < 15 kg/m^2 in those meeting DSM-V diagnostic criteria for AN. This study seeks to define the frequency of medical complications in this group of patients in order to help inform the care of individuals < 65% ideal body weight who seek treatment for their extreme eating disorders.

Methods: Through retrospective chart review and computerized data collection, we obtained the baseline characteristics and medical findings of 281 adult patients, with AN restricting and binge-purge subtypes, admitted to the ACUTE unit for medical stabilization between May 2013 and August 2018.

Results: In this population, with a mean admitting BMI of 12.1 kg/m^2 (range = 7.5–15.7), 56% admitted with bradycardia, 45% demonstrated increased liver function tests (LFTs) on admission, 64% admitted with leukopenia, 47% with anemia, and 20% presented with thrombocytopenia. During admission, 38% developed hypoglycemia, 35% developed refeeding hypophosphatemia, nearly 33% of patients developed edema, and low bone mineral density was diagnosed in almost 90% of the patients. Highly elevated LFTs (>3x upper limits of normal) predicted hypoglycemia, and low BMI predicted refeeding hypophosphatemia (p = .001).

Conclusions: Although conclusions drawn from the findings presented in this descriptive study must be tempered by relevant clinical judgement, these findings showcase that patients with extreme AN are at significantly increased risk for many serious medical complications secondary to their state of malnutrition and also with initial refeeding.

Keywords: Extreme anorexia nervosa, Medical complications, Malnutrition, Outcomes, Refeeding

Plain English summary

Extreme anorexia nervosa (AN) is defined as a BMI < 15 kg/m^2 in those meeting DSM-5 diagnostic criteria for AN. However, the frequency of medical complications specific to those meeting this greatest amount of weight loss is unknown. This retrospective study seeks to better define the frequency of medical complications in individuals < 65% ideal body weight admitting to an inpatient medical stabilization unit. We found that patients with extreme AN present with similar medical complications, although at a more frequent occurrence, to those at higher percent ideal body weights. Low bone mineral density is an almost universal finding in this population, with 45% of individuals presenting with osteopenia and 43% with osteoporosis. 35% of individuals developed hypophosphatemia and 38% developed hypoglycemia in this population, both more frequent in the restricting than binge-purge subtype of AN. Elevated liver function tests predict the development of

* Correspondence: Philip.mehler@dhha.org
[1]ACUTE Center for Eating Disorders at Denver Health, 723 Delaware St, Pav M 3rd floor, Denver, CO 80204, USA
[2]Department of Medicine, University of Colorado School of Medicine, 13001 E 17th Pl, Aurora, CO 80045, USA
Full list of author information is available at the end of the article

hypoglycemia. Patients with extreme AN are at a significantly increased risk for many serious medical complications secondary to their state of malnutrition and also with initial refeeding.

Background

Anorexia nervosa (AN) is a serious psychiatric illness that leads to medical complications which can adversely involve every organ system [1]. Mortality remains one of the highest of any psychiatric disorders [2] with cause of death often attributed to the medical complications of malnutrition [3, 4]. The prognosis for AN is somewhat guarded, with less than one-third of individuals recovered at 9 years and approximately two-thirds of individuals recovered when followed up to 22 years [5]. Correlational data suggest that full weight restoration is a predictor of a more favorable outcome at follow up [6, 7], but the lower the percentage of ideal body weight (%IBW) at presentation, the worse the prognosis due to more medical complications [8]. These patients may often undergo unnecessary evaluations for their medical complaints and languish in medical hospitals without definitive care.

The ACUTE Center for Eating Disorders at Denver Health (ACUTE), established in 2004, is a telemetry medical stabilization unit, with national and international draw, that singularly specializes in the care of the most medically compromised patients with eating disorders, as the typical patient admitted to ACUTE meets criteria for an extreme form of the illness per the DSM-V severity index for eating disorders [9]. In this article we present data from a series of 281 patients admitted to ACUTE, as the first study of a comprehensive evaluation of medical complications observed in patients with extreme AN.

Methods

Patients admitted to ACUTE are regularly transferred by air ambulance from medical hospitals where they had been admitted with various serious medical conditions such as syncope, cardiac arrhythmias, hypoglycemic seizures, failure to thrive, severe electrolyte imbalances and liver failure. Typical ACUTE patients have AN, restricting subtype (AN-R) or binge-purge subtype (AN-BP), with body weights less than 70% of ideal body weight (IBW), and with comorbid medical complications and marked physical deconditioning. Percent IBW is calculated using the Hamwi method [10]. Multidisciplinary expertise, in the medical complications of AN and refeeding, is exclusively provided by embedded full-time internal medicine physicians, psychiatrists, registered dietitians, clinical psychologists, physical therapists, occupational therapists, social workers, nurses, and certified nursing assistants. Standard blood tests, anthropometrics, 12-lead electrocardiograms (EKG), and vital signs with orthostatic blood pressures are obtained for all patients upon admission. Laboratory values, such as glucose, phosphorus, and liver function tests (LFTs) are closely monitored until stabilized. Daily blinded weights were also obtained at approximately the same time daily for each patient while wearing only a gown. The multidisciplinary team then facilitates the initiation of aggressive, albeit judicious, nutritional rehabilitation. Progressive oral (PO) kcals, increased until meeting our unit's expected weight trends of 0.2 kg/day, is provided with conversion to enteral nutrition (EN) only when patients are unable to tolerate PO intake; rarely, peripheral parenteral nutrition/total parental nutrition (PPN/TPN) is provided when unable to tolerate enteral feeds for significant physiologic reasons. In addition, all meal completion is monitored by a care patient safety aide with training in eating disorders. Once the patient has met ACUTE's discharge criteria, as well as meeting the accepting treatment program's admission criteria, they are discharged.

This retrospective study design involves 281 male and female adult patients who weighed less than 65% of IBW and admitted to ACUTE for medical stabilization, between May 18, 2013 and August 30, 2018. It compares baseline characteristics and medical complications between restricting and binge-purge subtypes. Patients were excluded if they were hospitalized for less than 72 h or if their percent IBW was above 65% on admission.

Patient demographics, anthropometric measurements, dietary intake, bone mineral density (BMD) tests, and EKG data were obtained from manual chart review. Nursing assessments and laboratory testing results were queried from the hospital database. Duration of illness and mode and frequency of purging behaviors were self-reported and recorded on admission. Hypothermia was defined as body temperature less than 36 °C and bradycardia was defined as heart rate less than 60 beats per minute (bpm). Severe hypoglycemia was defined as blood glucose < 2.2 mmol/L. Hypophosphatemia was defined as a serum value less than 0.87 mmol/L. Patients with hypophosphatemia on admission were excluded from the risk factor analysis for refeeding hypophosphatemia. Dual-energy X-ray absorptiometry (DXA) scans and lipodystrophy analysis/whole body scans were performed using the Hologic QDR Series model Discovery-W if not already completed within the previous 2 years. BMD was assessed using the lowest regional (hip, femoral neck, and lumbar spine) Z-score or T-score (if patient was 50 years old or older). On ACUTE, osteoporosis is diagnosed if the Z or T-score is less than − 2.5 and osteopenia is diagnosed when the lowest Z or T-score is between − 1 and − 2.5. Nadir body mass index (BMI) and percent IBW are listed to reflect the lowest body weight experienced during treatment. Admission and discharge caloric intake were based on those amounts consumed on the first and last day the patient was on the unit for 24 h. The study was reviewed and approved by the Colorado Multiple Institutional Review Board.

Statistical analysis

Univariate statistics were used to describe the cohort. Shapiro-Wilks test was used to determine the distribution of continuous variables. Depending on the distribution, patient characteristics, used to describe the medical complications on the ACUTE unit, were ascertained by Mann-Whitney *U* procedures, Pearson chi-square tests, and independent sample *t*-tests. When appropriate, degrees of freedom are shown in parentheses after the test statistic. Logistic regression analyses were used to investigate associations between medical complications with clinical or biochemical variables. Two-tailed *p* values < 0.05 were considered statistically significant, and all analyses were completed using SAS Enterprise Guide software version 7.1 (SAS Institute, Cary, NC).

Results

Baseline characteristics

Demographic characteristics and statistical comparisons between AN subtypes, in regard to percent IBW, BMI, and caloric intake, are listed in Table 1. A large majority of ACUTE patients (91%) were referrals from outside of Colorado. Most of the 281 study patients were female (91%), 62% were diagnosed as AN-R subtype, and the age range of the patients was 18–66 years with a median age of 28 years. The average BMI on admission was 12.1 kg/m^2 (SD = 1.3; range = 7.5–15.7) and average percent IBW was 57.7% (SD = 5.5; range = 34.8–65.0). The median duration of illness was 10 years (IQR = 5–20). For females, duration of illness was significantly higher with a median of 11 years (IQR = 6–21) and for males, the median was 4 years (IQR = 1–10), $p < .0001$. Out of the total cohort, 82 (29%) patients reported vomiting as a method of purging, 41 (15%) reported using laxatives, and 7 (2%) reported using diuretics. Many of these patients used just one method of purging, but some used two or even all three of the methods. However, many patients were unable to recall the frequency of their purging behaviors.

Patient care and discharge

Patients hospitalized at ACUTE had a median length of stay of 22 days (IQR = 15–30). The average percent IBW increased by 12% (SD = 8.4), and average BMI increased by 2.5 kg/m^2 (SD = 1.5) by time of discharge (Table 1). Patients with AN-BP gained 0.9 more kilograms per week compared to patients with AN-R ($p < .0001$). About one third of the patients developed edema during their hospital stay and half of those patients, almost entirely patients with AN-BP, were prescribed spironolactone to treat their excessive weight trends and/or edema. Patients with AN-BP, who were prescribed spironolactone, gained 0.7 kg more per week than patients with AN-BP who were not prescribed spironolactone.

Most of the patients discharged voluntarily ($n = 209$) with an average percent IBW of 69.4% (SD = 7.6); however, 37 patients discharged from ACUTE on a mental health hold (MHH), 21 discharged on a short-term certification (STC), and 14 discharged against medical advice (AMA).

All patients were medically stabilized prior to discharge. Two hundred forty-one patients (86%) discharged to an inpatient or residential program; however, 16 patients (6%) discharged to a partial hospitalization program (PHP), an outpatient team, or to another form of care, and the remaining 24 patients (9%) were discharged home due to mitigating circumstances. No patient died on the ACUTE unit during their medical stabilization and only 20 patients (7%) ever required brief transfer to the Denver Health medical intensive care unit (ICU) for conditions such as critical hyponatremia (< 116 mmol/L), critical hypokalemia (< 1.8 mmol/L), refractory hypoglycemia requiring intravenous (IV) glucose and frequent point of care glucose monitoring, small bowel obstructions requiring surgery, cardiogenic shock, upper gastrointestinal bleed requiring transfusion, and two with sustained ventricular tachycardia. Forty-three patients (15%) were deemed high fall risk upon admission, and 15 patients (5%) were initially incapable of ambulation. All received intensive physical therapy and were able to ambulate on their own at the time of discharge.

Nutrition

On admission, initial caloric intake for females ranged from 800 to 2450 kcals with an average of 1431 kcal/day (SD = 191) and initial caloric intake for males was significantly higher at 1714 kcal/day (SD = 507) ($p = .01$). The vast majority of patients were refed via progressive oral nutrition. There were 50 patients (18%) who required enteral feeds; 18 patients (6%) required some parenteral nutrition. Average daily caloric intake at the time of discharge for females was 3119 kcal/day (SD = 733) and 3744 kcal/day for males (SD = 829). During their ACUTE stay, patients gained 2 kg/wk. (SD = 1.5). There was not a significant difference in weight gain per week between genders ($p = .84$).

Medical findings

Patients were hypothermic during 35% of their total admission time at ACUTE with low percent IBW as a predictor of hypothermia ($p < .0001$). For patients with

Table 1 Characteristics of study participants

	Cohort (***N*** = 281)		AN-R (***N*** = 175)		AN-BP (***N*** = 106)			
Patient Characteristics	N	%	N	%	N	%		
Female	256	91	158	62	98	38		
Male	25	9	17	68	8	32		
Admitted from								
Home	219	78	128	58	91	42		
Hospital transfer	37	13	29	78	8	22		
Inpatient eating disorder program	23	8	17	74	6	26		
Other	2	< 1	1	50	1	50		
Referral from outside Colorado	257	91	161	63	96	37		
	Mean[a]	**SD**[a]	**Mean**[a]	**SD**[a]	**Mean**[a]	**SD**[a]	***t*-test**[b]	***p* value**
Age	28	22–37	27	22–38	31	22–37	15,900	0.15
Length of hospitalization (days)	22	15–30	23	16–33	21	13–28	13,754	0.07
Percent of IBW								
Admission	57.7	5.5	57.2	5.5	58.4	5.4	1.75	0.08
Nadir	57	6.2	56.5	6.1	57.9	6.5	1.81	0.07
Discharge	69	7.4	67.7	6.2	71.2	8.7	3.61	< .001
Change in %IBW	12	8.4	11.2	7.5	13.3	9.6	2.03	0.04
BMI (kg/m^2)								
Admission	12.1	1.3	12	1.3	12.2	1.3	1.01	0.31
Nadir	12	1.4	11.9	1.4	12.1	1.6	0.91	0.37
Discharge	14.5	1.5	14.2	1.3	14.9	1.7	3.5	< .001
Change in BMI	2.5	1.5	2.3	1.4	2.8	1.7	2.8	<.001
Weekly weight gain (kg)	2	1.5	1.7	0.9	2.6	2.0	4.26	< .0001
Daily caloric intake (kcal)								
Admission	1457	249	1477	269	1424	209	−1.74	0.06
Discharge	3175	762	3282	763	2996	728	−3.1	0.002

AN-R Anorexia nervosa restricting subtype, *AN-BP* Anorexia nervosa binge-purge subtype, *IBW* Ideal body weight, *BMI* Body mass index
[a]Median and IQR for not normally distributed variables
[b]Mann-Whitney *U* test

AN-R, the average percent IBW on the last hospital day of hypothermia was 61.5% (SD = 6.3) (Table 2).

There were 158 patients (56%) who were bradycardic on arrival to ACUTE, with the lowest recorded heart rate being 26 bpm, and the majority of those patients were diagnosed with AN-R. Admission BMI (r = .85, p < .0001) and percent IBW (r = .85, p < .0001) were highly correlated with bradycardia. For the patients with bradycardia, their heart rate had somewhat improved by median day 4 (IQR = 1–9). Findings from the admission EKG revealed that the average QTc was normal at 427 ms (SD = 34.4). Patients with AN-BP had significantly longer average admission QTc (436 ms, SD = 37.2) than patients with AN-R (421 ms, SD = 31.4), (p < .001).

Cardiac axis was mostly normal. There were 58 patients with right axis deviation but only 10 patients presented with left axis deviation. Five patients presented with a junctional rhythm. Admission BMI was not a significant predictor of either right axis deviation (p = .45) or of developing a junctional rhythm (p = .15).

Just over half of the patients admitted with low serum prealbumin values (< 0.2 g/L). Low serum prealbumin positively correlated with admission percent IBW (r = 0.6, p < .0001). Admission serum albumin and alkaline phosphatase levels were within normal ranges. However, 127 (45%) patients had elevated admission aspartate aminotransferase (AST) values (above 40 U/L) and 145 (52%) patients had elevated alanine aminotransferase (ALT) values (above 45 U/L). Patients with AN-R had significantly higher AST (p < .0001) and ALT (p < .0001) values compared to patients with AN-BP (Table 3).

The incidence of increased liver function tests (LFTs), on admission, is correlated with low BMI [$\chi^2(1) = 13.3$, p < .005]. Of the 281 study patients, only 85 (30%) had normal LFTs (AST < 41 U/L and ALT < 46 U/L) throughout their hospitalization. One hundred one (36%) had

Table 2 Medical complications between AN-R and AN-BP subtypes

	Cohort (**N** = 281)		AN-R (**N** = 175)				AN-BP (**N** = 106)					
	N	%	N	%	Mean[a]	SD[a]	N	%	Mean[a]	SD[a]	*t*-test[b]	***p*** value
Body Temperature												
Hypothermic during stay (< 36 °C)	168	60	110	65	35.8	0.1	58	35	35.8	0.2	1.59	0.11
Last hospital day < 36 °C					10	4–19			11	5–21	6084	0.85
%IBW on last day < 36 °C					61.5	6.3			65.8	7.2	4.12	< .0001
Heart Rate and EKG on Admission												
Heart rate (bpm)					55.3	13.1			60.7	12.5	3.37	0.0009
Nadir heart rate (bpm) during stay					50.1	11.8			54.3	3.9	3.06	0.002
QTc value (ms)					421	31.4			436	37.2	1.41	< .001
High QTc (480–500 ms)	7	3	2	29			5	71				
Critically high QTc (> 500 ms)	7	3	3	43			4	57				
Junctional rhythm	5	2	1	20			4	80				
Right axis	58	21	40	69			18	31				
Liver Function												
All normal LFTs (AST < 41; ALT < 46 U/L)	85	30	36	42			49	58				
Modestly Abnormal (up to 3x normal)	101	36	60	59			41	41				
Severely abnormal (> 3x normal)	95	34	79	83			16	17				
Highest AST					197	145–348			238	136–537	383	0.76
Highest ALT					270	197–485			261	196–518	618	0.65
Hospital day LFTs peaked					4	0–12			5	0–12	6381	0.21
Blood Glucose												
Hypoglycemia (< 3.3 mmol/L)	107	38	77	72	3.0	2.6–3.2	30	28	2.9	2.8–3.1	1637	0.45
Last hospital day glucose < 3.3 mmol/L					2	1–2			1	0–2	1963	0.06
Severe hypoglycemia (< 2.2 mmol/L)[c]	24	9	20	83	1.8	1.6–2.0	4	17	1.9	1.4–2.1		
Last hospital day glucose < 2.2 mmol/L					1	0–3			1	0–3		

AN-R Anorexia nervosa restricting subtype, *AN-BP* Anorexia nervosa binge-purge subtype, *IBW* Ideal body weight, *EKG* Electrocardiogram, *bpm* Beats per minute, *LFT* Liver function tests, *AST* Aspartate aminotransferase test, *ALT* Alanine aminotransferase test

[a]Median (IQR) for not normally distributed variables

[b]Mann-Whitney *U* test

[c]There were too few values for an analysis between AN subtypes and severe hypoglycemia

modestly elevated LFTs and 95 patients (34%) had LFTs of greater than three times normal during their hospitalization (Table 2). Modestly abnormal LFTs predicted thrombocytopenia (serum platelet count < 150 10^9 L^{-1}) on admission (p = .002) but did not predict hypoglycemia (p = 0.43). However, highly elevated LFTs (>3X normal) did predict the presence of hypoglycemia (p = .005).

More than one third (38%) of the patients experienced hypoglycemia while on ACUTE. Of these, 24 (9%) admitted with severe hypoglycemia (< 2.2 mmol/L.). Of the total 281 patients, 77 patients (27%) with AN-R developed hypoglycemia and 20 patients developed severe hypoglycemia. There were only 30 patients (11%) with AN-BP who developed hypoglycemia and only four developed severe hypoglycemia (Table 2).

Both admission sodium and potassium values, were lower in patients with AN-BP compared to patients with AN-R (M = 135 mmol/L, SD = 6.4 vs. M = 137.6 mmol/L, SD = 4.5, p < .0001). Hypokalemia was most commonly treated with a combination of oral potassium and IV fluids (47%), only oral potassium (28%), oral and IV potassium along with IV fluids (13%), combination oral and IV potassium (9%), or only IV fluids (3%). Only eight patients of those developing hypokalemia (n = 93) required transfer to the ICU for critically low values. Hyponatremia was most commonly treated with slow IV saline (50%), 34% were allowed to auto-correct without any particular intervention aside from nutrition and fluid intake, and 13% required fluid restriction due to a diagnosis of syndrome of inappropriate antidiuretic hormone (SIADH). Four (5%) of the total 82 patients, who developed hyponatremia, required transfer to the ICU for treatment of a critical value.

Table 3 Admission laboratory values between AN subtypes ($N = 281$)[a]

	AN-R		AN-BP		***t*-test**[b]	***p* value**
Laboratory Values (reference range)	Mean[c]	SD[c]	Mean[c]	SD[c]		
Sodium (135–143 mmol/L)	137.6	4.5	135	6.4	−4.01	<.0001
Potassium (3.6–5.1 mmol/L)	3.8	0.4	3.4	0.7	−6.39	<.0001
Carbon Dioxide (18–27 mmol/L)	27.7	3.3	29.3	7.3	2.57	0.01
Glucose (3.3–11.0 mmol/L)	4.57	3.91–5.89	5.26	4.29–6.0	16,507	0.009
Calcium (2.02–2.6 mmol/L)	2.1	0.1	2.2	0.2	5.11	<.001
Phosphorus (0.87–1.58 mmol/L)	1.03	0.2	1.1	0.4	1.69	0.09
Magnesium (0.65–1.1 mmol/L)	0.95	0.1	0.98	0.2	1.60	0.11
BUN (0.21–0.79 mmol/L)	0.57	0.36–0.86	0.50	0.32–0.75	13,987	0.07
Creatinine (44.2–122.9 μmol/L)	59.3	19.1	73.9	28.6	4.65	<.0001
AST (10–40 U/L)	49	26–113	27	21–42	11,730	<.0001
ALT (7–45 U/L)	73	37–194	32	24–50	10,671	<.0001
Total bilirubin (17.1–20.5 μmol/L)	8.6	6.8–12.0	6.8	5.1–15.4	14,294	0.16
Albumin (30–53 g/L)	38.5	4.9	37.9	5.9	−0.85	0.39
Alkaline phosphatase (35–137 U/L)	67	51–97	68	54–95	15,213	0.68
Total protein (60–82 g/L)	67.0	7.5	68.7	9.1	1.78	0.08
WBC (4.5–10.0 $10^9 L^{-1}$)	3.8	1.6	5.5	3.3	5.91	<.0001
Neutrophils (%) (48.0–69.0%)	56.9	12.6	57.4	14.5	0.27	0.79
Lymphocytes (%) (21.0–43.0%)	34.4	12.4	33.3	13.5	−0.71	0.48
Platelet count (150–400 $10^9 L^{-1}$)	192	142–250	271	201–387	19,308	<.0001
Hematocrit (%) (37.0–47.0%)	36.6	5.8	37.6	5.6	1.4	0.16
MCV (80–100 fL)	94.6	6.7	91.1	6.7	−4.27	<.0001
TSH (0.34–6.0 mU/L)	2	1.2–3.1	1.4	1–2.2	11,935	<.001
INR (0.83–1.19)	1.2	0.2	1.1	0.2	−3.49	<.001
1,25 Hydroxy vitamin D (74.9–199.7 nmol/L)	97.3	77.4–128.5	97.3	64.9–132.3	13,641	0.19
Testosterone (5.6–25.2 nmol/L)	5.9	2.1–11.7	5.9	4.4–14.6	74.0	0.39
Free T3 (4.0–7.4 pmol/L)[d]	3.1	2.0–3.7	2.3			
Free T4 (6.4–24.5 nmol/L)	11.1	9.1–12.9	13.1	11.8–16.3	632.0	0.01
Prealbumin (0.2–0.52 g/L)	0.18	0.06	0.21	0.07	3.61	<.001

AN-R Anorexia nervosa restricting subtype, *AN-BP* Anorexia nervosa binge-purge subtype, *BUN* Blood urea nitrogen, *AST* Aspartate aminotransferase test, *ALT* Alanine aminotransferase test, *WBC* White blood cell, *MCV* Mean corpuscular volume, *TSH* Thyroid stimulating hormone, *INR* International normalized ratio, *Free T3* Triiodothyronine, *Free T4* Thyroxine

[a]Magnesium and TSH were available on 274 admissions. Neutrophils, lymphocytes, and 1,25 Hydroxy Vitamin D were available on 275 admissions. INR was available on 280 admissions. Testosterone was available on 19 admissions. Free T3 was available on 7 admissions. Free T4 was available on 55 admissions. Prealbumin was available on 277 admissions

[b]Mann-Whitney *U* test

[c] Median (IQR) for not normally distributed variables

[d]There were too few values for an analysis between AN subtypes and Free T3 ($n = 7$)

There were 179 patients (64%) who admitted with low white blood cell counts (leukopenia), 47% with anemia and 20% with thrombocytopenia. Leukopenia and thrombocytopenia were more marked in patients with AN-R versus AN-BP ($M = 3.8\ 10^9 L^{-1}$, $SD = 1.6$ vs. $M = 5.5\ 10^9 L^{-1}$, $SD = 3.3$, $p < .0001$) and ($Mdn = 192\ 10^9 L^{-1}$, $IQR = 142–250$ vs. $Mdn = 271\ 10^9 L^{-1}$, $IQR = 210–387$, $p < .0001$), respectively (Table 3).

There were 60 patients on admission with a serum phosphorous level < 0.87 mmol/L and average %IBW was 55.3% ($SD = 6.4$). An additional 35% (5 males and 93 females) developed refeeding hypophosphatemia, as early as median day 2 ($IQR = 1–2$). Of those patients, 47% (3 males and 43 females) developed critical hypophosphatemia (serum phosphorus < 0.71 mmol/L). 49% of patients with critical hypophosphatemia required IV phosphorus for an average of 1.6 days ($SD = 0.8$), and all patients developing hypophosphatemia were treated for an average of 6.1 days ($SD = 5.1$) of oral phosphorous repletion. Patients maintained low serum phosphorous values <

0.87 mmol/L for a mean of 2.1 (SD = 1.3) days with use of supplement. When comparing the 98 patients who developed refeeding hypophosphatemia, with the 123 patients who never developed refeeding hypophosphatemia, there were more patients diagnosed with AN-R than patients diagnosed with AN-BP [23% vs. 21%, $\chi^2(1) = 5.44$, $p = .02$], but there were no significant differences between gender ($p = .14$). However, there was a significant difference in average nadir BMI between patients who developed refeeding hypophosphatemia (M = 11.8 kg/m^2, SD = 1.4) during their hospitalization compared to patients who did not (M = 12.4 kg/m^2, SD = 1.3, $p = .001$) (Table 4).

One hundred thirty-nine patients (49%) received DXA scans during their hospitalization. Only 12% had normal BMD (4% male), 45% osteopenia (6% male), and 43% osteoporosis (5% male). The average Z-score in males was − 1.8 (SD = 1.3) and in females, − 2.3 (SD = 1.2). There were no significant differences when comparing Z-scores between patients with AN-R and AN-BP ($p = .24$) (Table 5). The average T-score for males was − 3.9 (SD = 0.9), which was much worse than the average T-score for older females (M = -2.6, SD = 1.0).

Discussion

This is the largest study ever of severely malnourished adult patients with extreme AN, with percent IBW less than 65%, hospitalized on a medical stabilization unit. In comparison to our much smaller pilot study, AN patients are now more ill, manifested by an average admission BMI of 12.1 kg/m^2 (range = 7.5–15.7) compared to our previous 13.1 kg/m^2 (range = 9.5–15.4). Length of stay has increased from 19 to 22 days, but discharge BMI remained similar (14.5 kg/m^2 vs 14.4 kg/m^2). We have also become much more aggressive in our refeeding practices, with our admission kcals increasing from 990 to 1400 and discharge kcals increasing from 2000 kcal to approximately 3000 kcal [11].

When analyzed by type of eating disorder, patients with AN-R gained less weight per week than patients with AN-BP. We do not, however, believe that patients with AN-BP inherently gain weight faster than patients with AN-R, as previously suggested [12]. In that study, there was no mention of edema formation in the AN-BP group, nor how often the aldosterone antagonist spironolactone was utilized. Excessive purging behaviors lead to a secondary hyperaldosteronism (Pseudo Barter's syndrome) which makes these patients salt and water retentive, resulting in excessive weight trends and/or the development of edema [13, 14]. In our study, 89% of patients with AN-BP were treated with spironolactone for an average of 13 days.

Curiously, only 56% of the patients in this study were documented as having bradycardia, which is considered a universal finding in AN, especially in those patients with lower levels of body weight. Indeed, this study corroborated the correlation between bradycardia and percent IBW. Given this is a retrospective study, heart rates were obtained from the nurses' documented values, which are only obtained intermittently throughout the day; however, if 24-h telemetry values were instead used, it is likely the frequency of bradycardia would approach 100% especially with the known further lowering of heart rate at night.

Patients with AN-BP had a longer QTc interval than patients with AN-R, likely due to electrolyte imbalance. Indeed, patients with AN-BP had lower admission potassium levels which are known to prolong the QTc.

Table 4 Predictors of refeeding hypophosphatemia[a]

	Hypophosphatemia (**N** = 98)		Normal Phosphorus (**N** = 123)			
Factors	Mean[b]	SD[b]	Mean[b]	SD[b]	*t*-test[c]	*p* value
Nadir BMI	11.8	1.4	12.4	1.3	3.31	0.001
Nadir %IBW	56.7	6.3	58.5	5.5	2.21	0.03
Admission Glucose (mmol/L)	4.7	3.9–5.6	4.4	3.9–5.2	11,630	0.06
Admission Albumin (g/L)	36.8	6.8	38.0	6.3	− 1.41	0.16
Admission Prealbumin (g/L)	0.19	0.08	0.21	0.06	−1.87	0.06
Admission WBC (10^9 L^{-1})	4.8	2.5	4.3	2.7	−1.41	0.16
Lean Mass (g)[d]	27,597	4351	28,578	5702	−0.92	0.36
	N	**%**	**N**	**%**	**χ2**	***p* value**
Elevated admission AST (> 40 U/L)	41	42	45	37	0.63	0.42
Elevated admission ALT (> 45 U/L)	49	50	54	44	0.81	0.37

BMI Body mass index, *IBW* Ideal body weight, *WBC* White blood cell, *AST* Aspartate aminotransferase test, *ALT* Alanine aminotransferase test
[a]Hypophosphatemia defined as phosphorus < 0.87 mmol/L. 60 patients with hypophosphatemia on admission were excluded
[b]Median (IQR) for not normally distributed variables
[c]Mann-Whitney *U* test
[d]Data for lean mass (g) was available for 38 patients with refeeding hypophosphatemia and 66 patients with normal phosphorus

Table 5 Bone mineral density and lipodystrophy studies between AN subtypes

	Cohort (**N** = 139)	AN-R (**N** = 94)		AN-BP (**N** = 45)			
DXA scans		N	%	N	%		
Normal BMD (Z/T-score > −1)	17	11	65	6	35		
Osteopenia (Z/T-score − 1 to −2.5)	62	45	73	17	27		
Osteoporosis (Z/T-score < − 2.5)	60	38	63	22	37		
		Mean	**SD**	**Mean**	**SD**	***t*-test**	***p* value**
Z-score	127	−2.2	1.2	−2.4	1.1	−1.17	0.24
T-score[a]	12	−2.7	1.2	−3.7	0.4		
Lipodystrophy studies							
		Median	**IQR**	**Median**	**IQR**	**Mann-Whitney *U* test**	***p* value**
Body Fat (g)	134	3799	3398-4709	4329	3566-5317	3408	0.04
Body Fat (%)	134	11.6	10.8–13.4	12.8	11.2–16.1	3486	0.01
Lean Mass (%)	134	77.8	75.2–80.0	76.4	74.4–78.1	2465	0.02

AN-R Anorexia nervosa restricting subtype, *AN-BP* Anorexia nervosa binge-purge subtype, *DXA* Dual-energy X-ray absorptiometry, *BMD* Bone mineral density, *IQR* Interquartile range

[a]There were too few values for an analysis between AN subtypes and T-scores ($n = 12$)

Importantly, once again, no correlation was found between QTc and admission BMI thus reinforcing the fact that a prolonged QTc is not inherent to AN. Rather, when detected, a prolonged QTc is a consequence of electrolyte disturbances or the usage of QT-prolonging medications [15–17].

In our cohort, 70% of patients had abnormal LFTs which peaked on the fourth hospital day for patients with AN-R and day five for patients with AN-BP. On average, the ALT was greater than the AST across all subtypes of eating disorders with AN-R patients having higher transaminases than AN-BP patients. Elevations in transaminases are the most common kind of liver abnormality seen in patients with severe AN [18, 19]; bilirubin and alkaline phosphatase levels are almost never elevated. In our cohort, 40% of patients with a BMI < 12.1 kg/m^2 had elevated transaminases, thus supporting the relationship between severity of AN and likelihood of transaminitis. The most likely pathophysiologic mechanism is starvation-mediated autophagy [20, 21].

Hypoglycemia was more likely to develop in those with elevation of transaminases greater than three times normal and in those with greater severity of malnutrition, as evidenced by 27% of those with AN-R developing hypoglycemia vs. 11% of individuals with AN-BP. Thus, hypoglycemia as a surrogate of severity of illness was supported [22, 23]. This is very important because our experience suggests lean people do not typically have the customary adrenergic or neuroglycopenic warning symptoms typical of severe hypoglycemia [22].

Serum albumin levels were notably within the normal range, notwithstanding their marked malnutrition. However, more than 50% of our patients admitted with a low prealbumin level < 0.2 g/L, with AN-R patients having the lowest values. These findings are supported by an emerging literature that albumin is not considered a reliable indicator of the severity of AN [23, 24]. Rather, albumin is best viewed as an acute phase reactant that decreases predictably in critical illness such as sepsis [25]. The precise cause of low serum prealbumin levels in severe AN remains to be elucidated [24, 26]. Furthermore, low serum prealbumin is associated with both refeeding hypophosphatemia [27] as well as hypoglycemia in AN.

Patients with AN-R had more pronounced leukopenia and thrombocytopenia than those with AN-BP. In severe AN, the bone marrow shows signs of serous fat atrophy [28–30], which is directly related to duration of illness and BMI [31]. This corrects with a judicious nutritional plan.

The most common electrolyte abnormality on admission, in our cohort, was hypokalemia, with 33% of patients having a serum potassium level < 3.6 mmol/L, followed by hyponatremia. Hypernatremia was very rare. When examined by eating disorder sub-type, patients with AN-BP had, not surprisingly, statistically significant lower sodium and potassium levels on admission. The hyperaldosteronism resulting from the dehydration of purging along with loss of potassium and other electrolytes in emesis, stool, and urine contribute to hypokalemia [32, 33]. The ability to correct hypokalemia is improved with down-regulation of aldosterone secretion, which can be accomplished with intravascular volume repletion; hence the large number of patients that received IV fluids in the treatment of their hypokalemia.

Notably, only 21% of this cohort admitted with hypophosphatemia, but over one third of our patients subsequently developed refeeding hypophosphatemia by hospital day two. Compared to patients who did not develop hypophosphatemia, those who did, had lower admission BMI, thus representing a sicker patient population who is at greater risk for refeeding hypophosphatemia [34]. Studies have indeed shown that as BMI nears 12 kg/m^2, medical complications such as refeeding hypophosphatemia occur more frequently [27, 35, 36]. Based on this present study, patients who manifested a tendency towards developing refeeding hypophosphatemia had lower BMIs, higher transaminases, and lower serum prealbumin levels. Caloric intake during admission, per se, did not predict hypophosphatemia. However, notwithstanding the extremely ill population of patients cared for on ACUTE, 44% never developed refeeding hypophosphatemia. We therefore feel it unnecessary to prophylactically give phosphorus replacement to all patients at the time of admission given the possibility that it can cause diarrhea.

Lastly, 139 of our patients received a DXA scan during their admission and of those, 88% were found to have BMD loss [osteopenia (45%) and osteoporosis (43%)]. Although prior studies have shown rates of osteoporosis in males to be worse than females [37], in our current study, females had overall higher rates of osteoporosis (43% vs 5%). Weight restoration is the gold standard for treatment of osteoporosis [38, 39]. Further studies are needed to elucidate which available pharmaceutical options may also be valuable for this patient population [40].

While the strength of this article is that it describes the medical complications in the largest ever published cohort of male and female patients with extreme AN, there are limitations. First, it was based on retrospective data review, thereby somewhat limiting the conclusions that can be drawn from this descriptive study. Secondly, we included patients transferred from other hospitals as well as other eating disorder treatment facilities and we cannot account for the care and refeeding protocols the patients received there. Third, our sample size remains relatively small as our program focuses exclusively on the care of the extreme form of AN and may reduce the generalizability of our findings. Lastly, we did not include readmissions in this sample size.

In conclusion, this article methodically examines the many medical complications of patients with extreme AN-R and AN-BP in an effort to inform care providers of the multitude of medical issues which may be present in these patients with extreme forms of the illness.

Abbreviations

ACUTE: ACUTE Center for Eating Disorders at Denver Health; ALT: Alanine aminotransferase; AMA: Against medical advice; AN: Anorexia nervosa; AN-BP: Binge-purge subtype; AN-R: Restricting subtype; AST: Aspartate aminotransferase; BMD: Bone mineral density; BMI: Body mass index; BPM: Beats per minute; DSM: Diagnostic and Statistical Manual of Mental Disorders; DXA: Dual-energy X-ray absorptiometry; EKG: Electrocardiogram; IBW: Ideal body weight; ICU: Intensive care unit; IQR: Interquartile range; IV: Intravenous; LFT: Liver function test; M: Mean; MDN: Median; MHH: Mental health hold; PHP: Partial hospitalization program; SAS: Statistical analysis software; SD: Standard deviation; SIADH: Syndrome of inappropriate antidiuretic hormone; STC: Short-term certification

Acknowledgements

Not applicable.

Authors' contributions

DG interpreted data and was a major contributor to writing the manuscript. AW compiled and analyzed the data and was a major contributor to writing the manuscript. JC and MM were major contributors in writing the manuscript and in interpreting outcomes. PM conceptualized the study and contributed to writing of the manuscript. All authors read and approved the final manuscript.

Competing interests

PM and JC report equity in the Eating Recovery Center-Denver. DG, AW and MM declare that they have no competing interests.

Author details

[1]ACUTE Center for Eating Disorders at Denver Health, 723 Delaware St, Pav M 3rd floor, Denver, CO 80204, USA. [2]Department of Medicine, University of Colorado School of Medicine, 13001 E 17th Pl, Aurora, CO 80045, USA. [3]Eating Recovery Center, 7351 E Lowry Blvd, Denver, CO 80230, USA.

References

1. Mehler PS, Brown CA. Anorexia nervosa - medical complications. J Eat Disord. 2015;3:11.
2. Fichter MM, Quadflieg N. Mortality in eating disorders - results of a large prospective clinical longitudinal study. Int J Eat Disord. 2016;49(4):391–401.
3. Franko DL, Keshaviah A, Eddy KT, Krishna M, Davis MC, Keel PK, et al. A longitudinal investigation of mortality in anorexia nervosa and bulimia nervosa. Am J Psychiatry. 2013;170(8):917–25.
4. Pompili M, Mancinelli I, Girardi P, Ruberto A, Tatarelli R. Suicide in anorexia nervosa: a meta-analysis. Int J Eat Disord. 2004;36(1):99–103.
5. Eddy KT, Tabri N, Thomas JJ, Murray HB, Keshaviah A, Hastings E, et al. Recovery from anorexia nervosa and bulimia nervosa at 22-year follow-up. J Clin Psychiatry. 2017;78(2):184–9.
6. Baran SA, Weltzin TE, Kaye WH. Low discharge weight and outcome in anorexia nervosa. Am J Psychiatry. 1995;152(7):1070–2.
7. Rigaud D, Pennacchio H, Bizeul C, Reveillard V, Verges B. Outcome in AN adult patients: a 13-year follow-up in 484 patients. Diabetes Metab. 2011; 37(4):305–11.
8. Misra M, Aggarwal A, K Miller K, Almazan C, Worley M, Soyka L, et al. Effects of anorexia nervosa on clinical, hematologic, biochemical, and bone density parameters in community-dwelling adolescent girls. Pediatrics. 2005;114: 1574–83.
9. APA. Diagnostic and Statistical Manual of Mental Disorders. 5th ed. Washington: APA; 2013.
10. Hamwi GJ. Therapy: Changing dietary concepts. In: S Danowski T, editor. Diabetes mellitus: Diagnosis and treatment. New York: American Diabetes Association; 1964. p. 73–8.
11. Gaudiani JL, Sabel AL, Mascolo M, Mehler PS. Severe anorexia nervosa: outcomes from a medical stabilization unit. Int J Eat Disord. 2012;45(1):85–92.
12. Makhzoumi SH, Coughlin JW, Schreyer CC, Redgrave GW, Pitts SC, Guarda AS. Weight gain trajectories in hospital-based treatment of anorexia nervosa. Int J Eat Disord. 2017;50(3):266–74.
13. Bahia A, Mascolo M, Gaudiani JL, Mehler PS. PseudoBartter syndrome in eating disorders. Int J Eat Disord. 2012;45(1):150–3.
14. Mascolo M, Chu ES, Mehler PS. Abuse and clinical value of diuretics in eating disorders therapeutic applications. Int J Eat Disord. 2011;44(3):200–2.
15. Krantz MJ, Sabel AL, Sagar U, Long CS, Barbey JT, White KV, et al. Factors influencing QT prolongation in patients hospitalized with severe anorexia nervosa. Gen Hosp Psychiatry. 2011;34(2):173–7.

16. Facchini M, Sala L, Malfatto G, Bragato R, Redaelli G, Invitti C. Low-K+ dependent QT prolongation and risk for ventricular arrhythmia in anorexia nervosa. Int J Cardiol. 2006;106(2):170–6.
17. Mehler PS, Blalock DV, Walden K, Kaur S, McBride J, Walsh K, et al. Medical findings in 1,026 consecutive adult inpatient-residential eating disordered patients. Int J Eat Disord. 2018;51(4):305–13.
18. Rosen E, Sabel AL, Brinton JT, Catanach B, Gaudiani JL, Mehler PS. Liver dysfunction in patients with severe anorexia nervosa. Int J Eat Disord. 2016; 49(2):151–8.
19. Ozawa Y, Shimizu T, Shishiba Y. Elevation of serum aminotransferase as a sign of multiorgan-disorders in severely emaciated anorexia nervosa. Internal medicine (Tokyo, Japan). 1998;37(1):32–9.
20. Rautou PE, Cazals-Hatem D, Moreau R, Francoz C, Feldmann G, Lebrec D, et al. Acute liver cell damage in patients with anorexia nervosa: a possible role of starvation-induced hepatocyte autophagy. Gastroenterology. 2008; 135(3):840–8 8 e1–3.
21. Kheloufi M, Boulanger CM, Durand F, Rautou PE. Liver autophagy in anorexia nervosa and acute liver injury. Biomed Res Int. 2014;2014:701064.
22. Wexler DJ, Macias-Konstantopoulos W, Forcione DG, Xiong L, Cauley CE, Pierce KJ. Case 23-2018: a 36-year-old man with episodes of confusion and hypoglycemia. N Engl J Med. 2018;379(4):376–85.
23. Narayanan V, Gaudiani JL, Mehler PS. Serum albumin levels may not correlate with weight status in severe anorexia nervosa. Eat Disord. 2009; 17(4):322–6.
24. Huysentruyt K, De Schepper J, Vanbesien J, Vandenplas Y. Albumin and pre-albumin levels do not reflect the nutritional status of female adolescents with restrictive eating disorders. Acta Paediatr. 2016;105(4):e167–9.
25. Fuhrman MP, Charney P, Mueller CM. Hepatic proteins and nutrition assessment. J Am Diet Assoc. 2004;104(8):1258–64.
26. Gaudiani JL, Sabel AL, Mehler PS. Low prealbumin is a significant predictor of medical complications in severe anorexia nervosa. Int J Eat Disord. 2014; 47(2):148–56.
27. Brown CA, Sabel AL, Gaudiani JL, Mehler PS. Predictors of hypophosphatemia during refeeding of patients with severe anorexia nervosa. Int J Eat Disord. 2015;48(7):898–904.
28. Cleary BS, Gaudiani JL, Mehler PS. Interpreting the complete blood count in anorexia nervosa. Eat Disord. 2010;18(2):132–9.
29. Mohamed M, Khalafallah A. Gelatinous transformation of bone marrow in a patient with severe anorexia nervosa. Int J Hematol. 2013;97(2):157–8.
30. Hutter G, Ganepola S, Hofmann WK. The hematology of anorexia nervosa. Int J Eat Disord. 2009;42(4):293–300.
31. De Filippo E, Marra M, Alfinito F, Di Guglielmo ML, Majorano P, Cerciello G, et al. Hematological complications in anorexia nervosa. Eur J Clin Nutr. 2016;70(11):1305–8.
32. Imbierowicz K, Curkovic I, Braks K, Geiser F, Liedtke R, Jacoby GE. Effect of weight-regulating practices on potassium level in patients with anorexia or bulimia nervosa. Eur Eat Disord Rev. 2004;12(5):300–6.
33. Mascolo M, McBride J, Mehler PS. Effective medical treatment strategies to help cessation of purging behaviors. Int J Eat Disord. 2016;49(3):324–30.
34. National Institute for Health and Clinical Excellence. NICE quick reference guide: nutrition support in adults: oral nutrition support, enteral tube feeding and parenteral nutrition clinical guideline 32. London: National Institute for Health and Clinical Excellence; 2006.
35. Sachs KV, Andersen DM, Sommer J, Winkelman AB, Mehler PS. Avoiding medical complications during the refeeding of patients with anorexia nervosa. Eat Disord. 2015;23(5):411–21.
36. O'Connor G, Nicholls D. Refeeding hypophosphatemia in adolescents with anorexia nervosa: a systematic review. Nutr Clin Pract. 2013;28(3):358–64.
37. Mehler PS, Sabel AL, Watson TL, Andersen AE. High risk of osteoporosis in male patients with eating disorders. Int J Eat Disord. 2008;41(7):666–72.
38. El Ghoch M, Gatti D, Calugi S, Viapiana O, Bazzani PV, Dalle GR. The Association between Weight Gain/Restoration and Bone Mineral Density in Adolescents with Anorexia Nervosa: A Systematic Review. Nutrients. 2016; 8(12):769.
39. Misra M, Prabhakaran R, Miller KK, Goldstein MA, Mickley D, Clauss L, et al. Weight gain and restoration of menses as predictors of bone mineral density change in adolescent girls with anorexia nervosa-1. J Clin Endocrinol Metab. 2008;93(4):1231–7.
40. Drabkin A, Rothman MS, Wassenaar E, Mascolo M, Mehler PS. Assessment and clinical management of bone disease in adults with eating disorders: a review. J Eat Disord. 2017;5:42.

8

Experiences of patients with anorexia nervosa during the transition from child and adolescent mental health services to adult mental health services

Veronica Lockertsen[1,2*], Liv Nilsen[1], Lill Ann Wellhaven Holm[3], Øyvind Rø[4,2], Linn May Burger[5] and Jan Ivar Røssberg[1,2]

Abstract

Background: The transition between the Child and Adolescent Mental Health Services (CAMHS) and the Adult Mental Health Services (AMHS) is identified as an especially critical time for the continuity of care for patients with anorexia nervosa (AN). However, research on this topic is scarce. In the present study, we explore the patients' experiences of the transition between CAMHS and AMHS.

Methods: A qualitative explorative study was carried out based on recorded interviews from one multi-step focus group and six individual interviews with patients who experienced the transition from CAMHS to AHMS in Norway. This study is service user-initiated, meaning service users were involved in all steps of the research process.

Results: The adolescents' experiences are characterized by four overall themes regarding the transition process between CAMHS and AMHS: (1) "Being unprepared and alone in the transition process" describes how a lack of preparation for the transition between CAMHS and AMHS makes them feel alone and increases stress. (2) "It takes time to create a trusting relationship" describes how time influences patients' trust in therapists and motivation for treatment. (3) "We are not all the same" describes how adolescents develop differently but are not treated differently despite their diverse ability to be self-sufficient. (4) "How they see me and treat me affects my hope for the future" describes the interaction between adolescents and therapists.

Conclusions: Acknowledging the patients' needs during the transition period and considering their readiness for the transition is important. Taking into account the four dimensions described in the present study might improve the transition process and enhance the patients' self-sufficiency and maturity.

Keywords: Anorexia nervosa, Mental health transition, Adolescent, Patients' perspective, Qualitative research

* Correspondence: v.lockertsen@gmail.com
[1]Division of Mental Health and Addiction, Oslo University Hospital, P.O. Box 4959, Nydalen, Oslo, Norway
[2]Institute of Clinical Medicine, Faculty of Medicine, University of Oslo, 0318 Oslo, Norway
Full list of author information is available at the end of the article

Plain English summary

Adolescents with anorexia nervosa (AN) who receive care from Child and Adolescent Mental Health Services (CAHMS) often need further treatment from Adult Mental Health Services (AHMS). This study explored the transition between CAHMS and AHMS for patients with AN in a naturalistic public mental health-care setting. Our study identified four themes concerning the transition between CAMHS and AMHS, which patients considered influenced their transition and which demonstrated their lack of preparedness for the transition: The patients often felt alone in this period; time was considered an important element in developing trust in the therapeutic relationship; having the transition adapted to their individual needs and developmental stage is important for the transition outcome; how they were introduced to their new therapists and treated had an effect on their hope for recovery.

Introduction

As many patients experience the transition process between Child and Adolescent Mental Health Services (CAMHS) and Adult Mental Health Services (AMHS) as less than optimal, and many patients drop out of treatment [1], continuity of care in the transition from CAHMS to AMHS is of major importance. A qualitative meta-synthesis focusing on the transition of chronically ill adolescents found that adolescents are unprepared for the transition to AMHS and that the loss of a familiar surroundings and relationships they had at CAMHS creates anxiety [2]. Adolescents are vulnerable to the changes that occur during the transition process, and the inflexibility of the service systems puts many adolescents at risk of disengaging from further treatment [1]. Less than 5% of 154 adolescents with a mental health disorder experienced a satisfactory transition [3]. Research show that several mental health care systems, do not have satisfactory cooperation between the CAMHS and AMHS, which creates a lack of continuity for mental health patients [4, 5]. It is thus recommended that the transition process from CAMHS to AMHS should be carefully planned, taking into consideration the medical, psychosocial, and educational/vocational needs of the adolescents [6, 7]. The patients should be properly engaged at AMHS before their therapy at CAMHS is terminated, and they should view the transition period as a time to practice self-sufficiency and increase empowerment. A strong focus on family involvement in the transition period, is important [8, 9]. Anorexia nervosa (AN) is a severe psychiatric disorder that patients often struggle with for several years. The disorder often results in severe psychosocial and physical consequences for the individual and their family. Age of onset is typically between 14 and 19 years [10], and approximately 85% of the cases begin before the age of 20 [11]. Additionally, patients with AN often have comorbid disorders, such as substance abuse, depression, obsessive-compulsive disorder (OCD), anxiety, and post traumatic stress disorder (PTSD), which complicate the recovery process [12, 13]. Patients with AN often have a devastating fear of gaining weight; the nature of an eating disorder often implies that the patient does not consider themselves ill and has poor insights into the consequences of the illness, which frequently creates a struggle with motivation for recovery [14]. Patients claim that AN gives them a feeling of control and protection, making it difficult for them to let go of the disease and thus comply with treatment. As a result of the above, patients with AN often have complex needs in the transition period, and a thoughtful transition plan is necessary to maintain treatment progress [15]. Although there are variations between different local treatment cultures, CAMHS and AMHS have quite different approaches regarding the extent to which they engage the parents in the treatment [16]. The treatment approach at AMHS is based on individual responsibility. Dimitropoulos, Toulany [17] questioned these sudden changes in treatment approaches to determine whether the supporting surroundings at CAMHS offer adolescents the opportunities they need to practice self-sufficiency and eat independently without familial support. As patients with AN are thought to lag behind their peers both developmentally and psychologically, they typically require careful preparation to manage the transition process [18]. Professionals have underlined how a barrier is formed in the transition when age, rather than readiness, is set as a marker for timing the transition [18]. Most high-income countries divide their services between CAMHS and AMHS at around age 18 [19].

To increase the possibility of adolescents managing the transition, it is essential to have good collaboration between the two services. Nevertheless, a previous study found that the current lack of cooperation between CAMHS and AMHS makes it difficult for patients to navigate between the two services [20]. This gap seem to be present in several countries, regardless of how CAMHS and AMHS are organized [21]. There have been an increasingly awareness of the challenge's patients have in the transition process between CAMHS and AMHS. Based on equal input from relatives, professionals, and the patients, the Canadian Eating Disorder Priority Setting Partnership has prioritized research topics for female patients with AN [22]; they identified that one of the top priorities relates to gaps in treatment, suggesting that research should focus on the transition between services. "Integrated care" have also been identified by clinicians and service users, as a research priority in an Australian setting [23]. Although previous studies have investigated relatives', professionals', and patients' experiences of transitions in specialized eating disorder programs [17, 18, 24], few have focused solely on the patients' perspectives during this transition period, when treated in a naturalist public mental health-care setting. A greater understanding of how patients experience this transition through the different levels of organized health care could contribute to a more cohesive treatment process for patients. Thus, we interviewed patients with AN to understand their experiences of the transition from CAMHS to AMHS.

Methods

Design

The current study is part of a qualitative research project designed to investigate the experiences of the transition between CAMHS and AMHS for patients, parents, and professionals called Mind the Gap. To investigate the transition between CAMHS and AMHS from different perspectives, we used qualitative techniques, including semi-structured interviews and multi-step focus groups [25]. Mind the Gap is a user-initiated project, which implies that the experiences from a support group for relatives form the basis of the research questions. In the current study, the involvement of service users have influenced the research process from the start (designing the study) to the final version of the present manuscript. A former service user who has experience with AN (LMB) participated in the design of a semi-structured interview guide and moderated the interview in collaboration with the first author (VL). The research group also included a former service user with experience as a relative to a patient with AN (LAWH), two RN nurses (LN, VL), and two psychiatrists (JIR, ØR). We found this multi-perspective research group effective for forming the research questions, designing the interview guide, preparing and conducting the focus group interviews, and analyzing the transcriptions.

Recruitment and participants

A total of 10 participants were included in the study. All participants had experiences with the transition between CAMHS and AMHS in a specialized mental health care services. Six had experiences from inpatient units and three had been treated in a specialized eating disorder unit in CAMHS. Five of the participants had been treated in a specialized eating disorder unit in AMHS. All participants were women, with a median age of 22 (range; 19–29) years. The median time since the transition between CAMHS and AMHS was 4.5 years (range; 1–10 years). Six of the participants were working or studying at the time of the qualitative interview. Eight of the participants still received treatment. Six of the participants were invited to participate by current therapists who contacted participants they knew had experiences that could illuminate the research questions. The others made contact with the project manager after finding project information on an internet support site for eating disorders. Recruitment took place between February 2018 and May 2019. Written consent was obtained from all participants.

Data collection

Semi-structured interviews (lasting 60–90 min) were conducted by the fifth (LMB) and first (VL) authors as moderator and co-moderator, respectively. In addition to former user experiences, LMB has attended service user boards in hospitals and performed voluntary work in an interest group for eating disorders. We conducted five individual interviews and one multi-step focus group interview with four participants to explore the experiences of AN patients in the transition between CAMHS and AMHS. The individual and focus group interviews were both guided by our research question, and participants were encouraged to provide concrete examples of their experiences. Focus group interviews are described as a suitable technique in qualitative research because they elicit people's understandings and views of their experiences [26]. Focus groups can be stimulating environments, with co-participants positively triggering other participants' memories. Multi-step focus groups are considered a beneficial method when working with service users in research [27]. Repeated meetings give the participants an opportunity to inspect and challenge their own and others' experiences in a dialectic way. Between the focus group meetings, we handed out a summary of the first focus group interview, so the participants could prepare for the second meeting. This summary constructed the main themes we wanted to focus on in the second group meeting. The individual interviews supplied an in-depth answer of the research question. The first author recorded and transcribed the interviews verbatim. The interviews were conducted at the research clinic or in other neutral settings.

Data analysis

Data were analyzed using a systematic text condensation inspired by Giorgi [28, 29]. The method focused on presenting the patients' expressed experiences, rather than a possible underlying meaning of what was said. Using a method of de-contextualization and re-contextualization of the text, we analytically reduced the data and created a condensed text that represented the overall material [28]. The process comprised four steps: In the first step, the research group read the interviews several times to form an overall impression of the material. In step two, we started sorting the text. Text that belonged together was grouped and encoded. The codes were adjusted and organized so that themes with common content were collected under the same code. In step three, the meaning contents of the different codes were abstracted and collected across the interviews. Step four is the analytical text that represents the results of the research project. With our co-operative relationship, we managed to have a multi-perspective view of the data. To help organize and categorize the transcriptions, we used the computerized program NVivo 11 (QSR International Pty Ltd.)

Ethical aspects

The study was approved by the data protection authority at Oslo University Hospital OUS (2016/19732) and performed in accordance with the Declaration of Helsinki. The Regional Committee for Medical and Health Research Ethics for the Southeast Region of Norway (2016/1259) viewed the study not to be a medical or health-related research project regulated by the law of health research and was not therefore subject to presentation, cf. HFL. § 2.

Results

The participants' experiences are characterized by four overall themes regarding the transition process between CAMHS and AMHS: (1) "Being unprepared and alone in the transition process" describes how a lack of preparation for the transition between CAMHS and AMHS makes them feel alone and increases stress. (2) "It takes time to create a trusting relationship" describes how time influences patients' trust in therapists and motivation for treatment. (3) "We are not all the same" describes how participants develop differently but are not treated differently despite their diverse ability to be self-sufficient. (4) "How they see me and treat me affects my hope for the future" describes the interaction between participants and therapists.

Being unprepared and alone in the transition process

The participants described a feeling of being unprepared and alone during the transition between CAMHS and AMHS. Some patients described that their Primary Care Doctor (PCP) tried to compensate for the lack of follow-up by offering ad hoc support: "I went so many months on my own—without professional contact, just with a support-call from my PCP doctor." They felt overwhelmed when entering AMHS and were unprepared to handle the differences between CAMHS and AMHS. When treated at CAMHS, they felt they were followed up more closely during unstable periods. However, at AMHS, they were often discharged: "Here I got discharged when I was too ill to manage the treatment program." The participants believed they would feel less alone and stressed if CAMHS had a more active function in the transition process. "I remember my mom called CAMHS to ask if I could come back, just after turning 18, but they turned us down." Some participants explained that their parents became increasingly discouraged because they felt as if they had nowhere to turn to for help: "My parents lost hope after CAMHS because they thought that CAMHS had tried everything and that we had nowhere to turn to. So, my parents believed that this would last for the rest of our lives." Often when the participants felt alone and scared during the transition process, they turned to and focused more on their eating disorder to gain a sense of control in the situation. However, focusing on their AN ameliorated their internal chaos. Most of the participants said they were unprepared for the expectation at AMHS for them to be self-sufficient and for how their parent's role changed during the transition phase: "I went from being admitted with my parents in CAMHS to being transferred to a ward that treated my parents as distant relatives, with restrictions about when to call them and what to let them know." It was new for the patients to be responsible for passing information forward and managing the collaboration with their parents. Following the active role their parents had played in CAMHS, some participants felt it important to establish themselves as independent and maintain control. Therefore, many participants found it difficult to uphold an open dialog with their parents during the transition period. Differences in how parents were included in the treatment between CAMHS and AMHS made the patients concerned about their parents' well-being. They considered it important that their parents also received support and help from the therapists at AMHS.

It takes time to create a trusting relationship

Overall, the participants viewed their first meeting at AMHS as important for their adherence to the treatment. The participants often described themselves as being insecure when establishing a relationship at AMHS. They felt they were met with a preconception of what they were, and they were afraid that the new therapists would be unable to understand and acknowledge their situation. The participants were worried about being misinterpreted and were concerned that their story could turn into something they did not recognize as their own. Consequently, they held back, but they acknowledged that doing so made it difficult for the new therapist to help them. The participants stated that it would have been easier for them to connect if CAMHS had prepared them for the transition. Some participants believed that it would be easier to communicate with their new therapist at AMHS if their CAMHS therapist had been present for support in the first meetings. As one adolescent said, "I got scared in the first meeting because I was used to a warmer, more caring, and humble approach. At CAMHS, they often sat beside me, but at AMHS, I sat on the opposite side of a large table with a therapist that did not say much." When establishing a new relationship, the participants needed time to open up about their weight and food issues. They expected the therapists to understand this need, so it was difficult for the participants to understand why they rushed them into gaining weight, and why they—so early in the relationship—gave the responsibility for recovery back to the patients. They felt a need for more structure and time to feel safe and ready to work on their problems regarding food and their emotions. The participants often described how difficult it was to engage in treatment when entering AMHS. They mostly explained this in terms of how the treatment was carried out at CAMHS and how it ended. As they were defined as adults when they turned 18, CAMHS terminated the therapy. While some understood why the transition was timed as it was and felt included and ready for a change; others felt the timing to be arbitrary and felt ignored in the transition process. This made them feel let down by CAMHS, which led some to mistrust towards the treatment system.

The participants felt that the therapists failed to understand what state they were in and how long it could take to build a satisfactory relationship between them and the therapists; they expected too much, too fast. For the participants, this created an issue of mistrust and allowed room for misunderstandings between the therapist and patients: "Perhaps she just wanted to tell me that this is going to be all right, but that was not the way I understood it."

During the transition process to AMHS, the patients described many insecurities about who they were going to meet and how they would be met. They described how they were moved from person to person and how they were expected to follow and trust each new person they met. This was challenging for the participants because the information between CAMHS and AMHS was lacking, and the participants often had to repeat themselves, which made it difficult for the participants to develop motivation for their recovery. However, they managed to gain weight just by doing what they were told: "I realized that I needed the help—but I was never safe enough to choose to stay voluntary." The participants said it was important to have a therapist who showed that they cared about them and their problems. To find a way to trust their therapist, the participants described different ways to test the therapists' persistence and motivation. It could be as specific as in a meal situation or in evaluating the therapists' responses in conversations, e.g., what words they used. If therapists showed that they cared, and "passed their tests," the patients described that the motivation for recovery often increased, which gave them hope:

> It was really important for me to have them close and see their engagement. That was the first time I had my own desire for recovery. You get so tired of the fight between your own two voices that it has to be the people meeting you that figure it out.

The participants described how much easier it was to trust therapists that seemed to be transparent. Some of the patients had experiences with therapists at CAMHS who they felt misused their trust by hiding information from them and going behind their backs to talk to their parents. When they had met a therapist had helped them, they found that they were often the ones who had spent the most time with them and were authentic:

> It takes more time than a biweekly session. Now is the first time I have had a relationship with a therapist in almost a year. It is working now because we have passed the point of meeting each other with our assumptions, and I know he knows me—for me. I can be honest, and he knows my little signs of hurting.

We are not all the same

Some of the participants felt ready for the responsibility that AMHS expected of them, which was to based on AMHS's more individual, independent approach. Others found this shift in approach from that used at CAMHS too demanding. The participants missed being met with curiosity about what they viewed best for themselves during the transition process, including their ideas about how to recover. Despite having the same diagnosis, the participants were in different developmental stages and thus had different needs during the transition: "I was not ready—they wrote from CAMHS that I was eighteen on paper, but my mind was fourteen." The participants described a sense of lagging behind their peers because they had been ill for many years. Some participants explained that they felt almost developmentally disturbed because the years during which they lacked normal contact with school and friends had had a fundamental effect on their development and social skills. It can be painful being defined as an adult when you feel much younger. They felt that the mental health system has a rigid understanding of what an adult is, being defined by the age boundary of 18: "They have to look into the situation and the person. We are not the same." The participants agreed that the transition should be timed based on their developmental stage rather than their age.

While some described the transition to AMHS as something that prolonged their recovery process, others described it as vital for their improvement. They claimed that they were somewhat tired of CAMHS's more childish approach and were ready for the transfer at the age of 17. They felt they were emerging into adulthood and were treated with too much caution at CAMHS: "I had to solve some problems myself and could not depend on other grownups. I had to be a person in my own life." Although some of the participants had negative experiences of the transition, they thought it was important for their recovery process because it underlined the changes they had to make in regard to how they take responsibility. They claimed that "the transition can help reinforce that you are the most important person in your life and the only one who can change something. You're your mom or your therapist." They began to realize that they had to change, take control of their life, and become accountable to themselves, but they had to be ready to do so.

How they see me and treat me affects my hope for the future

The participants often underlined that they felt powerless during the transition; they were dependent on how the system and professionals related to them and perceived them during the transition process. These interactions not only had a practical meaning, but they were also deeply important to the participants. The participants described how the choice of words, spoken or written, influenced their motivation for recovery: "When you are met with 'this is chronic' at the age of 17, what is the point of trying? This just confirms that it is hopeless." For the adolescent patient, it was difficult to maintain motivation when they sensed that their surroundings did not envision their recovery. According to the participants, the difference between CAMHS and AMHS was evident in how they verbalized their visions and hope for the adolescent patient. While CAMHS focused on their future and the life they had in front of them, giving them hope, AMHS did not have the same focus in, for example, how they facilitated maintaining obligations to school or work. The participants perceived an attitude at AMHS that suggested they had to figure those things out on their own. Some participants were transferred from CAMHS to an adult acute psychiatric mental health ward, which they found particularly challenging. They described their mental state as being in crisis and could not understand why CAMHS refused to prolong their treatment. They thought that AMHS did not understand how frightening it could be to be admitted in an adult environment:

I had really nothing to say in that decision; they just let me know that I was going. I stayed for 8 months. I do not think that a 17–18-year-old is suited to an adult acute mental health care unit."

The powerlessness they felt during the transition underlined feelings of aloneness and being unvalued. They describe a sense of resignation—"so I lost interest"—mostly because they felt AMHS lacked an understanding of the difficulties they were experiencing during the transition period.

When treated in in-patient care, they were admitted with other patients who had been ill for a long time. These factors influenced the participants' hope for their recovery in the future: "At AMHS, I was admitted with patients that had been ill longer than I had been living." They described a system that met them with phrases like "early disability benefits," and their illness was described as "treatment resistant." They explained how such words affected their views of their future because such words would stick, influencing how the rest of the treatment system viewed them and contributing to misconceptions, which narrowed their room to change. As a result, the participants became more dependent on their relationships outside of the treatment system to maintain hope for them, as they found it challenging on their own.

When entering the transition phase, the participants often felt as though AMHS had more interest in their illness than in them. The therapist seemed to place more importance on evaluating and interpreting their symptoms and BMI than talking with them about their well-being and experiences of their condition. Some stated that everything in therapy at AMHS was oriented around food and weight, which made it difficult to create trusting relationships with the therapists, who interpreted their BMI as mental and emotional problems. There was a high focus on their somatic health, but little interest in their mental health: "If you eat your food, then you are OK. If your BMI is close to normal, you are good." They were asked if they wanted to have their parents with them, but when they responded negatively, they were never asked "why not." The participants felt that therapists at CAMHS seemed more interested in getting to know them as a person, while those at AMHS only wanted to understand their disease: "You become your symptoms and they just ask: how can we medicate that?" With the experienced alteration from being treated as an individual to being treated as an illness, the participants often felt like an object during the transition, dependent wholly on a relationship that was restricted more to the registration of symptoms and less to what they felt would help them. They verbalized a sense of no longer feeling like a human, just classified symptoms with associated expectations about what they should be struggling with. In their adolescent years, many of them only had social contact with people who were getting paid to be there. They had to protect themselves from becoming attached to the people surrounding them, which they felt changed how they related to people in their lives outside the mental health services. For some, that situation magnified the symptoms of the AN because of the safety they represented:

In the beginning, I got really attached to people, and when they got replaced, I was really affected. But now, it affects me less and less, and the AN has become more stable and safer—and it is always there for me.

Discussion

The findings of the current study provide a meaningful contribution to the research, which explores the experiences of participants with AN during the transition between CAMHS and AMHS. The qualitative analysis revealed four overall themes regarding the transition process: (1) "Being unprepared and alone in the transition process," (2) "It takes time to create a trusting relationship," (3) "We are not all the same," and (4) "How they see me and treat me affects my hope for the future." The themes are interrelated and display elements with the transition that positively and negatively influence the participants' experiences. These essential themes are discussed in the following paragraphs.

Being unprepared and alone in the transition process

The current study found that the participants were unprepared for the transition to AMHS, which led to increased feelings of being alone. Without an understanding of the differences in the treatment approaches between the services, they did not feel as though they were taken seriously at AMHS. They felt alone and without what they considered adequate support during the transition phase. Our study supports the findings of Newlove-Delgado, Ford [30], who found that participants with ADHD were unprepared and left alone during the transition. As in our study, only one of the seven participants included in the study experienced to be prepared for the transition. Good preparation was followed by less stress and fewer feelings of uncertainty. Exploring the transition from the perspectives of 21 participants treated by the mental health services, Cleverley, Lenters [31] described the transition as "objectively terrifying" and the lack of preparation as "overwhelmingly present." In the current study, it is unclear whether the experienced cultural and philosophical differences in approaches, was uncommunicated or not understood by the participants. Nonetheless, Winston, Paul [16] underlined the importance of discussing the differences between the services explicitly, with both the participants and their families. Consequently, the participants in current study lacked the ability to handle the sudden expectations of autonomy. Their destructive eating routine increased when in need for a feeling of safety they felt the illness (AN) provided them when the services did not. When exploring the transition of the patients with AN from the therapists' perspectives, Dimitropoulos, Tran [14] emphasized that for patients with AN, preparing for the transition is particularly important because they often display less self-sufficiency and have difficulties fully engaging in treatment. Similar to our study, Dimitropoulos, Toulany [17] found that it would be beneficial for the patients and their relatives to have a clearer understanding of the implications of the treatment methods used in AMHS. Since patients often are dependent on parents' external support in this phase, Dimitropoulos, Tran [14] underlined the importance of relatives being involved in the process. It could be argued that with more information and better preparation, parents would be better able to provide the support participants need during the transition process. As such, adequate support and preparation from the care system could decrease the patient's feelings of being alone during this time. Ideally, it should be a period of shared care between CAMHS and AMHS, giving the patients the opportunity to understand the way the adult team works to properly prepare them for the change.

It takes time to create a trusting relationship

In the current study, some patients had difficulty starting up a new relationship at AMHS with an open and trusting mind, and they supposed it would have been easier if they had received more support from CAMHS during the transition. The therapists' approach was considered vital when establishing a therapeutic alliance as the patients' social communication became more difficult when they felt unsafe. In accordance with our findings, previous studies have demonstrated that patients with AN are often particularly sensitive to other people's opinions about them [32]. Similarly, Sly, Morgan [33] found that the patients' first impressions of their new therapist often dictated if they would be open about themselves. They also found that young patients with AN needed a therapist that "talk[ed] straight" and required patients to be honest and open about their eating disordered behaviors; otherwise, the patients would disengage from the treatment.

The findings of this study underline the importance of the therapist's timing to address sensitive subjects. The current study found that the participants wanted their therapists to take more time to get to know them before talking about the elements that triggered them most. A major focus on food, weight, and body from the start of the therapeutic relation made it difficult to trust their therapist. Previous research has underlined the importance of the therapist's willingness to move slowly and collaborate on the therapeutic goals with the patients, especially in the earlier stages of therapy [34]. A trusting therapeutic relationship with patients with AN is considered a vital component of successful treatment, as these patients often are difficult to engage in treatment [16]. The participants often described how their ambivalent feelings toward recovery made it problematic to establish a new relationship with the therapists at AMHS. Ambivalence is described as one of the most challenging features of AN [35]. Swift and Greenberg [36] summarized 669 studies on dropout, and they found that studies with eating disorders, personality disorders, and higher proportions of young patients had higher dropout rates than other disorders. A stronger focus on building an alliance with the patient in these first meetings would influence the patients' experience and their compliance with treatment. One issue that emerges from these findings is the complexity of clinical settings. Although the therapists acknowledge that establishing an alliance with patients is essential, they also have to meet expectations concerning efficiency, which gives them little time to do so [20].

We are not all the same

In our study, the participants experienced the transition as an inflexible process. Some of the participants did not feel ready to be transferred to AMHS, but they had reached the age limit and were transferred anyway, which made them feel powerless. The participants viewed their developmental stage as more important for a successful transition than age. This is in line with findings of other studies conducted on transitions between CAMHS and AMHS [9, 17, 31] and in contrast to the clinical guidelines that guide therapists to collaborate with patients and relatives to find the optimal time for the transition [37]. The present study describes how the participants felt as though they were treated more as a patient than an individual when not included in the decisions made about their transition. This experience contrasts with the idea of the transition being a therapeutic process that empowers the patient's recovery process [38].

As in our study, Cleverley, Lenters [31] underlined how the participants already are in a stressful situation and in need of a more individually adapted transition. Many participants thought that the transition would be better in the early 20s, when their lives were more stable. These results reflect some of the discussion about the term "adolescence." The United Nations defines adolescence as the period of 10–19 years of age; however, Sawyer, Azzopardi [39] argued that this definition is outdated when considering contemporary patterns. They consider that extending the age group to 24 years corresponds more closely to adolescent growth and a contemporary understanding of this life phase. These ideas are consistent with other emerging literature on mental health transitions [40–42]. Raballo, Poletti [43] are concerned about the unwillingness to change the system to a more patient – oriented care that incorporates the full continuum of service response within a promotion and prevention framework for youth mental health. They are describing a more radical approach and suggest a substantial framework shift that reorient existing services towards youth- specific mental health care. With their proposition, the adolescent's developmental stage and readiness would determine the timing of the transition. We assume that with such an approach the negative experiences described in the current study, would have been reduced.

How they see me and treat me affects my hope for the future

The participants often described how they felt powerless, dependent on the system and the therapist's impression of them, and were repeatedly defined as an "anorectic patient." To maintain their motivation to recover, the participants needed to experience a therapist that perceived them as a person with unique qualities. Earlier research has described how patients with AN often feel treated as a diagnosis [44, 45]. Malson, Finn [46] found that both the patients and the therapists construct "the anorexic patient." Defined by their disorder, everything the "patient" says is part of the AN, not the person. This resonates with our study, where participants expressed that this objectification of themselves influenced not only their self-worth negatively but also often their commitment to the treatment. These results reflect earlier studies' claims that patients with AN associate negative treatment experiences with being treated as an anorexic, rather than an individual [47, 48].

One important finding in our study was how the participants emphasized the therapists' use of words that deprived them of motivation and hope for a better future. Words such as "chronic" and "treatment resistant" made them lose hope for further treatment progress and the future. In a previous study, the interviewed professionals treating patients with AN were aware of how patients appraised and interpreted words about themselves or their condition. The professionals thus set high standards for how they communicated with the participants [20], and they felt under high pressure to do so from the patients and themselves. They also described a high level of anxiety and uncertainty concerning their assessments, and they elaborated on the consequences of potential premature termination of treatment. Empirical research suggests that therapists tend to develop more feelings of frustration, hopelessness, and helplessness in therapy with AN patients than with patients with other eating disorders [49]. However, existing studies tend to focus on patients' characteristics when addressing dropout from treatment and fail to include systemic or therapist factors, implying that the high dropout rates are primarily the patients' responsibility [36, 50]. Some issues that emerged from the findings of our study relate to the rapid turnover of therapists and how this affected how they attach themselves in relationships with their therapists and in private relationships. Swift and Greenberg [36] examined the premature discontinuation of adult psychotherapy and suggested that future therapeutic relationships can be seriously impeded by a repeated loss of therapists. One hypothesis is that when patients are forced into new relationships that rapidly terminate, it has a negative influence on their own and their therapist's sense of achievement. This amplifies negatively both parties' abilities to create a therapeutic environment and form a basis for a future trusting relationship.

Strengths and limitations

The inclusion of experiences from a heterogenic patient group and the multi-perspective approach when analyzing the material may have provided validity to the study, otherwise missed [51–53] . This study has several limitations. The participants were a mix of self-selected and purposively selected participants, selected by a therapist or former therapist who viewed them as suitable for participating in the current study. The present study included only female participants; thus, a potentially different selection of participants may have emphasized other experiences. One obvious limitation is the retrospective nature of the interviews, which could represent a bias in material, as one often tends to remember the negative aspects better than the positive. The timespan of 0–10 years is wide; thus, participants could have been subject to recall biases. However, our study also had a thematic positive element. The participants connected meaningful elements from the transition to descriptions of consequences of the transition. Conducting qualitative interviews, the context as a phenomenon may influence the findings, here highlighted in two different ways. When trying to understand why and how particular experiences come into being, it can be a question of contextual factors. As we focus on patients' experience, these are generated from different contexts and from different parts of the country and treatment facilities [54]. The interviews in the current study were conducted in different contexts and the researchers held different roles in each interview. It is likely to assume the researcher's role as more active in the individual interviews compared to the focus group interviews. This, may have affected the contents of the interviews. At the same time, conducting individual interviews might also empower the participants by increasing their time frames to convey personal experiences without being influenced or modified by fellow participants.

Conclusion

To conclude, it is of major importance to acknowledge the patients' needs during the transition period and considering their readiness for the transition. To better the chances of a successful transition, both patient and relatives should be explained, in an explicit manner, the differences between the services. A stronger focus on building an alliance with the patient in the first meetings would influence the patients' experience and their compliance with treatment. Taking into account the four dimensions described in the present study might improve the transition process and enhance the patients' self-sufficiency and maturity.

Abbreviations

CAMHS: Child and adolescent mental health services; AMHS: Adult mental health services; AN: Anorexia Nervosa; OCD: Obsessive-compulsive disorder; PTSD: Post traumatic stress disorder; PCP: Primary Care Doctor

Acknowledgements

Thank you to all participants who supported this research study.

Authors' contributions

Design of the Mind the Gap study: LN, JIR, and LAWH. Data collection: VL and JIR. Drafting the article: VL, JIR, and LN. All authors contributed to data analysis, interpretation, and critical revision of the article as well as final approval of the version to be published.

Competing interests

The authors declare that they have no competing interests.

Author details

[1]Division of Mental Health and Addiction, Oslo University Hospital, P.O. Box 4959, Nydalen, Oslo, Norway. [2]Institute of Clinical Medicine, Faculty of Medicine, University of Oslo, 0318 Oslo, Norway. [3]Oslo, Norway. [4]Regional Department for Eating Disorders, Division of Mental Health and Addiction, Oslo University Hospital, Ullevål HF, Postboks 4950 Nydalen, 0424 Oslo, Norway. [5]Drammen, Norway.

References

1. Broad KL, Sandhu VK, Sunderji N, Charach A. Youth experiences of transition from child mental health services to adult mental health services: a qualitative thematic synthesis. BMC Psychiatry. 2017;17(1):380.
2. Fegran L, Hall EO, Uhrenfeldt L, Aagaard H, Ludvigsen MS. Adolescents' and young adults' transition experiences when transferring from paediatric to adult care: a qualitative metasynthesis. Int J Nurs Stud. 2014;51(1):123–35.
3. Singh SP, Paul M, Ford T, Kramer T, Weaver T, McLaren S, et al. Process, outcome and experience of transition from child to adult mental healthcare: multiperspective study. Br J Psychiatry. 2010;197(4):305–12.
4. Mulvale GM, Nguyen TD, Miatello AM, Embrett MG, Wakefield PA, Randall GE. Lost in transition or translation? Care philosophies and transitions between child and youth and adult mental health services: a systematic review. J Ment Health. 2019;28(4):1–10.
5. Paul M, Ford T, Kramer T, Islam Z, Harley K, Singh SP. Transfers and transitions between child and adult mental health services. Br J Psychiatry Suppl. 2013;54:s36–40.
6. Blum RG, D Hodgman C, et al. Transition from childcentered to adult health-care systems for adolescents with chronic conditions. J Adolesc Health. 1993;14:570–6.
7. Garland BH, Caldwell KL, Acosta AB, Wiemann CM, Gonzales SA, Wolfe RS. Clinical considerations for emerging adults with eating disorders and transition to adult-based care. Evid Based Pract Child Adolesc Mental Health. 2018:1–15.
8. Hergenroeder AC, Wiemann CM, Cohen MB. Current issues in transitioning from pediatric to adult-based care for youth with chronic health care needs. J Pediatr. 2015;167(6):1196–201.
9. Singh S, Paul M, Ford T, Kramer T, Weaver T, McLaren S, et al. Lost in transition: a multi-perspective study of process, outcome and experience of transition from child to adult mental health care (TRACK). Br J Psychiatry. 2010;197:305–12.
10. Pinhas L, Morris A, Crosby RD, Katzman DK. Incidence and age-specific presentation of restrictive eating disorders in children: a Canadian Paediatric surveillance program study. Arch Pediatr Adolesc Med. 2011; 165(10):895–9.
11. Herpertz-Dahlmann B. Adolescent eating disorders: definitions, symptomatology, epidemiology and comorbidity. Child Adolesc Psychiatr Clin N Am. 2009;18(1):31–47.

12. Arcelus J, Bouman WP, Morgan JF. Treating young people with eating disorders: transition from child mental health to specialist adult eating disorder services. Eur Eat Disord Rev. 2008;16(1):30–6.
13. Franko DL, Keshaviah A, Eddy KT, Krishna M, Davis MC, Keel PK, et al. A longitudinal investigation of mortality in anorexia nervosa and bulimia nervosa. Am J Psychiatr. 2013;170(8):917–25.
14. Dimitropoulos G, Tran AF, Agarwal P, Sheffield B, Woodside B. Navigating the transition from pediatric to adult eating disorder programs: perspectives of service providers. Int J Eat Disord. 2012;45(6):759–67.
15. Garland BH, Caldwell KL, Acosta AB, Wiemann CM, Gonzales SA, Wolfe RS. Clinical considerations for emerging adults with eating disorders and transition to adult-based care. Evid Based Pract Child Adolesc Mental Health. 2019;4(2):187–201.
16. Winston AP, Paul M, Juanola-Borrat Y. The same but different? Treatment of anorexia nervosa in adolescents and adults. Eur Eat Disord Rev. 2012;20(2): 89–93.
17. Dimitropoulos G, Toulany A, Herschman J, Kovacs A, Steinegger C, Bardsley J, et al. A qualitative study on the experiences of young adults with eating disorders transferring from pediatric to adult care. Eat Disord. 2015;23(2): 144–62.
18. Dimitropoulos G, Tran AF, Agarwal P, Sheffield B, Woodside B. Challenges in making the transition between pediatric and adult eating disorder programs: a qualitative study from the perspective of service providers. Eat Disord. 2013;21(1):1–15.
19. Signorini G, Singh SP, Marsanic VB, Dieleman G, Dodig-Curkovic K, Franic T, et al. The interface between child/adolescent and adult mental health services: results from a European 28-country survey. Eur Child Adolesc Psychiatry. 2018;27(4):501–11.
20. Lockertsen V, Nilsen L, Holm W, Lill A, Rø Ø, Burger LM, Røssberg JI. Mental health professionals' experience with the transition between the child and adolescent mental health system and the adult mental health system for patients with anorexia nervosa. Under review.
21. Signorini G, Singh SP, Boricevic-Marsanic V, Dieleman G, Dodig-Ćurković K, Franic T, et al. Architecture and functioning of child and adolescent mental health services: a 28-country survey in Europe. Lancet Psychiatry. 2017;4(9): 715–24.
22. Obeid N, McVey G, Seale E, Preskow W, Norris ML. Cocreating research priorities for anorexia nervosa: the Canadian eating disorder priority setting partnership. Int J Eat Disord. 2020;53(5):392–402.
23. Hart LM, Wade T. Identifying research priorities in eating disorders: a Delphi study building consensus across clinicians, researchers, consumers, and carers in Australia. Int J Eat Disord. 2020;53(1):31–40.
24. Anastasiadou D, Medina-Pradas C, Sepulveda A, Treasure J. A Systematic Review of Family Caregiving in Eating Disorders. Eat Behav. 2014;15(3): 464–77.
25. Stebbins RA. Exploratory research in the social sciences: Sage; 2001.
26. Wilkinson S. Focus groups. In: Smith JA, editor. Qual Psychol. London: SAGE Publications Ltd; 2015.
27. Hummelvoll JK. Kunnskapsdannelse i praksis: handlingsorientert forskningssamarbeid i akuttpsykiatrien [developing knowledge in practice: Co-operative inquery in acut psychiatry units]. Oslo: Universitetsforl; 2003. p. 286. s. fig. p.
28. Malterud K. Systematic text condensation: a strategy for qualitative analysis. Scand J Public Health. 2012;40(8):795–805.
29. Giorgi A. Sketch of a psychological phenomenological method. Phenomenol Psychol Res. 1985:8–22.
30. Newlove-Delgado T, Ford TJ, Stein K, Garside R. 'You're 18 now, goodbye': the experiences of young people with attention deficit hyperactivity disorder of the transition from child to adult services. Emot Behav Diffic. 2018;23(3):296–309.
31. Cleverley K, Lenters L, McCann E. "Objectively terrifying": a qualitative study of youth's experiences of transitions out of child and adolescent mental health services at age 18. BMC Psychiatry. 2020;20(1):147.
32. Nordbø RH, Espeset EM, Gulliksen KS, Skårderud F, Geller J, Holte A. Reluctance to recover in anorexia nervosa. Eur Eat Disord Rev. 2012; 20(1):60–7.
33. Sly R, Morgan JF, Mountford VA, Sawer F, Evans C, Lacey JH. Rules of engagement: qualitative experiences of therapeutic alliance when receiving in-patient treatment for anorexia nervosa. Eat Disord. 2014;22(3):233–43.
34. Oyer L, O'Halloran MS, Christoe-Frazier L. Understanding the working alliance with clients diagnosed with anorexia nervosa. Eat Disord. 2016;24(2): 121–37.
35. Vitousek K, Watson S, Wilson GT. Enhancing motivation for change in treatment-resistant eating disorders. Clin Psychol Rev. 1998;18(4):391–420.
36. Swift JK, Greenberg RP. Premature discontinuation in adult psychotherapy: a meta-analysis. J Consult Clin Psychol. 2012;80(4):547–59.
37. Eating disorders: Recognition and treatment. Full guideline [Internet]. 2017. Available from: https://www.nice.org.uk/guidance/ng69/evidence/full-guideline-pdf-161214767896. Accessed 13 Feb 2019.
38. Appleton R, Connell C, Fairclough E, Tuomainen H, Singh SP. Outcomes of young people who reach the transition boundary of child and adolescent mental health services: a systematic review. Eur Child Adolesc Psychiatry. 2019:1–16.
39. Sawyer SM, Azzopardi PS, Wickremarathne D, Patton GC. The age of adolescence. Lancet Child Adolesc Health. 2018;2(3):223–8.
40. Scott E, Naismith S, Whitwell B, Hamilton B, Chudleigh C, Hickie I. Delivering youth-specific mental health services: the advantages of a collaborative, multi-disciplinary system. Australas Psychiatry. 2009;17(3):189–94.
41. Malla A, Iyer S, Shah J, Joober R, Boksa P, Lal S, et al. Canadian response to need for transformation of youth mental health services: ACCESS open minds (Esprits ouverts). Early Interv Psychiatry. 2019;13(3): 697–706.
42. Hickie IB. Youth mental health: we know where we are and we can now say where we need to go next. Early Interv Psychiatry. 2011;5(s1):63–9.
43. Raballo A, Poletti M, McGorry P. Architecture of change: rethinking child and adolescent mental health. Lancet Psychiatry. 2017;4:656–8.
44. Tierney S. The individual within a condition: a qualitative study of young People's reflections on being treated for anorexia nervosa. J Am Psychiatric Nurs Assoc. 2008;13(6):368–75.
45. Offord A, Turner H, Cooper M. Adolescent inpatient treatment for anorexia nervosa: a qualitative study exploring young adults' retrospective views of treatment and discharge. Eur Eat Disord Rev. 2006;14(6):377–87.
46. Malson H, Finn D, Treasure J, Clarke S, Anderson G. Constructing 'the eating disordered Patient'1: a discourse analysis of accounts of treatment experiences. J Community Appl Soc Psychol. 2004;14(6):473–89.
47. Button EJ, Warren RL. Living with anorexia nervosa: the experience of a cohort of sufferers from anorexia nervosa 7.5 years after initial presentation to a specialized eating disorders service. Eur Eat Disord Rev. 2001;9(2):74–96.
48. Colton A, Pistrang N. Adolescents' experiences of inpatient treatment for anorexia nervosa. Eur Eat Disord Rev. 2004;12(5):307–16.
49. Colli A, Speranza AM, Lingiardi V, Gentile D, Nassisi V, Hilsenroth MJ. Eating disorders and therapist emotional responses. J Nerv Ment Dis. 2015;203(11): 843–9.
50. Werbart A, Andersson H, Sandell R. Dropout revisited: patient- and therapist-initiated discontinuation of psychotherapy as a function of organizational instability. Psychother Res. 2014;24(6):724–37.
51. Vostanis P. Patients as parents and young people approaching adulthood: how should we manage the interface between mental health services for young people and adults? Curr Opin Psychiatry. 2005;18(4):449–54.
52. Mjøsund NH, Eriksson M, Espnes GA, Haaland-Øverby M, Jensen SL, Norheim I, et al. Service user involvement enhanced the research quality in a study using interpretative phenomenological analysis–the power of multiple perspectives. J Adv Nurs. 2017;73(1):265–78.
53. Gillard S, Simons L, Turner K, Lucock M, Edwards C. Patient and public involvement in the coproduction of knowledge: reflection on the analysis of qualitative data in a mental health study. Qual Health Res. 2012;22(8): 1126–37.
54. Juritzen TI, Soberg HL, Roe C, Saebu M, Engen G, Bliksvaer T, et al. The one or the many: quantified subjectivity and aggregated uniqueness in qualitative rehabilitation research. Qual Health Res. 2017;27(1):51–9.

9

Earlier diagnosis in anorexia nervosa: better watch growth charts!

Morgane Marion[1*], Sylvie Lacroix[1], Marylène Caquard[1], Laurence Dreno[2], Pauline Scherdel[3], Christèle Gras Le Guen[3,4], Emmanuelle Caldagues[1] and Elise Launay[4]

Abstract

Background: A better understanding of the healthcare pathway of children and adolescents with anorexia nervosa (AN) may contribute to earlier detection and better disease management. Here we measured and compared the symptomatic time to diagnosis (TTD) (time between the first symptoms, as reported by parents, and the diagnosis) and the auxological TTD (time between the deviation in the weight growth curve and the diagnosis).

Methods: We performed a monocentric retrospective study including all patients age 9 years to 16 years who were hospitalized in Nantes University Hospital for AN between 2013 and 2016. We analysed the two TTDs by medical record review and growth curve investigation. TTDs were described by medians and Kaplan-Meier curves. Two profiles of patients were compared according to the kinetics of growth deviation and the occurrence of symptoms.

Results: Among the 137 patients included, the median symptomatic and auxological TTDs was 7.0 months (IQR: 4.0–12.0) and 7.2 months (IQR: 2.0–18.0). TTDs were significantly different but clinically similar. For 48% of the patients, a deviation in the growth curve could have been noted at a median of 9.7 months (IQR: 3.0–18.0) before the first symptoms were reported by parents. Those patients showed significantly slower weight loss than did patients with first symptoms reported before growth deviation (weight loss rate 0.41% vs 1.90% per month, $p < 0.0001$).

Conclusions: Careful study of growth curves remains an essential step in detecting eating disorders, possibly allowing for earlier detection of the disease in nearly half of these patients.

Keywords: Adolescent, Anorexia nervosa., Eating disorder., Feeding disorder., Time to diagnosis., Early diagnosis., Growth charts.

Plain English summary

Our study highlights the need for more meticulous analysis of growth charts to detect anorexia nervosa earlier in children and adolescents. Children and adolescents should be weighed and measured regularly and growth curves should be systematically constructed. Any deviation in the growth pathway (weight loss or stagnation) should be controlled and investigated if confirmed.

* Correspondence: marion.morgane@gmail.com
[1]CHU de Nantes, Department of adolescent medicine, Pédiatrie générale, 7 quai Moncousu, 44000 Nantes, France
Full list of author information is available at the end of the article

Introduction

The eating disorder (ED) anorexia nervosa (AN) is more common among girls than boys, with an estimated prevalence of 0.5 to 1% in adolescent girls [1, 2]. AN is responsible for substantial physical and psychological morbidity [1]. The main acute complication of malnutrition is death, but death can also occur over the long term, mainly because of suicide. Among adults, overall mortality with AN is estimated at about 5% [2].

One of the main somatic chronic complications in the pediatric age is the negative impact mainly on height growth and bone density [3, 4]. In fact, malnutrition during the pubertal growth spurt leads to stunted growth, which may not be caught up afterwards [5]. The major consequence is bone demineralization, which has multifactorial pathophysiologic causes (malnutrition, excessive exercise, hypo-estrogenism, hypogonadism with primary and secondary amenorrhoea) [6, 7]. Most of the time, anorexia occurs during adolescence around the menarche, between age 11 to 14 years for most girls. During this perimenarchal phase, 40 to 60% of bone density develops [8, 9]. Having an eating disorder during this critical phase for developing peak bone mass can have long-term implications [4].

The time to diagnosis (TTD), usually defined as the interval between the first symptoms and diagnosis, and its impact on prognosis are widely studied in paediatrics, particularly in pediatric oncology [10, 11]. Our clinical experience with patients with an ED led us to distinguish 2 different diagnostic processes. On one hand, major and fast weight loss in some adolescents will lead to an immediate alert in their family circle and quick access to treatment. On the other, some adolescents will have a slower disease course without or with slight weight loss but will show a deviation in their growth curve, which may lead to less of an alert in their family and longer TTD [12]. We hypothesize that these 2 types of patients have a differing TTD with differing determinants, which we need to consider in future research on the impact of TTD [13].

Studies of AN have included frequent reports of the positive impact of early treatments, particularly on weight restoration trajectories and risk of chronic disease [14–18]. In 2011, Forman et al. looked at predictors of weight outcomes at 1 year depending on the care program [18]. The authors showed that shorter duration of illness before intake and higher percentage of median body weight predicted improved weight outcomes at 1 year. In their study, the average duration of illness before intake in adolescents and young adults was 5.7 to 18.6 months depending on the center. The authors referred to the duration of illness before intake but did not define the TTD, as we propose. Some other studies showed that the median duration of illness before intake was 9 months (IQR: 5.0–16.0) [17] or 1.3 years (IQR: 0.7–4.1) in academic centers and 1.2 years (IQR: 0.5–2.0) in community hospitals [19]. However, these studies also did not clearly define the TTD and did not study the determinants of this delay. Regardless, the definition of TTD and considering the factors that could affect this delay (including the phenotype of the disease) are an important prior step for studying the frequently complex relation between TTD and outcome for a patient.

Our main objective was to describe and compare the symptomatic TTD and auxological TTD in children and adolescents with AN. Our secondary objective was to determine factors associated with the TTDs.

Methods

Study design

We conducted a monocentric and retrospective study including all children and adolescents aged 9 to 16 years old who were hospitalized in the day-hospital or had regular full-time hospitalization at Nantes University Hospital from January 2013 to December 2016. The protocol was approved by the local ethics committee of Nantes University Hospital. We relied on the REporting Studies on Time to diagnosis (REST) reporting guidelines to report this study [20].

Setting

Children and adolescents with AN in the 2 studied administrative French districts (Loire-Atlantique and Vendée) are mainly seen in Nantes University Hospital but can also consult in 2 pediatric psychiatry wards and 2 pediatric wards outside Nantes University Hospital. Adults and adolescents older than 16 years are usually seen in an adult ward (psychiatry or endocrinology) inside or outside Nantes University Hospital.

Patients with AN receiving treatment in Nantes University Hospital are usually referred by a general practitioner or pediatrician or, for children who are severely undernourished, are admitted to the emergency department at Nantes University Hospital. The care pathway for patients with AN is organized around a first step of consultation in the adolescent clinic, then hospitalization in the pediatric ward for diagnostic work-up and renutrition according to French recommendations [21]. The criteria for hospitalization of our patients also refers to the French national health authority recommendations (HAS) [21]. The recommendations consider somatic (e.g., a loss of > 2 kg per week, body mass index [BMI] < 13.2 kg/m^2 at age 15 years and 16 years or BMI < 12.7 kg/m^2 at age 13 years or 14 years, aphagia, dehydration, syncope, hypothermia, the existence of hemodynamic or electrolyte disorders, electrocardiography abnormalities), psychiatric (e.g., suicidal risk, co-morbidities) and environmental criteria. These criteria are close to those cited in an update of the medical management of eating disorders in adolescents by Golden et al. (2014) [22]. After hospital discharge, patients are followed in the adolescent clinic by adolescent medicine specialists and pediatric psychiatrists as outpatients or in the day-hospital depending on the disease severity. The proportion of patients who are followed at Nantes University Hospital adolescent clinics for ED but are never hospitalized is low, about 5%.

Participants

Patients were identified in an administrative database with the discharge diagnosis F50.0 according to the *International Classification of Diseases*, 10th revision. The diagnosis of AN was established after the first consultation in the adolescent clinic by using the *Diagnostic and Statistical Manual of Mental Disorders*, Fifth Edition (DSM-5), by 2 specialist physicians (pediatrician and pediatric psychiatrists) jointly caring for the patient. We included only patients treated as inpatients in Nantes University Hospital. We excluded patients who were hospitalized for a very short time but were not followed up at Nantes University Hospital.

Data collection

Data were collected on patients' age, puberty status, lifestyle (urban or rural residence, family composition, siblings), family history of ED, disease characteristics (date and age at diagnosis, weight loss at diagnosis, number and duration of hospitalizations) and patients' growth (weight, height and BMI expressed in standard deviation [SD] units) after age 8 years and up to 2 years after the diagnosis.

Outcome definition and measures

The auxological TTD was defined as the duration in months from the age at which the weight growth deviated by ≥0.5 SDs from the usual growth curve of the patient to the age at the first consultation in the adolescent clinic. The auxological TTD was obtained from studying the individual growth curve for each patient, which allowed for defining an age before growth curve deviation (last weight before the deviation from the curve) and an age at deviation (first weight deviating from the previous growth path) (Additional file 1). One of the authors (MM) determined the age at the weight-growth deviation by studying the patient's growth curve as follows: visual tracking, then checking by using the weight data and the corresponding SD for their age according to French growth charts routinely used in France at the time of the study [23]. Hence, the auxological TTD was obtained by calculating the age at first consultation at the adolescent clinic minus the age at weight-growth deviation.

The symptomatic TTD was defined by the duration in months from the age at which the first symptoms occurred (food restriction or sorting and/or change in behaviour) to the age at first consultation in the adolescent clinic. The question about first symptoms was routinely asked during the first interview with the patient and their family, and the response was noted in the medical file and considered the beginning of the symptoms. The symptomatic TTD was then obtained from the consultation reports, as the interval between the age at which parents and/or patients reported the occurrence of first symptoms and the age at first consultation at the adolescent clinic.

Then we compared the auxological and symptomatic TTDs and defined 2 diagnostic profiles of patients: those whose weight-growth deviation appeared before the first symptoms (longer auxological TTD than symptomatic TTD) and those whose weight-growth deviation appeared after the first symptoms (shorter auxological TTD than symptomatic TTD). We divided the patients into 2 groups — those with shorter symptomatic than auxological TTD and those with shorter auxological than symptomatic TTD — to investigate the determinants of delay.

We also calculated the interval from the age at which the first symptoms were noted to the age at weight-growth deviation and the interval from the age at the last consultation before weight-growth deviation to the age at weight-growth deviation (reflecting the interval between 2 weight measurements).

Statistical analysis

The characteristics of the population are described with median (interquartile range [IQR]) for quantitative data and frequency (%) with 95% confidence intervals (CIs) for categorical data. The auxological and symptomatic TTDs were represented by Kaplan-Meier curve and compared by log-rank test as appropriate for paired samples. Median auxological and symptomatic TTDs were also compared by Wilcoxon test for paired samples. To study the determinants of the auxological and symptomatic TTDs, we tested the association between the TTDs and rural or urban residence (according to the definition of the French national institute of statistics, a town has > 2500 inhabitants), parental situation (living together or separated), ED type (pubertal girls, prepubertal girls, boys), family history of ED, age at diagnosis, and weight-loss rate expressed as a percentage (percentage of total weight loss divided by duration of the weight loss in months). Factors associated with auxological and symptomatic TTD were independently analysed by a Cox proportional-hazards regression model including variables with $p < 0.2$ on univariate analysis. For these analyses, the deviance to linearity was tested (i.e., the relation between TTD and candidate variables) and the delay was transformed into a polynomial variable and classified by quartiles if there was deviation. We also compared the auxological and symptomatic TTDs and the characteristics between the 2 diagnostic profiles of patients (i.e., those with longer auxological than symptomatic TTD with reference to those with shorter auxological than symptomatic TTD). Factors associated with the diagnostic profile with $p < 0.2$ on univariate analysis were entered in the multivariate logistic regression analysis. Hazard ratios, odds ratios (ORs) and 95% CIs were estimated. $P < 0.05$ was considered statistically significant. Data were analysed by using Stata v11.

Results

Study population

We identified 146 patients hospitalized in Nantes University Hospital with a discharge code for AN in the medical record. For 7 patients, the diagnosis of AN was not confirmed in the medical record. In all, 139 patients were hospitalized for AN in the pediatric ward or in the pediatric day-hospital at Nantes University Hospital between January 2013 and December 2016. Two patients with a follow-up in another center were excluded (Fig. 1).

Among the 137 included patients were 88.3% girls (95% CI: 82.9–93.7) and 11.7% boys (95% CI: 6.3–17.1); the median age at diagnosis was 14 years (IQR: 12.6–14.8) (Table 1). Less than half of the families had 2 children [35% (95% CI: 27.0–43.0)]. The median weight loss at diagnosis was 8.0 kg (IQR: 4.0–11.0), which corresponds to 16.7% of total body mass. The maximum weight loss was 38 kg (52.7% of total body mass). Most patients (95%; 95% CI: 91.4–98.6) were hospitalized in the pediatric ward before receiving treatment in a day-hospital. The median time between the 2 weight measurements allowing to detect an absolute deviation of ≥0.5 SDs in the weight-growth curve was 9 months (IQR: 6.0–12.0). The median weight loss between the two weight measurements was 1.3 SDs (IQR: 0.9–2.0).

Half of the patients were hospitalized only once and 23% twice. The median duration of the first hospitalization was 44 days (IQR: 15–73). A weight gain contract was proposed to 67% (95% CI: 58.9–75.1) of patients during their first hospitalization. The median weight gain established in the contracts was 4.5 kg.

Description, comparison and determinants of TTDs

The median auxological TTD was 7.2 months (IQR: 2.0–18.0) and the median symptomatic TTD was 7.0 months (IQR: 4.0–12.0). The median auxological and symptomatic TTDs significantly differed ($p = 0.02$), but the probability of a diagnosis of AN did not significantly differ between the two TTDs ($p = 0.90$) (Additional file 2). On univariate analysis, we did not find any association between the symptomatic or auxological TTD and ED demographics by sex, parental situation, urban or rural residence, family history of ED, age at diagnosis, current

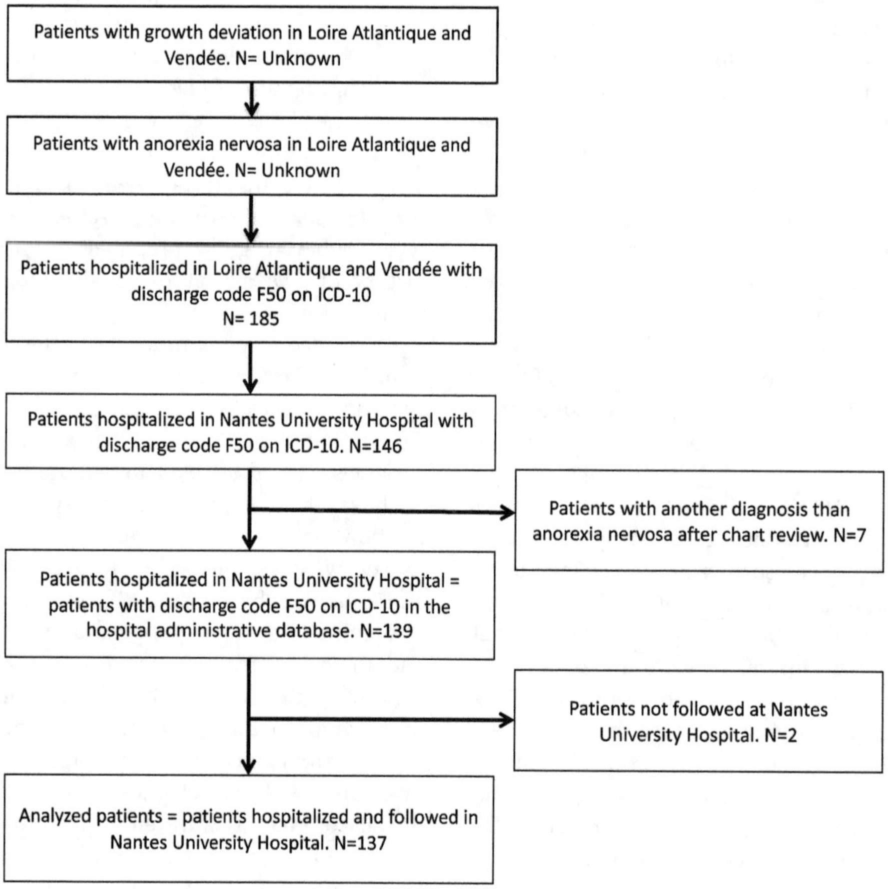

Fig. 1 Flowchart of the participants in the study according to the REporting Studies on Time to diagnosis (REST) reporting guidelines. ICD-10, *International Classification of Diseases*, 10th revision

Table 1 Characteristics of patients with anorexia nervosa who were hospitalized in Nantes University Hospital between 2013 and 2016 ($n = 137$)

	Number of patients	Percentage (95% CI)
Sex		
Girls	121	88.3 (82.9–93.7)
Boys	16	11.7 (6.3–17.1)
Girls puberty status		
Prepubertal girls	15	12,4 (6,5–18.3)
Pubertal girls	106	87.6 (81.7–93.5)
Residence		
Urban	126	92.0 (87.5–96.5)
Rural	11	8.0 (3.5–12.5)
Parental situation		
Together	111	81.0 (74.4–87.6)
Separated	26	19.0 (12.4–25.6)
A deceased parent	6	4.4 (1.0–7.8)
Family history of ED		
Yes	33	24.1 (16.9–31.3)
No	104	75.9 (68.7–83.1)
Obesity before AN (BMI > 2 SD)		
Yes	15	10.9 (5.7–16.1)
No	122	89.1 (83.9–94.3)
Associated bulimia		
Yes	20	14.6 (8.7–20.5)
No	117	85.4 (79.5–91.3)
	Median	**IQR**
Age at diagnosis (years)	14.0	12.6–14.8
Girls	14.1	12.6–14.9
Boys	13.2	12.7–14.1
Weight loss at diagnosis (kg)	8.0	4.0–11.0
Girls	8.0	5.0–12.0
Boys	4.8	1.0–6.5
Weight loss at diagnosis (%)	16.7	9.8–24.0
Girls	17.8	10.6–24.4
Boys	10.6	4.4–15.4
Highest BMI (SD)	0.3	−0.6–1.2
Girls	0.4	−0.4–1.2
Boys	0.0	−1.0–0.8
Lowest BMI (SD)	−2.3	−3.1– − 1.5
Girls	−2.2	−2.9– − 1.5
Boys	−3.1	− 3.2– − 1,9

AN anorexia nervosa, *BMI* body mass index, *CI* confidence interval, *ED* eating disorder, *IQR* interquartile range, *SD* standard deviation

BMI and weight loss rate (Table 2). TTDs (auxological and symptomatic) seemed longer in boys than girls, but probably owing to the small number of boys in our study, the results were not significant. The median auxological TTD was 9.2 months (IQR: 3.0–23.0) for boys and 6.6 months (IQR: 1.9–18.0) for girls ($p = 0.49$). Also, the median symptomatic TTD was 8.5 months (IQR: 3.5–12) and 7.0 months (IQR: 5–10), respectively ($p = 0.55$). On multivariate analysis, faster weight loss was associated with short TTD (i.e., greater risk of instantaneous diagnosis), regardless of type of TTD.

Comparison of groups of patients by diagnostic profile

Overall, 48% of patients had a growth deviation from the curve, with a median lapse time of 9.7 months (IQR: 3.0–18.0) before the first symptoms were noted by parents or patients (Fig. 2 B1). In this subgroup, patients had been weighed at a median lapse time of 12 months (IQR: 9.0–15.0) before growth deviation was noted (Fig. 2 B1). For the other subgroup (52% of patients), the first symptoms were noted at a median of 4 months [IQR 2.1–5.1] before the growth deviation appeared on growth charts (Fig. 2 B2). In this subgroup, patients had been weighed at a median lapse time of 11 months (IQR: 7.0–15.0) before growth deviation was noted. Symptomatic TTDs did not significantly differ between the 2 subgroups: 7.5 months (IQR: 4.0–10.0) with growth deviation detectable before symptoms were reported versus 7 months (IQR: 5.0–10.0) with growth deviation detectable after the first symptoms were reported ($p = 0.60$). Auxological TTDs significantly differed between the 2 groups: 18 months (IQR: 11.0–27.0) versus 3 months (IQR: 0–5) ($p < 0.001$).

On univariate analysis, weight loss rate was faster for patients with first symptoms reported by parents before the growth curve deviation than those with first symptoms identified after the growth curve deviation (1.9% vs 0.4% per month; OR 0.09 [95% CI: 0.04–0.2]) ($p < 0.0001$) (Table 3). The symptoms were noticed more frequently after the growth curve deviation if the patients were boys or prepubertal girls versus pubertal girls and to a lesser extent if parents were separated. On multivariate analysis, faster weight loss rate and parents living together were significantly associated with noticing the first symptoms before the growth-curve deviation.

Discussion

Main results and interpretation

In this first study focused on the TTD of AN in children and adolescents, the median symptomatic and auxological TTDs were significantly different but clinically similar: 7.0 and 7.2 months, respectively. The immediate probability of a diagnosis of AN did not differ between auxological and symptomatic criteria. However, for 48%

Table 2 Univariate and multivariate analysis of factors associated with the auxological and symptomatic time to diagnosis (TTD)

	Auxological TTD						Symptomatic TTD					
	Univariate analysis			Multivariate analysis			Univariate analysis			Multivariate analysis		
	HR	95% CI	p	aHR	95% CI	p	HR	95% CI	p	aHR	95% CI	p
ED demographic type												
Pubertal girls	1	–	–				1	–	–	1	–	–
Boys	0.8	0.5–1.5	0.5				0.6	0.4–1.1	0.1	0.7	0.4–1.3	0.3
Prepubertal girls	0.7	0.4–1.3	0.3				0.6	0.4–1.1	0.1	0.7	0.4–1.3	0.3
Parental situation												
Together	1	–	–				1	–	–			
Separated	0.9	0.6–1.6	0.9				0.8	0.5–1.3	0.3			
Residence												
Urban	1	–	–									
Rural	1.0	0.5–1.9	0.9									
Family history of ED												
No	1	–	–	1	–	–	1	–	–			
Yes	1.4	0.9–1.3	0.1	1.2	0.8–1.9	0.4	1.1	0.8–1.7	0.6			
Age at diagnosis (years)	0.9	0.8–1.1	0.4				0.9	0.9–1.1	0.7			
Current BMI (kg/m2)	0.9	0.8–1.1	0.3				0.9	0.9–1.1	0.9			
Weight loss rate (% of body mass/month)	1.9	1.7–2.2	< 0.001	1.9	1.6–2.2	< 0.001	1.2	1.1–1.3	< 0.001	1.2	1.1–1.3	< 0.001

BMI body mass index, *ED* eating disorder, *HR* hazard ratio, *aHR* adjusted hazard ratio, *CI* confidence interval

of our patients, the growth-curve deviation was detectable at a median of 9.7 months before the first symptoms occurred. Therefore, the diagnosis could have been established earlier in nearly half of our cases. Fast weight loss rate appeared to be a key factor affecting the TTD and was associated with short auxological and symptomatic TTD.

This study confirmed our clinical impression of 2 different diagnostic processes for patients with AN: 1) patients with "noisy" symptoms and fast weight loss that would alert caregivers and result in an early diagnosis and 2) patients with insidious weight stagnation, whose symptoms remain unnoticed for longer. Symptoms triggered a diagnosis, as opposed to growth-chart deviation leading to an avoidable long time of weight-growth stagnation in half of our patients. In fact, symptomatic TTD was about 7.0 months in both groups (those with symptoms noticed after growth deviation and those with symptoms noticed before growth deviation), whereas auxological TTD was much longer when symptoms were noticed after growth deviation was detectable on growth charts (18 vs 3 months). Our hypothesis is that parents alerted by symptoms brought their children to a medical consultation, during which weight stagnation or loss was then interpreted as pathological, whereas a deviation on growth deviation noted before symptoms were reported by parents did not lead to a systematic search for these symptoms and was not interpreted as pathological by clinicians. Moreover, patients were weighed in both groups at a comparable median interval of 11 and 12 months before weight growth deviation was detectable. The diagnostic delay was then due to suboptimal analysis of the growth chart by physicians and not lack of consultation or delay in seeking care by parents.

The symptoms were identified more often after the growth curve deviation in prepubertal versus pubertal girls. This observation is consistent with the literature, in which younger patients are described to more frequently have unusual clinical presentations than older youths. Instead of a fast weight loss rate, they may present a weight stagnation or an inability to gain weight. Moreover, dysmorphophobia is often more undetectable in the first stage for younger than older adolescents. These atypical presentations may be responsible for a late diagnosis [16, 24].

We did not find any sex differences in TTDs. In contrast to the study of Strandjord et al. [25], TTD (symptomatic and auxological) was longer for the boys than girls in our cohort but was not significant perhaps because of the low number of boys.

Internal validity

To establish a definition of the TTD, we referred to the well-known diagnostic triad of AN: anorexia, weight loss, amenorrhoea [2]. For evaluating symptomatic TTD, we used symptoms of food restriction and sorting detected by parents and patients as reported at the first consultation at the adolescent clinic. However, the real duration

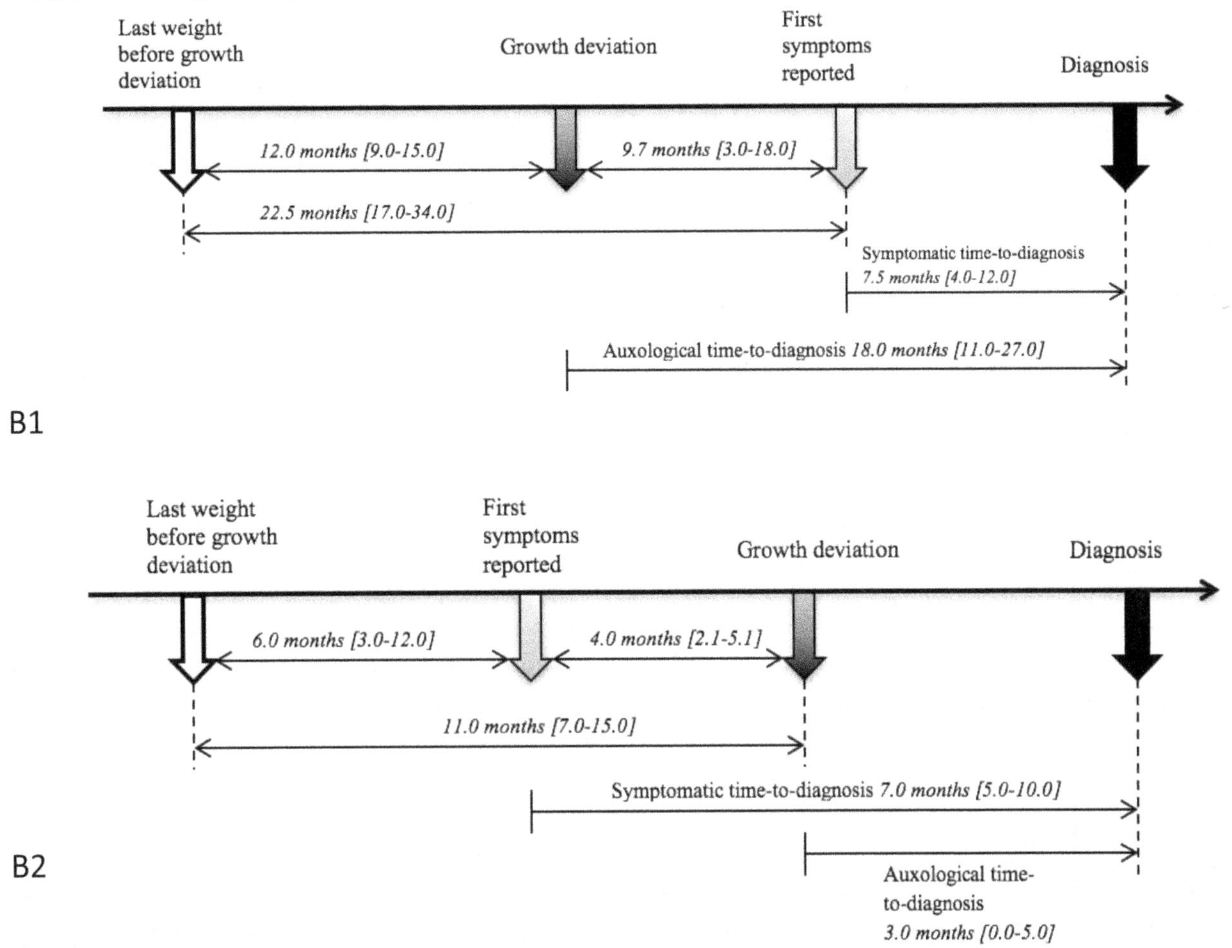

Fig. 2 B1) Schema of the diagnostic process for patients with the earliest auxological time to diagnosis ($N = 66$); B2) Schema of the diagnostic process for patients with the earliest symptomatic time to diagnosis ($N = 71$). Data are mean (interquartile range)

of symptom evolution may be underestimated by this method. Indeed, a 2014 study showed that parents frequently attributed the early signs of AN to the normal development of adolescents and expected the weight loss to be short-lasting, which delayed the first medical consultation [26]. We did not retain the amenorrhoea criterion to study TTD. Indeed, this piece of data was not relevant in our population composed partly of boys and prepubertal girls and was shown to be invalid in children and adolescent populations [16]. Moreover, in the 2013 DSM-5 update, the presence of amenorrhoea is no longer necessary for a diagnosis of AN [2]. For the symptomatic diagnosis of AN, tools available for primary care are poor. Only the SCOFF questionnaire is available, but it was validated in French only for an adult population [16, 27].

Auxological TTD was defined by a meticulous analysis of growth charts. The definition of weight growth deviation as ≥0.5 SDs of the usual growth path was arbitrarily chosen and may have overestimated auxological TTD, but, as in other fields of pediatrics, we lack consensus on defining the abnormal growth curve for early detection of AN [13]. Comparison with growth charts of "safe" controls may be helpful to test the specificity of this weight-growth deviation.

Strengths and limitations

We present detailed data and auxological characteristics of a large population of children and adolescents with AN. Because of the pediatric nature of our hospital, which admits patients under age 16 years only, the population of our study is younger than in studies from other countries and therefore not representative of all patients with AN. However, our study has some limitations, the first of which is recruitment bias. The adolescents followed at Nantes University Hospital, a referral center for ED, probably have more severe somatic and psychiatric presentation with greater weight loss or longer TTD than other adolescents. Besides, the definition method of TTD implies a memory recall bias concerning

Table 3 Comparison of patients by diagnostic profile on univariate and multivariate analysis

	Growth curve deviation before first symptoms [a] *N* = 66	Growth curve deviation after first symptoms *N* = 71	Univariate analysis[a]			Multivariate analysis[a]		
			OR	95% CI	p	aOR	95% CI	p
ED demographic type								
Pubertal girls	45 (68.2%)	61 (85.9%)	1.0	–	–	1.0	–	–
Prepubertal girls	10 (15.2%)	5 (7.1%)	2.7	0.9–8.7	0.08	0.6	0.1–2.6	0.5
Boys	11 (16.6%)	5 (7.1%)	2.9	0.9–9.4	0.05	1.8	0.2–13.3	0.6
Parental situation								
Together	50 (75.8%)	61 (85.9%)	0.5	0.2–1.2	0.1	0.2	0.04–0.8	0.03
Separated	16 (24.2%)	10 (14.1%)	1.0	–	–	1.0	–	–
Residence								
Rural	8 (12.1%)	3 (4.2%)	3.1	0.8–12.6	0.09	2.5	0.3–21.8	0.4
Urban	58 (87.9%)	68 (95.8%)	1.0	–	–	1.0	–	–
Family history of ED								
Yes	15 (22.7%)	18 (25.4%)	0.9	0.4–1.9	0.7			
No	51 (77.3%)	53 (74.6%)	1.0	–	–			
Age at diagnosis (years), median (IQR)	14.0 (12.7–14.8)	14.0 (12.5–14.9)	0.9	0.8–1.1	0.5			
Current BMI (kg/m^2) (SD), median (IQR)	0.3 (−0.7–1.1)	0.4 (−0.2–1.1)	0.9	0.7–1.2	0.5			
Weight loss rate (% body mass/month), median (IQR)	0.4 (0.2–0.8)	1.90 (1.1–3)	0.09	0.04–0.2	< 0.0001	0.07	0.03–0.2	< 0.0001

[a] Reference group: Patients with growth curve deviation before first symptoms, i.e., longer auxological TTD than symptomatic TTD
BMI body mass index, *ED* eating disorder, *OR* odds ratio, *aOR* adjusted odds ratio, *CI* confidence interval

the symptoms detected by parents, especially due to the denial inherent in AN. Symptoms more detailed than restrictions such as occasionally skipping a meal or discrete dietary changes could not be detected in our study because of the retrospective approach. We would have gained accuracy by using a standardized questionnaire. This could be a great contribution in future studies. Finally, the definition of the diagnosis date is questionable. The choice of the first specialized consultation is pragmatic and corresponds to the beginning of the specific management of the disease. Moreover, confirmation of the diagnosis often occurs after this consultation. However, this choice does not account for previous consultations with the physician for the same reason, nor treatment in primary care, which could have been initiated before the specialized consultation. Because of the retrospective data collection and the occasionally incomplete data in medical files, the choice of the first hospital consultation date ensured an objective and constant definition of TTD among patients.

Conclusion

Our study highlights the need for a more meticulous analysis of growth curves to detect AN earlier. Children and adolescents should be weighed and measured regularly, and growth curves should be systematically constructed. Any deviation in the growth pathway (weight loss or stagnation) should be controlled and investigated if confirmed. Consequences of the TTD for adolescents with AN have not been studied in a large population. Long TTD and particularly long auxological TTD may have consequences on bone mineralisation and adult size. A multicentric prospective study should be performed to better define auxological TTD and better evaluate its consequences and bone mineralisation [28]. Comparison of growth curves for healthy children and adolescents and those with AN could also help define a screening algorithm.

Abbreviations

AN: Anorexia nervosa; BMI: Body mass index; CI: Confidence interval; ED: Eating disorder; IQR: Interquartile range; OR: Odds ratio; SD: Standard deviation; TTD: Time to diagnosis

Authors' contributions

MM, SL, MC, LD, PS, CGL, EC and EL designed the study. MM collected the patient data. EL, PS and MM analyzed and interpreted the patient data. MM wrote the manuscript. EL and PS were major contributors to writing and correcting the manuscript. All authors read and approved the final manuscript.

Competing interests

The authors declare that they have no competing interests.

Author details

[1]CHU de Nantes, Department of adolescent medicine, Pédiatrie générale, 7 quai Moncousu, 44000 Nantes, France. [2]CHU de Nantes Department of child psychiatry, University of Hospital Nantes, Nantes, France. [3]CHU de Nantes, Centre d'Investigation Clinique (CIC004), Nantes, France. [4]CHU de Nantes, Department of Pediatrics, Nantes, France.

References

1. Zipfel S, Giel KE, Bulik CM, Hay P, Schmidt U. Anorexia nervosa: aetiology, assessment, and treatment. Lancet Psychiatry. 2015;2(12):1099–111.
2. Alvin P. Anorexie et boulimie à l'adolescence. 4th ed; 2013. (collection conduites).
3. Modan-Moses D, Yaroslavsky A, Kochavi B, Toledano A, Segev S, Balawi F, et al. Linear Growth and Final Height Characteristics in Adolescent Females with Anorexia Nervosa. Milanese S, editor. PLoS One. 2012;7(9):e45504.
4. Mumford J, Kohn M, Briody J, Miskovic-Wheatley J, Madden S, Clarke S, et al. Long-term outcomes of adolescent anorexia nervosa on bone. J Adolesc Health. 2019;64(3):305–10.
5. Alvin P, Marcelli D. Medecine de l'adolescent. 2nd ed. Masson; 2005. (Pour le praticien).
6. Nicaise D, Beaumesnil M, Chaillou E, Wagner A-C, Avarello G, Audran M, et al. Anorexie mentale de l'adolescent : conséquences sur la minéralisation osseuse. Arch Pédiatrie. 2012;19(1):17–21.
7. Hofman M, Landewé-Cleuren S, Wojciechowski F, Kruseman AN. Prevalence and clinical determinants of low bone mineral density in anorexia nervosa. Eur J Intern Med. 2009;20(1):80–4.
8. Bonjour J-P, Theintz G, Buchs B, Slosman D, Clavien H, Rizzoli R. Variation in spinal and femoral bone mass gain, energy and calcium intake during adolescence. Osteoporos Int. 1993;3:67–8.
9. Bailey DA, Martin AD, McKay HA, Whiting S, Mirwald R. Calcium accretion in girls and boys during puberty: a longitudinal analysis. J Bone Miner Res. 2000;15(11):2245–50.
10. Brasme J-F, Grill J, Gaspar N, Oberlin O, Valteau-Couanet D, Chalumeau M. Evidence of increasing mortality with longer time to diagnosis of cancer: is there a paediatric exception? Eur J Cancer. 2014;50(4):864–6.
11. Launay E, Morfouace M, Deneux-Tharaux C. Gras le-Guen C, Ravaud P, Chalumeau M. quality of reporting of studies evaluating time to diagnosis: a systematic review in paediatrics. Arch Dis Child. 2014;99(3):244–50.
12. Treasure J, Stein D, Maguire S. Has the time come for a staging model to map the course of eating disorders from high risk to severe enduring illness? An examination of the evidence: a staging model for eating disorders. Early Interv Psychiatry. 2015;9(3):173–84.
13. Scherdel P, Dunkel L, van Dommelen P, Goulet O, Salaün J-F, Brauner R, et al. Growth monitoring as an early detection tool: a systematic review. Lancet Diabetes Endocrinol. 2016;4(5):447–56.
14. Mairs R, Nicholls D. Assessment and treatment of eating disorders in children and adolescents. Arch Dis Child. 2016;101(12):1168–75.
15. Cadwallader JS, Godart N, Chastang J, Falissard B, Huas C. Detecting eating disorder patients in a general practice setting: a systematic review of heterogeneous data on clinical outcomes and care trajectories. Eat Weight Disord - Stud Anorex Bulim Obes. 2016;21(3):365–81.
16. Campbell K, Peebles R. Eating disorders in children and adolescents: state of the art review. PEDIATRICS. 2014;134(3):582–92.
17. Forman SF, McKenzie N, Hehn R, Monge MC, Kapphahn CJ, Mammel KA, et al. Predictors of outcome at 1 year in adolescents with DSM-5 restrictive eating disorders: report of the National Eating Disorders Quality Improvement Collaborative. J Adolesc Health. 2014;55(6):750–6.
18. Forman SF, Grodin LF, Graham DA, Sylvester CJ, Rosen DS, Kapphahn CJ, et al. An eleven site National Quality Improvement Evaluation of adolescent medicine-based eating disorder programs: predictors of weight outcomes at one year and risk adjustment analyses. J Adolesc Health. 2011;49(6):594–600.
19. Strandjord SE, Sieke EH, Richmond M, Khadilkar A, Rome ES. Medical stabilization of adolescents with nutritional insufficiency: a clinical care path. Eat Weight Disord. 2016;21(3):403–10.
20. Launay E, Cohen J, Bossuyt P, Chalumeau M. Studies on time to diagnosis : proposal of reporting guideline by an international panel. BMC Med. 2016.
21. Anorexie mentale: prise en charge. Recommandations juin 2010. Juin: Recomm HAS; 2010.
22. Golden NH, Katzman DK, Sawyer SM, Ornstein RM, Rome ES, Garber AK, et al. Update on the medical Management of Eating Disorders in adolescents. J Adolesc Health. 2015;56(4):370–5.
23. Rolland-Cachera MF, Cole TJ, Sempé M, Tichet J, Rossignol C, Charraud A. Body mass index variations: centiles from birth to 87 years. Eur J Clin Nutr. 1991;45(1):13–21.
24. Walker T, Watson HJ, Leach DJ, McCormack J, Tobias K, Hamilton MJ, et al. Comparative study of children and adolescents referred for eating disorder treatment at a specialist tertiary setting: eating disorders among children and adolescents. Int J Eat Disord. 2014;47(1):47–53.
25. Strandjord SE, Sieke EH, Richmond M, Rome ES. Refeeding hospitalized patients with eating disorders: does gender matter? J Nutr health food Sci. 2016.
26. Thomson S, Marriott M, Telford K, Law H, McLaughlin J, Sayal K. Adolescents with a diagnosis of anorexia nervosa: parents' experience of recognition and deciding to seek help. Clin Child Psychol Psychiatry. 2014;19(1):43–57.
27. Garcia FD, Grigioni S, Allais E, Houy-Durand E, Thibaut F, Déchelotte P. Detection of eating disorders in patients: validity and reliability of the French version of the SCOFF questionnaire. Clin Nutr. 2011;30(2):178–81.
28. Position Paper of the Society for Adolescent Health and Medicine. Medical Management of Restrictive Eating Disorders in adolescents and young adults. J Adolesc Health. 2015;56(1):121–5.

Evaluation of cognitive function in patients with severe anorexia nervosa before and after medical stabilization

Melanie Rylander[1*], Gillian Taylor[2], Susan Bennett[2], Christopher Pierce[2], Angela Keniston[3] and Philip S. Mehler[4]

Abstract

Background: The purpose of this study was to quantify cognitive deficits in severe anorexia nervosa (AN) before and after medical stabilization.

Methods: This was a prospective study of 40 females between the ages of 18 and 50 admitted to a medical stabilization unit with severe AN (%IBW < 70). The primary outcome of the study was change in test scores on the Repeatable Battery for the Assessment of Neuropsychological Status (RBANS) at baseline and after medical stabilization.

Results: There were no statistically significant differences in baseline RBANS scores between AN patients overall and controls ($p = 0.0940$). There was a statistically significant change in RBANS from baseline 94.1 $\pm$ 12.7 to medical stabilization 97.1 $\pm$ 10.6 ($p = 0.0173$), although notably both mean values fell within the average range. There were no significant differences in baseline RBANS scores between controls and AN-BP patients ($p = 0.3320$) but significant differences were found between controls and AN-R patients ($p = 0.0434$).

Conclusions: No baseline deficits in cognition were found in this sample of women with severe AN.

Keywords: Anorexia nervosa, Malnutrition, Cognition, Refeeding, Starved brain

Plain English summary

This study sought to identify impairments in cognition in women suffering from severe anorexia nervosa (AN), binge purge subtypes (AN-BP) and restricting subtype (AN-R), relative to healthy volunteers. All subjects were patients on a medical refeeding unit with severe illness. Cognitive testing occurred upon entry into the program and at exit. Surprisingly, our study did not find any difference in baseline cognition between patients with AN as a whole and health volunteers. Patients with AN-R had significant improvements in cognition, but this is likely not clinically relevant.

* Correspondence: melanie.rylander@dhha.org
[1]Departments of Internal Medicine and Psychiatry, Denver Health Medical Center, University of Colorado School of Medicine, 777 Bannock St, Denver, CO 80204, USA
Full list of author information is available at the end of the article

Background

Anorexia nervosa (AN) is associated with adverse effects on cognitive functioning in the domains of attention, processing speed, visual and verbal memory, and visuo-spatial construction [1–5], as well as high rates of co-morbid anxiety, depression, and obsessive compulsive disorder [1, 6, 7]. Both mental and physical stabilization are essential for full recovery from AN [8–10]. Several neuropsychological studies that have reported cognitive impairment in individuals with anorexia nervosa before formal treatment subsequently noted improvement in many facets of cognitive functioning following weight restoration [2–5]. However, the findings noted above have been discordant from those of other studies. Two studies found no change in cognitive functioning with weight restoration [11, 12]. Another study found differences in baseline cognition between patients with AN and healthy controls, but no improvement in cognition with weight restoration [13]. Additionally, investigators have found that impairments in the cognitive domain of memory performance persist after weight restoration [14]. The inconsistencies in findings may be due to different patient populations, study designsvarying assessment tools, and patients being studied at different stages of weight recovery. No studies have examined the cognitive function of a patient population with severe AN defined as an ideal body weight less than 70% (%IBW < 70) before and after medical stabilization. The degree to which cognitive function is variably compromised in patients with severe forms of AN remains unknown.

Only two other studies have quantified the difference in change of cognitive function between patients with the two distinct subtypes of AN, the restricting subtype and the binge-purge subtype (R and BP) [3, 14]. These studies report contrasting results. Since medical treatments, lengths of stay, and course of recovery differ for the two groups, compromised cognitive functions in the two populations are likely to differ. No prior studies have examined differences between AN-R and AN-BP in highly medically compromised populations of patients with AN.

The prognosis of AN in adults is poor, with less than half of patients reaching recovery [15]. Standardized mortality ratios for patients with AN range from 4.4–14 [8, 16–18], suggesting that current therapies for AN do not facilitate recovery in the majority of patients. Potentially contributing to poor outcomes, severely ill patients may not be able to fully participate in current standard of care psychotherapies because they are largely cognitive based.

Leptin is an adipokine traditionally thought to be involved in energy regulation [19]. Several studies have found leptin deficiencies in patients with AN and subsequent increases in leptin with refeeding [20–24]. Recently, animal studies have demonstrated that leptin has a role in synaptogensis and neurogenesis in the hippocampus [25–28]. Furthermore, deficits in learning and memory in leptin deficient mice have been corrected with leptin administration [25]. Leptin's observed role in neurogenesis and learning raises questions about whether leptin deficiency is a mediator of cognitive deficits observed in AN.

The primary aims of this study were four-fold:

1) Quantify baseline cognitive deficits in patients with severe AN in the domains of immediate memory, delayed memory visuospatial/constructional, language, and attention. We hypothesized that patients with severe AN would have deficits in these domains relative to healthy controls.
2) Evaluate changes in immediate memory, delayed memory visuospatial/constructional, language, and attention from baseline through the end of acute refeeding and medical stabilization in patients with severe AN. We hypothesized that after medical stabilization performance in the cognitive domains tested in patients with AN would significantly improve.
3) Evaluate and compare baseline and change in immediate memory, delayed memory visuospatial/constructional, language, and attention by AN subtype (binge-purge (BP) vs. restricting (R) after medical stabilization. We hypothesized that cognitive rebound after medical stabilization would be greater in the BP subtype compared to the R subtype in the domains tested.
4) Evaluate correlations between changes in immediate memory, delayed memory, visuospatial/constructional, language, and attention from baseline to medical stabilization with changes in serum leptin levels from baseline to medical stabilization after controlling for changes in weight. We hypothesized there would be a positive correlation between changes in cognitive domains and changes in serum leptin levels after controlling for changes in weight.

This is the first study to evaluate change in cognitive deficits in patients with severe AN, compare differences in cognitive function between AN subtypes, and evaluate leptin as a possible mediator of cognitive impairment in severe malnutrition.

Materials and methods

Patient population

This prospective, single-center, non-randomized design was conducted between July 2016 and October of 2018. All patients (n = 510) between the ages of 18 years and 50 years who presented to the ACUTE Center for Eating Disorders at Denver Health Medical Center were screened for inclusion. Inclusion criteria were chosen to minimize confounders of older age on cognitive function and barriers inherent to conducting cognitive testing in non-English speaking patients. Exclusion criteria were chosen to eliminate patients in whom cognitive testing would not be possible or the results of such testing would be rendered invalid because of comorbid factors known to negatively impact cognition.

Inclusion Criteria included English speaking women between the ages of 18 and 50, a DSM 5 diagnosis of AN-R or AN-BP, and an IBW < 70%. Exclusion criteria included inability to give informed consent, inability to follow study protocol, neurologic disorders including multiple sclerosis, seizure disorders, dementias or mild cognitive impairment, delirium, history of traumatic brain injury, use of anti-epileptic medications, use of lithium, documented or self reported history of intellectual disability, active alcohol/substance use disorder, or alcohol/substance intoxication or withdrawal.

Age and gender matched controls were recruited from electronic and written advertisements sent to university and hospital list serves and posted around campus to match study subjects. Controls were screened for substance use disorders, neurologic disorders, seizure disorders, intellectual disabilities, and use of medications that might impair performance on cognitive testing via interview with a study team member. Controls were screened for eating disorders using Module H of the SCID as well a weight history to rule out those with a history of extreme weights or BMIs.

Study assessments

All patients admitted to ACUTE were given standard of care treatment. Standard of care on the ACUTE unit includes collecting the following information upon admission and throughout hospitalization:

- Demographics
- Medical/Medication History
- Physical Exam
- Standard of Care ACUTE blood work
- Body Height
- Body Weight
- Vital Signs (blood pressure, heart rate, respiratory rate, temperature)
- Concomitant Medications (monitored routinely as per care standard)

Diagnosis of anorexia nervosa was made upon admission using DSM 5 diagnostic criteria by a licensed psychologist who specializes in diagnosis and treatment of eating disorders as per standard work flow on ACUTE [29]. Restricting and binge-purge subtypes were diagnosed upon admission based on current self-reported purging behavior, collateral history from outside sources, physical exam, and routine laboratory data.

Outcomes

The primary outcome of the study was change in test scores on the Repeatable Battery for the Assessment of Neuropsychological Status (RBANS) at baseline and after medical stabilization.

Secondary outcomes included:

- Change in Trail Making Test, Part B/D (TMT-B/D) scores from baseline to medical stabilization
- Wide Range Achievement Test, (W-RAT 4) Word Reading Subtest at baseline
- Change in Beck Depression Inventory (BDI) scores from baseline to medical stabilization
- Change in Beck Anxiety Inventory (BAI) scores from baseline to medical stabilization
- Change in the Obsessive-Compulsive Inventory - Revised (OCI-R) scores from baseline to medical stabilization
- Changes in serum leptin levels and RBANS scores from baseline to medical stabilization after controlling for changes in weight.

Standardized measures

Cognitive function:

- The RBANS [30] is a brief cognitive battery comprised of 12 subtests measuring 5 cognitive domains: immediate memory, delayed memory visuospatial/constructional, language, and attention. Four alternate forms of the RBANS are available, assessing the same cognitive domains with slightly different content. Two versions (Forms A and B) were administered in a counterbalanced fashion to control for order effects when doing longitudinal assessments. For half the patients RBANS A was administered within 3 days of admission to the ACUTE unit and RBANS B was administered once medical stabilization was achieved; the other half were first assessed with RBANS B followed by A.
- TMT-B [31] is a neuropsychological test of visual attention and task switching. TMT-D is an alternative form of TMT-B that can be used to minimize practice effect when doing longitudinal assessments [32].
- WRAT-4 [33] Word Reading Subtest was used to measure cognitive reserve, which is a predication of cognitive capacity before injury or illness, to control for baseline intelligence.
- The BDI [34], BAI [35], and OCI-R [36] were used to control for comorbid psychiatric symptoms that can impact cognition.

Medical stabilization: defined based on ACUTE protocol:

a) The patient is consuming 2000–3000 kcal/day.
b) Laboratory values indicate that end organ failure is resolved or resolving, and refeeding syndrome is no longer a concern.
c) The patient has minimal edema and is physically strong enough to progress to eating disorder treatment programs.
d) The patient is deemed medically stable for discharge by the treating physician.

Sample size

The study required 20 patients in the AN BP group, 20 patients in the AN R group, and 10 controls for a total of 50 participants to test all study hypotheses and detect the pre-stated differences in outcomes. All power calculations assumed a type I error rate of 0.05, standard deviation of 9.4 for baseline RBANS test scores, standard deviation of 15.3 for post medical stabilization RBANS tests scores and a pooled standard deviation of 11.0 for the change in RBANS tests scores. A clinically meaningful difference in RBANS between independent groups was set at 13.1 [3]. A clinically meaningful difference in change in RBANS was set at 5.3 [5].

Sample sizes for testable hypotheses in the research aims were calculated such that the hypothesis test attained 95% power. Depending on the hypothesis, an independent samples t-tests or paired t-tests was used as the test statistic. The largest study sample size was taken as the sample size required to attain 95% power for all testable hypotheses.

Test administration

Psychometric tests were administered within 3 days of admission by a licensed psychologist trained in neuropsychological assessments. Repeat psychometrics were performed by a licensed psychologist trained in neuropsychological assessments upon medical stabilization. All psychological testing was administered the same day as RBANS before and after medical stabilization. Alternate forms of the RBANS and TMT were administered in a counterbalanced manner at baseline and following medical stabilization to minimize any concern for administration order effects.

Quantitative serum leptin levels were obtained via chemiluminescent immunoassay performed by ARUP Laboratories. Leptin levels were obtained upon study entry and medical stabilization. Leptin levels were obtained the same day as psychometric tests were administered. Table 1 outlines the timeline of study specific events. Controls completed baseline psychometric testing and repeat psychometric testing within the same time frame as study patients. Controls did not undergo repeat leptin levels.

Statistical analysis

Patients were categorized by DSM 5 diagnosis of anorexia nervosa (AN) subtype, either binge-purge (AN-BP) or restricting (AN-R). Continuous variables were described using means and standard deviations (SD) or medians and interquartile ranges (IQR) based on tests of normality. Categorical variables were described using counts and frequencies.

Baseline data, specifically height, weight, BMI, and percent ideal body weight, were compared between cases and controls as well as between case subtypes using a Student's t-test. W-RAT 4 for AN patients were compared to control participants using a Student's t-test.

A paired t-test was used to test changes in the TMT-B/D score and Wilcoxon signed rank sum tests were used to evaluate changes in BDI-II total scores, BAI total scores, and OCI-R scores for checking, hoarding,

Table 1 Study Timeline (Testing occurs within 3 days of admission)

Baseline	Medical Stabilization
Standard of Care Covariate information · Demographics · Medical/Medication History · Psychiatric History · Physical Exam · Body Height · Body Weight · BMI · Vital Signs · Complete metabolic panel and blood counts · Serum Prealbumin · Informed Consent	**Standard of Care Covariate information** · Medical/Medication History · Physical Exam · Body Height · Body Weight · BMI · Vital Signs · Complete metabolic panel and blood counts
Psychometric tests: · Wide Range Achievement Test 4, Word Reading Subtest · Repeatable Battery for the Assessment of Neuropsychological Status A or B · Beck Depression Inventory · Beck Anxiety Inventory · Obsessive Compulsive Inventory-Revised · Trail Making Test, Part B or D	**Psychometric tests:** · Repeatable Battery for the Assessment of Neuropsychological Status A or B · Beck Depression Inventory · Beck Anxiety Inventory · Obsessive Compulsive Inventory-Revised · Trail Making Test, Part B or D
Additional biomarker tests: · Serum Leptin	**Additional biomarker tests:** · Serum Leptin
AN-R = 20, AN-BP = 20, Controls = 10	AN-R = 20, AN-BP = 20, Controls = 10 (Psychometric tests only)

neutralizing, obsessing, ordering, and washing from baseline to medical stabilization.

Linear regression modeling was used to assess the correlation between change in RBANS score and change in leptin values from baseline to after medical stabilization for AN patients, after controlling for changes in weight. Pearson Correlation Coefficients were used to assess correlations between improvements in RBANS score and improvements in the BDI-II total score, BAI total score, and OCI-R scores for checking, hoarding, neutralizing, obsessing, ordering, and washing for AN patients and for AN-BP and AN-R patients separately.

P values of < 0.05 were considered statistically significant, and all analyses were done using SAS Enterprise Guide software version 7.1 (SAS Institute, Cary, NC).

Results

During the study period 510 patients were screened for eligibility. Fifty-seven patients met eligibility criteria and 39 patients completed the protocol. Four patients declined to participate in the study (one AN-BP patient and three AN-R patients), five patients were screen failures (four AN-BP patients and one AN-R patient), and nine patients withdrew from the study (five AN-BP patients and four AN-R patients). The average age of patients who did not participate in the study was 29 ± 9 years of age.

Demographic characteristics of cases and controls are listed in Table 2, and anthropometric measurements are displayed in Table 3. There were no statistically significant differences in baseline weight, BMI or percent ideal body weight between AN-BP patients and AN-R patients. Baseline weights, BMI and percent ideal body weight differed significantly between AN-R and AN-BP patients and controls ($p < 0.0001$).

Aim 1: quantify baseline cognitive deficits in patients with severe AN

Results from neuropsychiatric assessments are presented in Table 4. W-RAT 4 scores at baseline for AN patients were compared to control participants using a Student's t-test. No statistically significant differences were found (62.3 ± 4.4 vs. 64.0 ± 4.0, $p = 0.2708$) suggesting no differences in premorbid intelligence. There were no statistically significant difference in baseline RBANS scores between AN patients overall and controls ($p = 0.0940$) or in baseline TMT B/D scores between controls and AN patients overall ($p = 0.125$).

Table 2 Demographic Characteristics of Patients and Controls

	Patients			Controls
	N = 39	AN-BP **N** = 19	AN-R **N** = 20	**N** = 10
Age, Mean ± SD	33 ± 12	35 ± 15	31 ± 10	35 ± 9
Caucasian, N (%)	39 (100)	19 (100)	20 (100)	9 (90)
Hispanic, N (%)	0 (0)	0 (0)	0 (0)	3 (30)
Days Treatment ± SD		15 ± 9	21 ± 10	n/a

Aim 2: evaluate changes in cognitive functions from baseline through the end of acute refeeding and medical stabilization in patients with severe AN

For AN patients overall, there was a statistically significant change in RBANS from baseline (94.1 ± 12.6) to medical stabilization (97.1 ± 10.6) ($p = 0.0173$), although notably both mean values fell within the average range. When RBANS subscores were analyzed, only coding, story memory, and story recall showed statistically significant increases from baseline in AN patients as a whole ($p < 0.004$) (Table 5). No statistically significant change was found for control patients from baseline to post testing ($p = 0.1955$). No statistically significant change was found in TMT B/D scores from baseline through medical stabilization for AN patients as a whole.

Statistically significant decreases in BDI and BAI scores were found for all AN patients ($p < .0001$). No statistically significant correlations were found between increases in RBANS score and changes in BDI or BAI scores for AN patients overall. Overall, AN patients showed significant decreases from baseline to medical stabilization in the OCI-R domains of checking ($p < 0.05$), obsessing ($p < 0.05$), hoarding ($p < 0.02$), neutralizing ($p < 0.02$), and washing ($p < 0.02$). No correlations between changes in RBANS score and OCI-R domains were found for AN patients overall. Controls did not show significant changes in OCI-R domains.

Aim 3: evaluate and compare baseline and change in cognitive functions by AN subtype (binge-purge (BP) vs. restricting (R) after medical stabilization

There were no significant differences in baseline RBANS scores between controls (101.6 ± 11.7) and AN-BP patients (97.2 ± 11.4) ($p = 0.3320$) but significant differences were found between controls (101.6 ± 11.7) and AN-R patients (91.1 ± 13.3) ($p = 0.0434$). There were no significant differences between baseline TMT B/D scores in control versus AN-BP ($p = 0.3881$) or AN-R patients ($p = 0.0628$). In subgroup analysis, statistically significant changes in RBANS score from baseline to medical stabilization were found for AN-R patients ($p = 0.0091$) but not AN-BP patients ($p = 0.4862$). In addition, statistically significant changes in TMT B/D scores from baseline to medical stabilization were found for AN-R patients but not AN-BP patients ($p = 0.0094$ and $p = 0.0995$, respectively).

Statistically significant improvements in BDI and BAI scores were found for both AN-BP and AN-R patients

Table 3 Anthropometric Measurements of Patients and Controls

	Patients						Controls
	N = 39		AN-BP **N** = 19		AN-R **N** = 20		**N** = 10
	Pre	Post	Pre	Post	Pre	Post	Pre
Height, Mean ± SD	64.7 ± 2.7		64.2 ± 2.6		65.0 ± 2.7		64.2 ± 2.7
Weight (kgs), Mean ± SD	34.4 ± 4.8	41.0 ± 4.9	34.7 ± 5.0	41.3 ± 5.4	34.1 ± 4.8	40.7 ± 4.5	63.8 ± 9.0
BMI, Mean ± SD	12.7 ± 1.1	14.6 ± 1.2	12.9 ± 1.2	14.8 ± 1.2	12.5 ± 1.1	14.4 ± 1.3	24.0 ± 3.6*
% Ideal Body Weight	61 ± 5*	73 ± 4*	62 ± 5*	75 ± 5*	60 ± 5*	72 ± 3*	117 ± 20

*$P < 0.0001$difference relative to controls

($p < 0.001$). No statistically significant correlations were found between improvements in RBANS score and changes in BDI or BAI scores for AN-BP or AN-R patients. For OCI-R domains, subgroup analysis showed significant changes in AN-R patients in the domains of checking ($p < 0.05$), obsessing ($p < 0.05$), hoarding ($p < 0.001$, and neutralizing ($p < 0.0035$). AN-BP patients showed significant reductions in checking ($p < 0.05$) and obsessing ($p < 0.05$). Across domains of the OCI-R (checking, hoarding, neutralizing, obsessing, ordering,

Table 4 Neuropsychiatric Assessments

	Patients						Controls	
	N = 39		AN-BP **N** = 19		AN-R **N** = 20		**N** = 10	
	Baseline	Post	Baseline	Post	Baseline	Post	Baseline	Post
Wide Range Achievement Test (W-RAT 4) Word Reading Subtest, Mean ± SD	62.3 ± 4.4		62.4 ± 4.5		62.3 ± 4.5		64.0 ± 4.0	
Repeatable Battery for the Assessment of Neuropsychological Status (RBANS) Total Score, Mean ± SD	94.1 ± 12.6	97.1 ± 10.6*	97.2 ± 11.4	98.4 ± 11.4	91.1 ± 13.3**	95.8 ± 10.0*	101.6 ± 11.7	105.3 ± 8.8
Beck Depression Inventory (BDI-II) Total Score, Median (IQR)	35 (30, 42)	20 (13, 28)*	33 (30, 39)	20 (15, 29)*	38 (29.5, 45)	19.5 (10, 26)*	3.5 (1, 5)	1 (0, 3)
Beck Anxiety Inventory (BAI) Total Score, Median (IQR)	25 (17, 33)	19 (12, 24)*	23 (14, 31)	19 (10, 21)*	29 (18.5, 40)	17.5 (14, 26.5)*	3 (1, 4)	1.5 (0, 4)
Trail Making Test, Part B Score, Mean ± SD	34.7 ± 10.5	39.5 ± 10.5	37.4 ± 8.6	40.8 ± 10.1	32.2 ± 11.7	38.2 ± 10.9*	40.4 ± 9.2	44.2 ± 6.1
Obsessive Compulsive Inventory – Revised (OCI-R), Median (IQR)								
Checking	3 (2, 4)	2 (0, 3)*	3 (2, 6)	1 (0, 4) *	2 (1.5, 4)	2 (0.5, 2.5) *	0 (0, 0)	0 (0, 0)
Hoarding	4 (1, 6)	2 (0, 4)*	3 (0, 6)	2 (0, 6)	5 (1, 6)	2 (0, 2.5)*	1.5 (0, 3)	1 (0, 3)
Neutralizing	3 (1, 7)	1 (0, 6)*	1 (0, 6)	1 (0, 6)	5 (2, 7.5)	1.5 (0.5, 3.5)*	0 (0, 0)	0 (0, 0)
Obsessing	7 (3, 10)	3 (2, 7)*	6 (2, 10)	4 (1, 7)*	7 (3, 9.5)	3 (2, 7.5)*	1 (0, 3)	0 (0, 2)
Ordering	7 (5, 11)	6 (4, 9)	8 (5, 11)	7 (3, 9)	7 (4, 11)	6 (4, 11)	1.5 (0, 3)	2.5 (0, 3)
Washing	2 (0, 7)	1 (0, 4)*	2 (0, 7)	1 (0, 6)	1.5 (1, 7)	1.5 (0, 3.5)	0 (0, 0)	0 (0, 0)
Leptin Level (ng/mL), N (%)								
< 0.4	**31 (79)**	**19 (49)**	**16 (84)**	**10 (53)**	**15 (75)**	**9 (45)**		
0.4–1.0	7 (18)	10 (26)	3 (16)	6 (32)	4 (20)	7 (35)		
> 1.0	1 (3)	7 (18)	0 (0)	2 (11)	1 (5)	2 (10)		
< 6.0							4 (40)	
6.0–10.0							2 (20)	
> 11.0							3 (30)	
Increase in Leptin Level, N (%)	14 (36)		6 (32)		8 (40)			

*$P < 0.05$ change from baseline
**$P < 0.05$ relative to baseline of controls

Table 5 RBANS Subscores

	Cases						Controls	
	N = 39		AN-BP **N** = 19		AN-R **N** = 20		Controls **N** = 10	
	Pre	Post	Pre	Post	Pre	Post	Pre	Post
Repeatable Battery for the Assessment of Neuropsychological Status (RBANS), Mean ± SD								
List Learning Total Score	30 ± 5	31 ± 3	31 ± 5	32 ± 3	30 ± 5	30 ± 4	31 ± 3	31 ± 3
Story Memory Total Score	15 ± 4	18 ± 3*	16 ± 4	19 ± 3*	15 ± 4	17 ± 3	19 ± 3	19.5 ± 2
Figure Cope Total Score	19 ± 2	19 ± 1	19 ± 1	19 ± 1	19 ± 2	19 ± 2	19 ± 1	19 ± 1
Line Orientation Total Score	17 ± 3	18 ± 2	17 ± 3	17 ± 2	17 ± 3	18 ± 2	18 ± 2	17.5 ± 2
Picture Naming Total Score	10 ± 1	10 ± 1	9 ± 1	10 ± 1	10 ± 1	10 ± 1	10 ± 0	10 ± 1
Semantic Fluency Total Score	24 ± 5	24 ± 6	25 ± 5	23 ± 6	23 ± 5	25 ± 5	23 ± 4	23 ± 2
Digit Span Total Score	10 ± 2	10 ± 2	10 ± 2	10 ± 2	10 ± 2	10 ± 2	11 ± 2	12 ± 2
Coding Total Score	50 ± 10	54 ± 10*	51 ± 8	55 ± 9	49 ± 13	54 ± 11	55 ± 10	61 ± 9
List Recall Total Score	7 ± 2	7 ± 2	7 ± 2	7 ± 1	8 ± 2	7 ± 2	8 ± 2	8 ± 3
List Recognition Total Score	20 ± 1	19 ± 1	19 ± 1	19 ± 1	20 ± 1	19 ± 1	20 ± 1	19.5 ± 1
Story Recall Total Score	9 ± 2	10 ± 2*	10 ± 2	10 ± 2	8 ± 2	10 ± 2*	10 ± 1	11 ± 1
Figure Recall Total Score	15 ± 4	16 ± 3	16 ± 2	17 ± 2	15 ± 4	15 ± 3	15.5 ± 4	17 ± 2

*$P < 0.004$, adjusted for multiple comparisons

and washing), we found a statistically significant correlation between improvements in RBANS and improvement in the washing domain ($p = 0.0432$) for AN-R patients only. No other correlations between changes in RBANS score and all other OCI-R domains were found in subgroup analysis.

Aim 4: evaluate the correlation between changes in cognition from baseline to medical stabilization with changes in serum leptin levels from baseline to medical stabilization after controlling for changes in weight

Comparing AN patients and controls, there was no statistically significant difference in change in leptin from baseline to medical stabilization ($p = 0.1573$). Subgroup analysis showed similar findings. There was no difference in the proportion of AN-BP patients relative to control with change in leptin levels ($p = 0.1266$) or between controls and AN-R patients ($p = 0.4197$). After controlling for changes in weight, increases in RBANS score from baseline to after medical stabilization were not significantly associated with increases in leptin from baseline to medical stabilization for AN patients overall ($p = 0.9661$) or for either AN-BP patients ($p = 0.9437$) or AN-R ($p = 0.9608$) patients.

Discussion

General

This is the first study to examine cognitive deficits in patients with severe AN before and after medical stabilization. Our population is unique in the severity of malnutrition as evident in their admission %IBW as well as their stage of treatment at the time of enrollment. No prior studies have examined patients during acute refeeding on a medical inpatient setting.

Our study has several noteworthy findings. We found significantly lower admission cognitive scores in patients with severe AN-R relative to healthy controls and statistically significant increases in cognition after refeeding. The clinical significance of these differences is questionable. Normative data indicates RBANS Index scores of 90–109 are within the average range [37]. Both subgroups of patients and controls fell into this range at baseline and post testing. Although we hypothesized that cognitive deficits would interfere with the ability of patients in acute stages of illness to participate in cognitive based therapies, our data provides only limited support at best for this possibility. Analysis of subscores also did not show significant baseline deficits between patients and controls.

We found no differences in cognition between patients with AN-BP and healthy controls as measured by RBANS and TMT. Several previous studies demonstrating cognitive impairment in patients with AN have not investigated potential differences in diagnostic subtypes [2, 4, 11]. The lack of observed difference in baseline cognition between AN-BP and healthy controls was surprising given the significant differences in body weight. As we discuss below, body weight is likely not a complete proxy for nutritional status.

Though cognitive scores improved in our total patient cohort, subgroup analysis revealed that these improvements were only observed in patients with AN-R. The lack of significant improvement in AN-BP patients was not unexpected given the absence of significant baseline impairments. The improvements in AN-R patients remained significant after controlling for changes in BAI, BDI, and OCI-R scores suggesting improvement in comorbid psychiatric symptoms did not account for improvements in cognition. The noted improvement in AN-R patients cannot be attributed to poorer nutritional status at baseline as measured by body weight as we found no significant difference between patients with AN-R and AN-BP in admission BMI or %IBW.

These findings suggest that weight is not a complete proxy for malnutrition, and other factors beyond simple weight or broader nutritional status likely impact cognition. Other potentially important physiological differences may exist between these two subgroups. Restrictors tend to have long and enduring periods of starvation whereas those with binge-purge patterns often weather peaks and valleys of nutritional intake; they might not be subjected to the chronicity and intensity of deprivation experienced by AN-R patients. Regular caloric consumption that occurs during acute refeeding might constitute larger deviations from baseline for patients with AN-R compared to AN-BP, and might thereby facilitate more rapid improvement in cognitive status.

Though several prior studies have examined cognitive deficits in AN, many used adolescent populations, cross sectional designs, or different assessment methods [2, 4, 11–14, 38]. Three previous studies examined cognitive impairment in adults with AN using RBANS [3, 5, 39]. However, Keifer et al. [3] and [5] used the same patient cohort. Since Keifer et al. [3] broke the cohort into AN subtypes we will further examine their results in reference to ours in addition to evaluating those of Mikos et al. (2008) [39].

Keifer et al. found improvements in RBANS scores after treatment only in patients with AN-BP, which our opposite to our findings. However, our studies differ in several ways. Our patients were tested at significantly lower BMIs (BMI at baseline 12.7 ± 1.1 and stabilization 14.6 ± 1.2 compared to baseline 16.58 ± 2.49 and post treatment 19.28 ± 1.49 in [3]). Unexpectedly, both our AN-R and AN-BP patients had higher baseline RBANS scores than those of Keifer et al. [3]. Since the opposite would be expected given poorer nutritional status observed in our population as measured by BMI and %IBW it is difficult to account for the differences observed between our study and that of Keifer et al. [3].

Mikos et al. (2008) [39] did not show significant improvements in RBANS scores from admission to discharge though they did not break their population into subtypes and their admission BMI was much higher than our's at 17.09. They did find significant differences in admission RBANS scores and scores at 2 year follow up. We have not followed our cohort long enough to determine if we would see similar findings. Despite lower BMI, our AN-BP patients had higher RBANS scores than the cohort of Mikos et al. (2008) [39] though our AN-R patient's showed similar scores. These results again come as suprising given differences in BMI in our respective populations.

We found no relationship between changes in cognition and serum leptin levels, suggesting the adipokine does not mediate the measured cognitive domains assessed in this study. However, our study was not designed or powered to specifically detect this outcome and our conclusions in this regard are therefore limited.

Limitations

Our study has several limitations. First, to measure cognition we used RBANS rather than more comprehensive and perhaps more sensitive assessments. However, our patient population would have had difficulty tolerating lengthier and comprehensive testing batteries given significant weakness and fatigue observed for BMIs averaging 12.7. The time between initial testing and repeat testing for our patients was generally between 1 and 3 weeks, significantly shorter than testing intervals in previous studies which have ranged from 1 to 12 months ([2–4, 11]). However, we were interested in the impact of acute refeeding, a shorter process than residential or outpatient treatment. The study most consistent with ours regarding timeframe is that of Keifer et al. [3], although our results differed as discussed above. Our final study population included only 39 patients as opposed to the original power calculation requiring 40 patients. However, inclusion of one additional patient is unlikely to have majorly altered our findings.

Strengths of our study include our unique patient population with regard to low weights and medical acuities. We also employed a control group which was not used by Keifer et al. [3]. Our analyses looked at differences in diagnostic subgroups and controlled for comorbid symptoms of anxiety and depression which previous studies have neglected ([2–4, 11]).

Conclusion

In summary, our study showed no clinically meaningful decrements in cognitive functioning in a large cohort of significantly malnourished patients with anorexia nervosa. We found statistically significant increases in cognitive test scores amongst patients with AN-R relative to healthy controls after acute refeeding that were independent of improvements in comorbid psychiatric symptoms and unrelated to changes in serum leptin levels. These findings argue against theoretical concerns regarding cognitive function in severely ill patients.

Abbreviations

AN: Anorexia nervosa; AN-BP: Anorexia nervosa, binge purge subtype; AN-R: Anorexia nervosa, restrincting subtype; BAI: Beck Anxiety Inventory; BDI: Beck Depression Inventory; BMI: Body mass index; DSM: Diagnostic and Statistical Manual; IBW: Ideal body weight; OCI: Obsessive compulsive inventory; RBANS: Repeatable Battery for the Assessment of Neuropsychological Status; TMT – B/D: Trail Making Test, Part B/D; WRAT: Wide range achievement test

Acknowledgments

The authors would like to acknowledge the assistance of the following individuals: Tiffany Bendelow, BA, MPH,, Jodie Benabe, PsyD, John Brinton, PhD, Hilde Heyn, Robert M. House, MD, Lauren McBeth, BA, MD, David S. Resch, MD, Joel Yager, MD, Jodi B. Zik, MD.

Authors' contributions

MR was involved in study conceptualization, design, data curation, data analysis and/or interpretation, manuscript preparation and revisions, and have approved this draft. GL was involved in study conceptualization, design, data curation, data analysis and/or interpretation, manuscript preparation and revisions, and have approved this draft. SB was involved in study conceptualization, design, data curation, data analysis and/or interpretation, manuscript preparation and revisions, and have approved this draft. CP was involved in study conceptualization, design, data curation, data analysis and/ or interpretation, manuscript preparation and revisions, and have approved this draft. AK was involved in study conceptualization, design, data curation, data analysis and/or interpretation, manuscript preparation and revisions, and have approved this draft. PM was involved in study conceptualization, design, data curation, data analysis and/or interpretation, manuscript preparation and revisions, and have approved this draft.

Competing interests

The authors have no competing interests to declare.

Author details

[1]Departments of Internal Medicine and Psychiatry, Denver Health Medical Center, University of Colorado School of Medicine, 777 Bannock St, Denver, CO 80204, USA. [2]Department of Psychiatry, Denver Health Medical Center, University of Colorado School of Medicine, Denver, CO 80204, USA. [3]Department of Internal Medicine, University of Colorado School of Medicine, Denver, CO 80204, USA. [4]ACUTE Center for Eating Disorders, Denver Health Medical Center, University of Colorado School of Medicine, Denver, CO 80204, USA.

References

1. Brand-Gothelf A, Leor S, Apter A, Fennig S. The impact of comorbid depressive and anxiety disorders on severity of anorexia nervosa in adolescent girls. J Nerv Ment Dis. 2014;202(10):759–62. https://doi.org/10.1097/NMD.0000000000000194.
2. Hatch A, Madden S, Kohn MR, Clarke S, Touyz S, Gordon E, Williams LM. In first presentation adolescent anorexia nervosa, do cognitive markers of underweight status change with weight gain following a refeeding intervention? Int J Eat Disord. 2010;43(4):295–306. https://doi.org/10.1002/eat.20695.
3. Keifer E, Duff K, Beglinger LJ, Barstow E, Andersen A, Moser DJ. Predictors of neuropsychological recovery in treatment for anorexia nervosa. Eat Disord. 2010;18(4):302–17. https://doi.org/10.1080/10640266.2010.490120.
4. Lozano-Serra E, Andres-Perpina S, Lazaro-Garcia L, Castro-Fornieles J. Adolescent anorexia nervosa: cognitive performance after weight recovery. J Psychosom Res. 2014;76(1):6–11. https://doi.org/10.1016/j.jpsychores.2013.10.009.
5. Moser DJ, Benjamin ML, Bayless JD, McDowell BD, Paulsen JS, Bowers WA, et al. Neuropsychological functioning pretreatment and posttreatment in an inpatient eating disorders program. Int J Eat Disord. 2003;33(1):64–70. https://doi.org/10.1002/eat.10108.
6. Halmi KA, Eckert E, Marchi P, Sampugnaro V, Apple R, Cohen J. Comorbidity of psychiatric diagnoses in anorexia nervosa. Arch Gen Psychiatry. 1991; 48(8):712–8.
7. Kaye WH, Bulik CM, Thornton L, Barbarich N, Masters K. Comorbidity of anxiety disorders with anorexia and bulimia nervosa. Am J Psychiatry. 2004; 161(12):2215–21. https://doi.org/10.1176/appi.ajp.161.12.2215.
8. Franko DL, Keshaviah A, Eddy KT, Krishna M, Davis MC, Keel PK, Herzog DB. A longitudinal investigation of mortality in anorexia nervosa and bulimia nervosa. Am J Psychiatry. 2013;170(8):917–25.
9. Long CG, Fitzgerald KA, Hollin CR. Treatment of chronic anorexia nervosa: a 4-year follow-up of adult patients treated in an acute inpatient setting. Clin Psychol Psychother. 2012;19(1):1–13. https://doi.org/10.1002/cpp.738.
10. Wentz E, Gillberg IC, Anckarsäter H, Gillberg C, Råstam M. Adolescent-onset anorexia nervosa: 18-year outcome. Br J Psychiatry. 2009;194(2):168–74.
11. Green MW, Elliman NA, Wakeling A, Rogers PJ. Cognitive functioning, weight change and therapy in anorexia nervosa. J Psychiatr Res. 1996;30(5): 401–10.
12. Kingston K, Szmukler G, Andrewes D, Tress B, Desmond P. Neuropsychological and structural brain changes in anorexia nervosa before and after refeeding. Psychol Med. 1996;26(1):15–28.
13. Kjaersdam TG, Fagerlund B, Jepsen JR, Bentz M, Christiansen E, Valentin JB, Thomsen PH. Are weight status and cognition associated? An examinatin of cognitive development in children and adolescents with anorexia nervosa 1 year after first hospitalization. Eur Eat Disord Rev. 2016;24(5):366–76. https://doi.org/10.1002/erv.2445.
14. Nikendei C, Funiok C, Pfuller U, Zastrow A, Aschenbrenner S, Weisbrod M, et al. Memory performance in acute and weight-restored anorexia nervosa patients. Psychol Med. 2011;41(4):829–38. https://doi.org/10.1017/S0033291710001121.
15. Steinhausen HC. The outcome of anorexia nervosa in the 20th century. Am J Psychiatr. 2002;159(8):1284–93.
16. Arcelus J, Mitchell AJ, Wales J, Nielsen S. Mortality rates in patients with anorexia nervosa and other eating disorders. A meta-analysis of 36 studies. Arch Gen Psychiatry. 2011;68(7):724–31. https://doi.org/10.1001/archgenpsychiatry.2011.74.
17. Hoang U, Goldacre M, James A. Mortality following hospital discharge with a diagnosis of eating disorder: national record linkage study, England, 2001-2009. Int J Eating Disord. 2014;47(5):507–15.
18. Huas C, Caille A, Godart N, Foulon C, Pham-Scottez A, Divac S, et al. Factors predictive of ten-year mortality in severe anorexia nervosa patients. Acta Psychiatr Scand. 2011;123(1):62–70.
19. Ahima RS, Flier JS. Leptin. Annu Rev Physiol. 2000;62:413–37. https://doi.org/10.1146/annurev.physiol.62.1.413.
20. Eckert ED, Pomeroy C, Raymond N, Kohler PF, Thuras P, Bowers CY. Leptin in anorexia nervosa. J Clin Endocrinol Metab. 1998;83:791–5. https://doi.org/10.1210/jc.83.3.791.
21. Haas V, Onur S, Paul T, Nutzinger DO, Bosy-Westphal A, Hauer M, et al. Leptin and body weight regulation in patients with anorexia nervosa before and during weight recovery. Am J Clin Nutr. 2005;81:889–96 doi:81/4/889 [pii].
22. Haluzík M, Papežová H, Nedvídková J, Kábrt J. Serum leptin levels in patients with anorexia nervosa before and after partial refeeding, relationships to serum lipids and biochemical nutritional parameters. Physiol Res. 1999;48: 197–202.
23. Hebebrand J, Blum WF, Barth N, Coners H, Englaro P, Juul A, et al. Leptin levels in patients with anorexia nervosa are reduced in the acute stage and elevated upon short-term weight restoration. Mol Psychiatry. 1997;2:330–4. https://doi.org/10.1038/sj.mp.4000282.
24. Monteleone P, Di Lieto A, Tortorella A, Longobardi N, Maj M. Circulating leptin in patients with anorexia nervosa, bulimia nervosa or binge-eating disorder: relationship to body weight, eating patterns, psychopathology and endocrine changes. Psychiatry Res. 2000;94:121–9. https://doi.org/10.1016/S0165-1781(00)00144-X.
25. Dagon Y, Avraham Y, Magen I, Gertler A, Ben-Hur T, Berry EM. Nutritional status, cognition, and survival: a new role for leptin and AMP kinase. J Biol Chem. 2005;280:42142–8. https://doi.org/10.1074/jbc.M507607200.
26. Dhar M, Wayman G a, Zhu M, Lambert TJ, Davare M a, Appleyard SM. Leptin-induced spine formation requires TrpC channels and the CaM kinase Cascade in the Hippocampus. J Neurosci. 2014a;34:10022–33. https://doi.org/10.1523/JNEUROSCI.2868-13.2014.
27. Dhar, M., Zhu, M., Impey, S., Lambert, T. J., Bland, T., Karatsoreos, I. N., … Wayman, G. A. (2014b). Leptin induces hippocampal synaptogenesis via CREB-regulated MicroRNA-132 suppression of p250GAP. Mol Endocrinol (Baltimore, Md.), 28, 1073–87. doi:https://doi.org/10.1210/me.2013-1332.
28. Morrison CD. Leptin signaling in brain: a link between nutrition and cognition? Biochim Biophys Acta Mol basis Dis. 2009. https://doi.org/10.1016/j.bbadis.2008.12.004.

29. American Psychiatric, A., & Force, D. S. M. T. (2013). Diagnostic and statistical manual of mental disorders : DSM-5. Retrieved from http://dsm.psychiatryonline.org/book.aspx?bookid=556.
30. Randolph C. Repeatable battery for the assessment of neuropsychological status update (RBANS update). San Antonio: Psychological Corporation; 2012.
31. Reitan R. The relation of the trail making test to organic brain damage. J Consult Psychol. 1955;19(5):393–4.
32. DesRosiers G, Kavanagh D. Cognitive assessment in closed head injury: stability, validity and parallel forms for two neuropsychological measures of recovery. Int J Clin Neuropsychol. 1987;9:162–73.
33. Wilkinson GS, Robertson GJ. Wide range achievement test 4: professional manual. Lutz, FL: Psychological Assessment Resources; 2006.
34. Beck AT, Steer RA, Brown GK. Beck depression inventory–second edition: manual. San Antonio: Psychological Corporation; 1996.
35. Beck AT, Steer RA. Beck anxiety inventory: manual. San Antonio: Psychological Corporation; 1990.
36. Foa EB, Kozak MJ, Salkovskis PM, Coles ME, Amir N. The validation of a new obsessive-compulsive disorder scale: the obsessive-compulsive inventory. Psychol Assess. 1998;10(3):206–14.
37. Randolph C, Tierney MC, Mohr E, Chase TN. The repeatable battery for the assessment of neuropsychological status (RBANS): preliminary clinical validity. J Clin Exp Neuropsychol. 1998;20(3):310–9. https://doi.org/10.1076/jcen.20.3.310.823.
38. Harper JA, Broderick B, Van Enkevort E, McAdams CJ. Neuropsycholigcal and cognitive correlates of recovery in anorexia nervosa. Eur Eat Disorder Rev. 2017;25(6):491–500.
39. Mikos A, McDowell B, Moser D, Bayless J, Bowers W, ANserson A, Paulson J. Stability of neuropsychological performance in anorexia nervosa. Ann.Clin Psychiatry. 2008;20(1):9–13.

11

Echocardiographic abnormalities in 124 severely malnourished adult anorexia nervosa patients: frequency and relationship with body composition and biological features

Mouna Hanachi[1,2*], Annabel Pleple[1], Caroline Barry[3], Marika Dicembre[1], Emilie Latour[1], Maeva Duquesnoy[1], Jean-Claude Melchior[1,2,3] and Abdallah Fayssoil[4]

Abstract

Background: Anorexia Nervosa (AN) is a complex psychiatric disorder that can lead to specific somatic complications. Heart abnormalities are frequently reported, while their frequency and associated factors in severely malnourished AN patients remain poorly defined.

Objectives: This study aimed to characterize echocardiographic abnormalities in severely malnourished AN patients and to assess associated clinical, biological and related body composition features.

Methods: Between January 2013 and January 2015, all severely malnourished adult patients with AN (Mental Disorders, 4th Edn.-DSM IVr) were included in a monocentric study performed in in a highly specialized AN inpatient unit. Electrocardiogram (ECG) and echocardiography were used to assess both heart rhythm and function. All inpatients underwent a Doppler echocardiography procedure after undergoing combined blood volume adjustment, micronutrients deficiencies supplementation and electrolyte disorders correction. Right Ventricular (RV) and Left Ventricular (LV) systolic and diastolic functions were collected and compared to 29 healthy normal subjects in a control group.

Results: One hundred and 24 patients (119 (96%) women, 5 (4%) men) with a mean age of 30.1 ± 11 years old and an average Body Mass Index (BMI) of 12 kg/m^2 were included. Ninety patients (73%) had been diagnosed with AN Restrictive type (AN-R), 34 (27%) an AN Binge eating/Purging type (AN-BP). Eighteen patients (15%) disclosed an abnormal Left Ventricular Ejection Fraction (LVEF) (< 52% for male and < 54% for female). LVEF impairment was associated with AN-BP patients ($p < 0.017$) and hypertransaminasemia (AST and/or ALT ≥2 N) ($p < 0.05$). Left Ventricular mass (LV mass) and Left Ventricular End Diastolic Diameter (LVEDD) were significantly reduced in patients ($p < 0.001$, $p < 0.001$). Left and right ventricular tissue Doppler Imaging Velocities (TDI) peak were reduced
(Continued on next page)

* Correspondence: mouna.hanachi@aphp.fr
[1]Clinical Nutrition Unit, Raymond Poincaré Hospital (AP-HP), Garches, France
[2]Université de Versailles, Saint-Quentin-en-Yvelines, Montigny-le-Bretonneux, Versailles, France
Full list of author information is available at the end of the article

(Continued from previous page)
in patients: Septal and Lateral LV Sm velocities peaks respectively 10 ± 2 cm/s (vs 14 ± 2 cm/s in controls, $p < 0.001$), 12 ± 3 cm/s (vs 16 ± 3 cm/s in controls, $p < 0.001$), basal RV Sm velocity peaks at 14 ± 3 cm/s (vs 19 ± 3 cm/s in controls, $p < 0.001$). Additionally, LV and RV diastolic velocity peaks were reduced: LV septal and lateral velocity peaks were respectively 13 ± 3 cm/s (vs 18 ± 2 cm/s $p < 0.001$), 12 ± 3 cm/s (vs 22 ± 4 cm/s, $p < 0.001$) and RV diastolic velocity peaks at 14 ± 3 cm/s (vs 21 ± 4 cm/s $p < 0.001$). LV diastolic velocity TDI peaks were significantly associated with hypertransaminasemia ($p < 0.05$) and tended to be associated with a low all body Fat-Free Mass Index (FFMI) (using Dual-energy X- ray Absorptiometry (DXA) (HOLOGICQDR 4500) ($p = 0.056$). Thirty-four patients (27%) had a pericardial effusion and were significantly associated with a decreased all body FFMI ($p < 0.036$).

Conclusion: Heart abnormalities are frequent in malnourished patients with AN, particularly in AN-BP type. Both liver enzymes and body composition abnormalities tended to be associated with heart dysfunction (non-significant association). Prospective studies are needed to better characterize and describe the evolution of cardiac abnormalities during the refeeding period and subsequent weight restoration.

Keywords: Heart abnormalities, Anorexia nervosa, Malnutrition, Echocardiography, Body composition

Plain English summary

AN is a complex and severe eating disorder that affects 1–2.2% of young women. Its mortality rate is high, up to 12 times compared that of the general population. AN is defined as either an inability to maintain adequate dietary intakes associated with an intense fear of gaining weight or becoming fat, or a persistent behavior preventing weight gain and causing interference with body image.

Dietary restriction can cause undernutrition and serious medical complications such as heart abnormalities, which are frequent yet poorly defined.

We aimed to characterize echocardiographic abnormalities in severely malnourished patients suffering from AN and to assess associated clinical, biological and related body composition features. Results support that heart abnormalities are frequent in malnourished patients with AN (BMI < 12), particularly in the AN-BP type. Liver enzyme levels were associated with heart dysfunction. Body composition abnormalities tended to be associated with heart dysfunction. Our outcomes suggested that echocardiography may be performed in all severe malnourished AN-BP type patients on presentation, in order to diagnose and manage heart-related abnormalities, thereby reducing potential complications.

Prospective studies are needed to describe the evolution of these abnormalities after weight recovery.

Introduction

Anorexia Nervosa (AN) currently affects 1% of young women [1]. With a mortality rate of 12 times that of the general population [2], AN is considered to be one of the most serious psychiatric eating disorders [1]. AN is defined as an inability to maintain adequate dietary intakes, to maintain normal weight for age, associated with an intense fear of gaining weight or becoming fat, or persistent behavior that interferes with weight gain and disturbances of the body image [3]. Two sub-types of AN are described, the pure restricting sub-type (AN-R), and the binge-eating/purging sub-type (AN-BP), combined with cycles of large meals that are followed by purging behaviors (vomiting and/or laxative abuse [3].

Serious medical complications have been reported, including electrolyte disorders, hematologic disorders [4], severe bone loss, fractures [5] and liver abnormalities [6]. Clinical and biological severity factors have been identified [7], including the reported complication of abnormalities affecting heart function [8]. The frequency of heart abnormalities varied between 0 and 76% depending on studies and may include myocardial dysfunction [9], arrhythmia, prolongation of the QT interval and sudden death [10]. The risk factors, pathophysiology and the cause for heart abnormalities observed in patients with AN remain under-investigated [11, 12].

In this study, we aimed to characterize echocardiographic abnormalities in extremely severe malnourished patients suffering from AN and to assess associated clinical, biological and related body composition features.

Materials and methods

We conducted a retrospective study of all malnourished patients with AN (according to DSM IVr) [13] hospitalized for nutritional rehabilitation at Raymond Poincaré University Hospital, Garches; the largest specialized nutrition unit in France.

Data were collected for the time period between January 2013 and January 2015 and included patients with the following criteria: AN patients aged ≥16 years-old, BMI < 16 [14] with either a AN-R or AN-BP type. We excluded all patients with pre-existing heart or thromboembolic disease, inflammatory or septic disorders, hyper or hypothyroidism, and any pathology that might be associated with heart disease such as diabetes, infectious diseases and/or chronic inflammatory disease. ECG and echocardiography were used as tests of heart rhythm and function. Patients were compared to a control group of 29 healthy subjects, and were selected from the medical and paramedical staff in nutrition unit of Raymond Poincaré University Hospital (Garches, France). The control group underwent Doppler echocardiography performed by the same operator (AF) as for AN patients to reduce operator error.

Patient management

During the first 48 h after admission, all patients underwent standard progressive enteral feeding, using standard polymeric enteral nutrition products, combined with initial intravenous supplementation of vitamins, phosphorus and trace elements. This therapeutic protocol was initially recommended by the NICE (National Institute for Health and Clinical Excellence) in the UK [7] and was subsequently confirmed by French National Health Authority (HAS) guidelines [15].

In cases where the BMI was below 12 and the patient exhibited hypophosphatemia at admission, patients were fasted, hydrated intravenously and given micronutrient supplements for the first 24 h. After the hydration period, enteral nutrition was initiated according HAS (France) and NICE (UK) recommendations, to avoid the occurrence of refeeding syndrome (RS) [16].

Enteral feeding was started gradually with the administration of 10 kcal / kilogram of body weight / day, followed by a gradual increase depending on clinical status and phosphatemia [17, 18]. No patients received parenteral nutrition. Oral nutrition was initiated gradually depending on the evolution of body weight under enteral refeeding by nasogastric tube. Clinical and biological data were collected weekly for 1 month.

Studied parameters

For each patient the following clinical data were collected at admission: age, gender, AN types, height and weight. Blood biological parameters collected were as follows: Aspartate Transaminase (AST), Alanine Transaminase (ALT), Gamma Glutamyl- Transpeptidase (GGT), Alkaline Phosphatase (ALP), Prothrombin Rate (PR), and other biological parameters, such as: serum electrolytes, Urea, Creatinine, Phosphorus, Calcium, Magnesium, Calcifediol (25- OHD3), Thyroid-Stimulating Hormone (TSH) free Thyroxine (T4), Triiodothyronine (T3), Brain Natriuretic Peptide (BNP), Selenium, Thiamine, total Cholesterol and LDL (Low Density Lipoprotein), Triglycerides (TG), Albumin, Thransthyretin (TTR) and C-Reactive Protein (CRP).

Body composition Fat Mass (FM), Fat-Free Mass (FFM) and calculated Fat-Free Mass Index (FFMI) were studied using Dual-energy X-ray Absorptiometry (DXA) (HOLOGIC QDR 4500) measurements collected at admission.

Healthy normal weight (BMI between 18.5 and 25) volunteers were enrolled consecutively after a medical interview, among hospital's medical and paramedical staff. Past and actual overweight (BMI $\geq$ 25) volunteers were excluded. Controls did not undergo DXA or blood tests.

Doppler echocardiography

After blood volume, electrolyte and/or micronutrient disorder correction, Doppler echocardiography were performed during the first week of hospitalization (median: 3 days) by an experienced AF, with a specialization in childhood and adult myopathic diseases, during the. Heart parameters were determined and interpreted according to the guidelines issued by the American Society of Echocardiography [19]. We recorded the following parameters: end-diastolic septal wall thickness (IVS), end-diastolic posterior wall (PW) thickness and end-diastolic LVdiameter (LVEDD), LV mass and left ventricular ejection fraction (LVEF). LVEF was considered normal if greater than 52% for male and 54% for female [20]. Tissue Doppler Imaging (TDI) was used to assess sub-clinical heart impairment, which allowed us to record, LV and RV systolic (Sm) and diastolic peak velocities (Ea) from the apical four chamber view. The tricuspid annular plane systolic displacement (TAPSE) recorded from the apical four chamber view using the M- mode cursor positioned at the free wall angle of the tricuspid valve annulus was used for the RV systolic function assessment [21].

RV systolic dysfunction was defined if TAPSE < 17 mm or peak RV systolic velocity (RV Sm) < 9.5 cm/s [20].

Statistical analysis

Study results were analyzed using SPSS 11.0 (Chicago, Illinois, USA) software.

Student's *t* test, chi-square test and Fisher's test were used for univariate analysis. The risk factors identified using univariate analyses were tested using a multivariate logistic regression. A *p* value lower or equal to 0.05, was considered statistically significant.

Results

Patient characteristics at admission

One hundred and 27 inpatients were screened, 3 patients were excluded for concomitant comorbidities (one hypothyroidism, one diabetes and one pulmonary infection). One hundred and 24 were ultimately enrolled: 119 women (96%) and 5 men (4%). Ninety patients (73%) were suffering from AN-R type as defined by the DSM-IVr, while the other 34 (27%) presented AN with associated purgative behaviors (AN-BP). The mean age of patients was 30.1 ± 11 years old, with an average BMI of 12.3 ± 2.5 kg/m^2 (BMI: 18.5–24.9 kg/ m^2). Clinical and biological characteristics of the study population are summarized in Table 1. Twenty-nine healthy subjects, 28 women (97%) and 1 man (3%), aged 32 ± 10 years, represented the control group; their heart parameters were used for comparison to patients.

Heart findings in patients and controls

A comparison of patients' heart parameters and controls is presented in Table 2. At admission, 18 patients (15%) had a left ventricular systolic function < 52% (vs 0 subject in control group, $p < 0.05$). LV mass and LVEDD was reduced in patients (74.8 ± 23.4 g vs 110.77 ± 32.17 g, $p < 0.001$; 38 ± 5 mm vs. 44 ± 5 mm, $p < 0.001$ respectively). Left and right ventricular TDI systolic velocity peaks were significantly reduced in patients: LV septal and lateral Sm velocity peaks respectively 10 ± 2 cm/s (vs 14 ± 2 cm/s $p < 0.001$), 12 ± 3 cm/s vs 16 ± 3 cm/s $p < 0.001$), basal RV Sm velocity peak 14 ± 3 cm/s (vs 19 ± 3 cm/s). In addition, LV and RV diastolic velocity peaks were both reduced: septal and lateral LV Ea velocity peaks respectively 13 ± 3 cm/s (vs 18 ± 2 cm/s $p < 0.001$), 12 ± 3 cm/s (vs 22 ± 4 cm/s, $p < 0.001$) and RV Ea diastolic velocity peak at 14 ± 3 cm/s (vs 21 ± 4 cm/s $p < 0.001$). TAPSE was significantly reduced in patients compared to controls (16.66 ± 3.95 mm vs. 22.8 ± 2.8 mm, $p = 0.0002$) (Table 2). Thirty-three patients (27%) presented mild to moderate pericardial effusion without heart impairment nor clinical signs of pericarditis. Two groups were identified according to their LVEF parameters: group A with an abnormal LVEF defined in males as < 52% and in females < 54%; group B with a normal LVEF ≥ 52% in males and ≥ 54% in females) [20] (Table 3).

Factors associated with heart function abnormalities

Using univariate analysis, patients with AN-BP had a higher incidence of LV dysfunction compared to patients with AN-R ($p < 0.017$). Patients with LV systolic dysfunction frequently displayed hypertransaminasemia in comparison to patients with normal systolic function ($p < 0.05$). Using multivariate analysis, hypertransaminasemia and AN-BP were independently associated with LVEF alteration ($p = 0.016$; $p < 0.05$). LV TDI diastolic peak velocities (Ea septal peak and Ea lateral peak) were significantly associated with hypertransaminasemia ($p = 0.05$); there was an additional trend toward an association with FFMI, ($p = 0.056$). TDI Right ventricular diastolic velocity peaks ʿRV Ea peak) were above the lower limit of normal in all AN patients. Considering an elevated BNP value (> 100 pg/ml) as a parameter indicative of altered left ventricular function, abnormal BNP values (> 100 pg/l)

Table 1 Clinical and biological characteristics of patients at admission

	***N* = 124 patients**
Age (Y)	32 ± 2.8
Gender (M/F)	5 / 119
AN-R type	90 (73%)
AN-BP type	34 (27%)
Duration of AN since diagnostic (Y)	7.9 ± 5.7
BMI	12.3 ± 2,5
HR (bpm)	61.6 ± 17.2
SBP (mm Hg)	99.2 ± 12
DBP (mmHg)	65.6 ± 10.6
Body composition (DEXA)	
FFM (Kg)	***28.8*** ± 4.8
FM (%)	8.8 ± 3.8
FFMI (%)	10.8 ± 1.4
Cardiac findings	
QT interval (mm)	406 ± 54
QTc interval (mm)	385 ± 31
QT/QTc	1 ± 0.1
Pericardial effusion	34 (27%)
LVEF (%)	63 ± 10
LV mass (g)	80 ± 22
Biological findings	
Albumin (38–52 g/l)	36.9 ± 7.1
Transthyretin (0.21–0.45 g/l)	0.248 ± 0.102
CRP (< 5 mg/l)	6.5 ± 23.7
BNP (< 100 pg /l)	54 ± 70
Potassium (3.7–4.7 mmol/l)	3.8 ± 0.6
Calcium (2.12–2.52 mmol/l)	2.2 ± 0.1
Phosphorus (0.8–1.45 mmol/l)	1.1 ± 0.3
Magnesium (0.70–1.00 mmol/l)	0.8 ± 0,1
Patients with Hypertransaminasemia[a]	34 (27%)
AST (15–37 UI/l)	137.6 ± 425.8
ALT (12–78 UI/l)	170.1 ± 371.4
Total Cholesterol (C) (3.00–6.00 mmol/l)	4.2 ± 1.4
HDL-C (0.8–1.9 mmol/l)	1.8 ± 0.7
LDL-C (< 4.1 mmol/l)	2.1 ± 1.1
Total TG (< 1.7 mmol/l)	0.9 ± 0.7

Data are expressed as mean ± SD or number (percentage)
Y Years, *M* Men, *F* Females, *AN-R* Anorexia Nervosa Restrictive type, *AN-BP* Anorexia Nervosa Binge Eating/Purging type, *BMI* Body Mass Index, *HR* Heart Rate, *SBD* Systolic Blood Pressure, *DBP* Diastolic Blood Pressure, *FFM* Free Fat Mass, *FM* Fat Mass, *FFMI* Free Fat Mass Index, *QTc* corrected QT interval, *LVEF* Left Ventricular ejection fraction, *LV* Left Ventricle, *CRP* C-Reactive Protein, *BNP* Brain Natriuretic Peptid, *AST* Aspartate Transaminase, *ALT* Alanine Transaminase, *HDL* High Density Lipoprotein, *LDL* Low Density Lipoprotein, *TG* triglycerides
[a] = (AST and/or ALT> 2 N)

Table 2 Echocardiographic data between patients and controls at admission

	Patients (n = 124)	Controls (n = 29)	p
BMI (kg/m²)	12 ± 2	21 ± 3	< 0.001
Age (Y)	32 ± 3	32 ± 10	NS
LVEF (%)	63 ± 10	66 ± 7	0.03
LV Mass (g)	74.8 ± 23.4	110.77 ± 32.17	< 0.001
LV Mass Indexed(g/m²)	43.20 ± 12.22	46.83 ± 10.77	0.07
LVEDD (mm)	38 ± 5	44 ± 5	< 0.001
IVS (mm)	6.92 ± 1.39	7.73 ± 1.39	0.08
PW (mm)	7.3 ± 1.34	8.31 ± 1.38	0.07
TAPSE (mm)	16.66 ± 3.95	22.8 ± 2.8	< 0.001
Peak RV Sm velocity (cm/s)	14 ± 3	19 ± 3	< 0.001
Peak LV septal Sm velocity (cm/s)	10 ± 2	14 ± 2	< 0.001
Peak LV lateral Sm velocity (cm/s)	12 ± 3	16 ± 3	< 0.001
Peak RV Ea velocity (cm/s)	14 ± 3	21 ± 4	< 0.001
Peak LV septal Ea velocity (cm/s)	13 ± 3	18 ± 2	< 0.001
Peak LV lateral Ea velocity (cm/s)	12 ± 3	22 ± 4	< 0.001

Data are expressed as mean ± SD or number (percentage)
p p-value, *NS* Not Significant, *BMI* Body Mass Index, *Y* Years, *LVEF* Left Ventricular ejection fraction, *LV mass* Left Ventricular Mass, *LV Mass Indexed* Left Ventricular Mass Indexed, *LVEDD* Left Ventricular End Diastolic Diameter, *IVS* End Diastolic Left Ventricular Septal Thickness, *PW* End-Diastolic Posterior Wall Tickness, *TAPSE* Tricuspid Annular Planeystolic Displacement, *RV* Right Ventricle, *LV* Left Ventricle, *Sm* Systolic Myocardial Velocity recorded withTissue Doppler Imaging; Ea: Early Diastolic Myocardial Velocity recorded with Tissue Doppler Imaging

were significantly associated with older age (38 vs. 29 years old, $p < 0.05$) and with hypertransaminasemia ($p = 0.001$). A decreased FM was significantly associated with pericardial effusion (FM 2.4 kg in patients with pericardial effusion, vs. 3.1 kg in patients without pericardial effusion; $p = 0.036$).

Discussion

In this study, we found that all severely undernourished AN patients had sub-clinical myocardial impairments and 15% of them displayed LV systolic dysfunction.

Cardiac abnormalities were associated with AN-BP type and hypertransaminasemia.

Free Fat Mass tends to be associated with LV diastolic function. Pericardial effusion was frequent and its presence was associated with a low FM.

Our results highlight the relationship between both heart and liver functions.

Characterization of heart abnormalities may lead to a better understanding for anticipating morbi-mortality in the future; though to our knowledge, no studies so far have focused on heart function (right and left, systolic and diastolic function) in AN patients. As for other disease settings, myocardial function may be altered in the context of metabolic disorders, such as acid-base disorders, hyperkalemia, hypomagnesaemia and hypocalcaemia [22]. These alterations, frequent in the context of AN, may also be associated with arrhythmia, and even with sudden death [23] though mitigating metabolic disorders can restore heart function [9]. This type of heart disorder was not studied and was therefore not covered by the present report. As for heart dysfunctions specific to AN, eight studies were published between 1994 and 2017, including seven comparing patients versus a control group. The number of patients included in these studies ranged from 11 to 91 [24, 25], mainly teenagers or very young adults with an average BMI 15 kg/m². Overall four studies provided data on LV systolic function especially in very young patients, with outcomes within the normal ranges in all cases. The other studies reported a difference in structural parameters, but only two studies [25, 26] discussed subclinical systolic alterations, observed in 23 patients. Authors included structural parameters and LVEF in AN patients when echocardiographic assessment was performed. *Kastner* et al [11] carried out a large study of 173 children and adolescent patients with AN (age ranged from 12 to 17 years) and reported a frequency of pericardial effusion at 34.7% and reduced LVEDD in observed patients. Our study is one of the few that have addressed adult patients (mean age: 32 years old), with the largest number of patients having severe undernutrition (average BMI at 12 kg/m²). The Doppler-echocardiographic analysis was the most thorough compared with all others studies, focusing not only on the LVEF but also on subclinical systolic and diastolic function assessment. Our study was thus able to identify risk factors for subclinical heart alterations (FFMI, hypertransaminasemia, AN-BP type and elevated BNP). One of the major risk factors identified in this study was AN-BP type which is characterized by

Table 3 Comparison patients with and without heart failure (defined by LVEF Fraction < 52% for male and 54% for female)

	Patients heart failure (n = 18)	Patients without heart failure(n = 107)	p
Age (Y)	28 ± 5	32 ± 3	NS
BMI (kg/m^2)	11.4 ± 1.6	12.3 ± 2.5	NS
FFMI (kg)/weight^2)	10.49 ± 1.0	10.18 ± 1.2	NS
FM (%)	9 ± 2	8.8 ± 4	NS
AN types:			
AN-R	7 (50%)	84 (76%)	NS
AN-BP	7 (50%)	27 (24%)	0.16
Years of evolution of AN since AN diagnosis	11 ± 5	9 ± 7	NS
Selenium (mmol/l)	1 ± 0.1	1.4 ± 0.1	NS
Potassium (mmol/l)	4 ± 0.6	3.8 ± 0,6	NS
Calcium (mmol/l)	2 ± 0.2	2.2 ± 0.1	NS
Magnesium (mmol/l)	1 ± 0.2	0.8 ± 0.1	NS
BNP (pg/l)	60 ± 63	54 ± 63	NS
Albumin (g/l)	34 ± 9	37 ± 7	NS
Transthyretin (mg/l)	0.218 ± 0.096	0.248 ± 0.102	NS
CRP (mg/l)	5 ± 8	7 ± 23	NS
Hypertransaminasemia (% patients)	71%	43%	< 0.05
AST (UI)	290 ± 577.4	137.6 ± 425.8	
ALT (UI)	280 ± 439.7	170.1 ± 371.4	
HR (bpm)	70 ± 25	61 ± 17	NS
QT (ms)	402 ± 59	405 ± 54	NS
QTc (ms)	397 ± 30	388 ± 33	NS
QT/QTc	1.0 ± 0.1	1 ± 0.2	NS

Data are expressed as mean ± SD or number (percentage)
p p-value, *NS* Not Significant, *Y* Years, *BMI* Body Mass Index, *FFMI* Free Fat Mass Indexed, *FM* Fat Mass, *AN* Anorexia Nervosa, *AN-R* Anorexia Nervosa Restrictive type, *AN-BP* Anorexia Nervosa Binge Eating/Purging type, *BNP* Brain Natriuretic Peptide, *CRP* C-Reactive Protein, *AST* Aspartate Transaminase, *ALT* Alanine Transaminase, *HR* Heart Rate, *QTc* corrected QT interval

vomiting and laxative misuse potentially leading to hypokalemia, hypomagnesaemia and metabolic alkalosis. However these electrolyte disorders were not observed in our study because they were corrected intravenously in the early days of hospitalization, before refeeding. One can suppose that chronic metabolic disorders may alter myocardial fibers and that the damage remains even after micronutrient deficiency correction and subsequent recovery. This hypothesis was supported by both Romano et al. and Oflaz et al. [24, 26]. It would be interesting to perform heart evaluation a few weeks after undernutrition recovery to confirm or reject this hypothesis. Finally, particular focus should be on the heart function of AN-BP patients. *Rautou* et al reported on the liver biopsy of 12 malnourished AN patients with acute liver insufficiency, hepatocyte autophagia, liver hypoxia and decreased portal pressure. These microscopic abnormalities were associated with heart output. This low heart output appeared to be related to heart muscle atrophy and heart arrhythmia, which had been enhanced by electrolyte disorders, leading to hypokalemia and hypocalcaemia, and inducing QT prolongation and impairment of the autonomic nervous system [27]. Hypertransaminasemia was significantly associated with subclinical diastolic function impairment. In addition, a low FFMI tended to be associated with subclinical impairment of heart diastolic function. Hypertransaminasemia is usually frequent when the patients' BMI is low [6]; this was our observation in this present study, and is corroborated by a research study carried out within our working group [6]. as well as in other literature [12].

Our study found a relationship between the level of severe undernutrition and heart alterations, highlighting the potential specific association between muscle mass and hepatic and cardiac impairment as a consequence of severe undernutrition.

The results of our study suggest that cardiac assessment for AN patients with hypertransaminasemia may be warranted prior to refeeding (or early in the refeeding algorithm) in order to prevent complications such as heart failure.

Conclusion

Heart abnormalities are frequent in severely malnourished AN patients. LV function can be altered especially in AN-BP patients. Subclinical heart abnormalities are also frequent and tend to be associated to body composition abnormalities. Prospective studies are needed to determine and to describe the evolution of these heart abnormalities during refeeding and after weight restoration.

Abbreviations

AN: Anorexia Nervosa; DSM: Diagnostic and Statistical Manual of Mental Disorders; RV: Right Ventricular; LV: Left Ventricular; BMI: Body Mass Index; AN-R: Restrictive type; AN-BP: Binge eating/purging type; LVEF: Left Ventricular Ejection Fraction; AST: Aspartate Transaminase; ALT: Alanine Transaminase; LV mass: Left Ventricular mass; LVEDD: Left Ventricular end-Diastolic Diameter; TDI: Tissue Doppler Imaging; NICE: National Institute for Health and Clinical Excellence; HAS: French National Health Authority; RS: Refeeding Syndrome; GGT: Gamma Glutamyl-Transpeptidase; ALP: Alkaline Phosphatase; PR: Prothrombin Rate; 25-OHD3: Calcitriol; TSH: Thyroid-Stimulating Hormone; T4: Thyroxine; T3: Triiodothyronin; BNP: Brain Natriuretic Peptide; CRP: C-Reactive Protein; FM: Fat Mass; FFM: Fat Free Mass; DXA: Dual-Energy X- Ray Absorptiometry; IVS: Septal Wall Thickness; PW: Posterior Wall Thickness; TAPSE: Tricuspid Annular Plane Systolic Displacement

Authors' contributions

MH performed the study design and wrote the article, AP and CB contribute to the study design and the statistical analyses. MD and JCM reviewed the manuscript final version and the study design; EL contributed mainly in the methodology section and reviewed the manuscript and AF contributed significantly to the study design. He also was a major contributor of the article writing and reviewing. The author(s) read and approved the final manuscript.

Competing interests

The authors declare that they have no competing interests.

Author details

[1]Clinical Nutrition Unit, Raymond Poincaré Hospital (AP-HP), Garches, France. [2]Université de Versailles, Saint-Quentin-en-Yvelines, Montigny-le-Bretonneux, Versailles, France. [3]France INSERM, U1178 Paris, VI, France. [4]Institut de Myologie, Groupe Hospitalier Pitié-Salpêtrière, APHP, Paris, France.

References

1. Hudson JI, Hiripi E, Pope HG, Kessler RC. The prevalence and correlates of eating disorders in the National Comorbidity Survey Replication. Biol Psychiatry. 2007;61(3):348–58 Available from: http://www.ncbi.nlm.nih.gov/pubmed/16815322.
2. Huas C, Caille A, Godart N, Foulon C, Pham-Scottez A, Divac S, et al. Factors predictive of ten-year mortality in severe anorexia nervosa patients. Acta Psychiatr Scand. 2011;123(1):62–70 Available from: http://www.ncbi.nlm.nih.gov/pubmed/20958272.
3. De Filippo E, Marra M, Alfinito F, Di Guglielmo ML, Majorano P, Cerciello G, et al. American Psychiatric Association. Mental Disorders, 5th Edn., (DSM-5). Washington, DC: American Psychiatric Publishing; 2013.
4. De Filippo E, Marra M, Alfinito F, Di Guglielmo ML, Majorano P, Cerciello G, De Caprio C, Contaldo F, Pasanisi F. Hematological complications in anorexia nervosa. Eur J Clin Nutr. 2016; 70(11):1305–8. Available from: http://www.ncbi.nlm.nih.gov/pubmed/27436150.
5. Baranowska B, Kochanowski J. Neuroendocrine aspects of anorexia nervosa and bulimia nervosa. Neuro Endocrinol Lett. 2018;39(3):172–8 Available from: http://www.ncbi.nlm.nih.gov/pubmed/30431742.
6. Hanachi M, Melchior JC, Crenn P. Hypertransaminasemia in severely malnourished adult anorexia nervosa patients: Risk factors and evolution under enteral nutrition. Clin Nutr. 2013;32(3):391–5. https://doi.org/10.1016/j.clnu.2012.08.020.
7. Wilson GT, Shafran R. Eating disorders guidelines from NICE. Lancet (London, England). 2005;365(9453):79–81 Available from: http://www.ncbi.nlm.nih.gov/pubmed/15639682.
8. Casiero D, Frishman WH, et al. Cardiovascular complications of eating disorders. Cardiol Rev. 2006;14(5):227–31.
9. Escudero CA, Potts JE, Lam P-Y, De Souza AM, Mugford GJ, Sandor GGS. An Echocardiographic Study of Left Ventricular Size and Cardiac Function in Adolescent Females with Anorexia Nervosa. Eur Eat Disord Rev. 2016;24(1): 26–33 Available from: http://www.ncbi.nlm.nih.gov/pubmed/26449643 J Eat Disord Assoc Internet] 2015.
10. Facchini M, Sala L, Malfatto G, Bragato R, Redaelli G, Invitti C. Low-K+ dependent QT prolongation and risk for ventricular arrhythmia in anorexia nervosa. Int J Cardiol. 2006;106(2):170–6 Available from: http://www.ncbi.nlm.nih.gov/pubmed/16321688.
11. Kastner S, Salbach-Andrae H, Renneberg B, Pfeiffer E, Lehmkuhl U, Schmitz L. Echocardiographic findings in adolescents with anorexia nervosa at beginning of treatment and after weight recovery. Eur Child Adolesc Psychiatry. 2012;21(1):15–21 Available from: http://www.ncbi.nlm.nih.gov/pubmed/22086424.
12. Meczekalski B, Podfigurna-Stopa A, Katulski K. Long-term consequences of anorexia nervosa. Maturitas. 2013;75(3):215–20 Available from: http://www.ncbi.nlm.nih.gov/pubmed/23706279.
13. Battle DE. Diagnostic and Statistical Manual of Mental Disorders (DSM) Codas. 2013;25:191–2.
14. Physical status: the use and interpretation of anthropometry. Report of a WHO Expert Committee. World Health Organ Tech Rep Ser. 1995;854:1–452.
15. Haute Autorité de Santé. Prise en charge de l'anorexie mentale. Available from: https://www.has-sante.fr/portail/jcms/c_985715/fr/anorexie-mentale-prise-en-charge. Accessed 5 Apr 2019.
16. Hofer M, Pozzi A, Joray M, Ott R, Hähni F, Leuenberger M, et al. Safe refeeding management of anorexia nervosa inpatients: an evidence-based protocol. Nutrition. 2014;30(5):524–30 Available from: http://www.ncbi.nlm.nih.gov/pubmed/24698345.
17. Melchior JC. From malnutrition to refeeding during anorexia nervosa. Curr Opin Clin Nutr Metab Care. 1998;1(6):481–5 Available from http://www.ncbi.nlm.nih.gov/pubmed/10565398.
18. Cheitlin MD, Armstrong WF, Aurigemma GP, Beller GA, Bierman FZ, Davis JL, et al. ACC/AHA/ASE 2003 Guideline Update for the Clinical Application of Echocardiography: summary article. A report of the American College of Cardiology/American Heart Association Task Force on Practice Guidelines (ACC/AHA/ASE Committee to Update the 1997 Guidelines for the Clinical Application of Echocardiography). J Am Soc Echocardiogr Off Publ Am Soc Echocardiogr. 2003;16(10):1091–110 Available from: http://www.ncbi.nlm.nih.gov/pubmed/14566308.
19. Lang RM, Badano LP, Mor-Avi V, Afilalo J, Armstrong A, Ernande L, et al. Recommendations for cardiac chamber quantification by echocardiography in adults: an update from the American Society of Echocardiography and the European Association of Cardiovascular Imaging. Eur Heart J Cardiovasc Imaging. 2015;16(3):233–70 Available from: http://www.ncbi.nlm.nih.gov/pubmed/25712077.
20. Jurcut R, Giusca S, La Gerche A, Vasile S, Ginghina C, Voigt J-U. The echocardiographic assessment of the right ventricle: what to do in 2010? Eur J Echocardiogr J Work Gr Echocardiogr Eur Soc Cardiol. 2010;11(2):81–96 Available from: http://www.ncbi.nlm.nih.gov/pubmed/20124362.
21. Brown C, Mehler PS. Medical complications of anorexia nervosa and their treatments: an update on some critical aspects. Eat Weight Disord EWD. 2015;20(4):419–25 Available from: http://www.ncbi.nlm.nih.gov/pubmed/26138740 XXXXX.
22. Ratcliffe PJ, Bevan JS. Severe hypoglycaemia and sudden death in anorexia nervosa. Psychol Med. 1985;15(3):679–81 Available from: http://www.ncbi.nlm.nih.gov/pubmed/4048325.
23. Ulger Z, Gürses D, Ozyurek AR, Arikan C, Levent E, Aydoğdu S. Follow-up of cardiac abnormalities in female adolescents with anorexia nervosa after refeeding. Acta Cardiol. 2006;61(1):43–9 Available from: http://www.ncbi.nlm.nih.gov/pubmed/16485732.
24. Romano C, Chinali M, Pasanisi F, Greco R, Celentano A, Rocco A, et al. Reduced hemodynamic load and cardiac hypotrophy in patients with anorexia nervosa. Am J Clin Nutr. 2003;77(2):308–12 Available from: http://www.ncbi.nlm.nih.gov/pubmed/12540387.
25. Galetta F, Franzoni F, Cupisti A, Morelli E, Santoro G, Pentimone F. Early detection of cardiac dysfunction in patients with anorexia nervosa by tissue Doppler imaging. Int J Cardiol. 101(1):2005, 33–7 Available from: http://www.ncbi.nlm.nih.gov/pubmed/15860380.

12

Body mass index and blood urea nitrogen to creatinine ratio predicts refeeding hypophosphatemia of anorexia nervosa patients with severe malnutrition

Michitaka Funayama[1*], Yu Mimura[1,2], Taketo Takata[1], Akihiro Koreki[1,3], Satoyuki Ogino[1,4] and Shin Kurose[1]

Abstract

Aim: To investigate development of refeeding hypophosphatemia during the refeeding period and the extent of the decrease in the serum phosphorus level among anorexia nervosa patients with severe malnutrition.

Objective: The accurate prediction of the severity of refeeding hypophosphatemia in patients with anorexia nervosa during acute treatment is of great importance. Although some predictors were found in previous reports, these studies used binominal data—the presence or absence of hypophosphatemia—as an outcome indicator but not the extent of serum phosphorus level decrease. It is crucial in clinical settings to predict the extent of the serum phosphorus level decrease as well as development of refeeding hypophosphatemia, in particular, for patients with severe malnutrition, who has a higher risk of death.

Methods: We investigated 63 admissions from 37 patients with anorexia nervosa who had severe malnutrition (admission body mass index 11.5 ± 1.6) and carried out a linear discriminant regression analysis for the development of refeeding hypophosphatemia. The extent of the decrease in the serum phosphorus level were investigated using multiple linear regression analysis. Explanatory variables included data upon admission (age, sex, body mass index, blood urea nitrogen to creatinine ratio, albumin, initial serum phosphorus level, anorexia nervosa type, i.e., restrictive or binge-purge) as well as treatment-related indicators (calorie intake, amount of phosphate administered, and rate of weight gain).

Results: Development of refeeding hypophosphatemia and a change in serum phosphorus levels were predicted by body mass index and elevated blood urea nitrogen to creatinine ratio.

Conclusions: Our study found that refeeding hypophosphatemia among patients with severe malnutrition was predicted by a lower body mass index and elevated blood urea nitrogen to creatinine ratio.

Keywords: Anorexia nervosa, Hypophosphatemia, Refeeding, Blood urea nitrogen to creatinine ratio, Body mass index (BMI), Phosphorus

* Correspondence: mctkfnym@gmail.com
[1]Department of Neuropsychiatry, Ashikaga Red Cross Hospital, 284-1 Yobe, Ashikaga-city, Tochigi 326-0843, Japan
Full list of author information is available at the end of the article

Plain English summary

Refeeding hypophosphatemia is a life-threatening condition that occurs in patients with severe malnutrition, in particular, anorexia nervosa. It is of great importance to predict the risk of refeeding hypophosphatemia in patients with anorexia nervosa during acute treatment. Although some predictors were found in previous reports, these studies used binominal data—the presence or absence of hypophosphatemia—as an outcome indicator but not the extent of serum phosphorus level decrease. Our study found that development of refeeding hypophosphatemia and a change in serum phosphorus levels were related to elevated blood urea nitrogen to creatinine ratio and body mass index.

Introduction

Refeeding hypophosphatemia is a life-threatening condition that occurs in patients with severe malnutrition, in particular, anorexia nervosa. It is of great importance to predict the risk of refeeding hypophosphatemia in patients with anorexia nervosa during acute treatment. Recently, researchers have identified some risk factors regarding refeeding hypophosphatemia for patients with anorexia nervosa [1–4]. Golden et al. (2013) [1] found that the incidence of hypophosphatemia is associated with body mass index and rate of weight loss prior to admission, but not with caloric intake after admission. Similarly, Redgrave et al. (2015) [2] showed that body mass index, but not the rate of weight gain after admission, predicts development of refeeding hypophosphatemia. Brown et al. (2015) [3] reported that body mass index and levels of serum potassium, albumin, and hemoglobin are predictors of hypophosphatemia during refeeding of patients with severe malnutrition. Meanwhile, Kameoka et al. (2016) [4] reported that elevated blood urea nitrogen to creatinine ratio (BUN/Cr ratio) at admission predicts the incidence of refeeding hypophosphatemia. These studies suggest that data upon admission, i.e., body mass index, the rate of weight loss, hemoglobin, albumin, potassium, and BUN/Cr ratio, could be used to predict the incidence of hypophosphatemia, rather than indicators related to treatment, i.e., caloric intake or the rate of weight gain. These previous studies focused on the development of refeeding hypophosphatemia, that is, whether patients had hypophosphatemia or not as an outcome indicator, and the threshold of hypophosphatemia varies among these reports, ranging from 2.3 mg/dl to 3.0 mg/dl [1–4].

In the clinical setting, it is also important to predict the extent of reduction in the serum phosphorus level during the refeeding period, in particular, for patients at the highest risk for severe malnutrition, who have a risk of death [5]. In the previous studies, the prescribed calorie was used as an indicator of caloric intake after hospitalization, but not the actual amount of caloric intake. In addition, they did not include phosphorus administration as a variable that might be accountable for development of refeeding hypophosphatemia. To address these issues, we conducted a retrospective study using 63 anorexia nervosa patients with severe malnutrition and investigated predictors for the decrease in the serum phosphorus level during the refeeding period, as well as development of refeeding hypophosphatemia. We hypothesized that some of the above-mentioned variables predict the extent of reduction in the serum phosphorus level as well as development of refeeding hypophosphatemia.

Materials and methods

Participants

Ethical aspects of this study were reviewed and approved by the Human Research Ethics Committee at the Ashikaga Red Cross Hospital. This study was performed after obtaining informed consent from all participants upon admission. For a patient below the age of 18 years, informed parental consent was also obtained. Diagnosis was based on criteria in the ICD-10, and each patient was diagnosed by two of the three psychiatrists (MF, AK, and TT), each of whom had > 10 years of experience in psychiatry at the time of the study. Participants were recruited from the neuropsychiatric unit in Ashikaga Red Cross Hospital during the period from April 1999 to March 2018. Among 96 admissions with eating disorders that were managed in our unit (F50.0, anorexia nervosa; F50.2, bulimia nervosa), only those with a body mass index of < 16 (68 admissions) were included to investigate refeeding hypophosphatemia, which are considered severe malnutrition among patients with anorexia nervosa [6]. The five patients who discharged themselves from the hospital against medical advice or declined repeated blood tests were excluded. Thus, 63 admissions met the abovementioned criteria and were included in this study. Consecutive admissions with recurrences of anorexia nervosa were included as separate admissions [2, 4] because weight and nutritional status, and thus risk of refeeding syndrome, changed with each admission [2]. In this study, among a total of 37 patients, all of whom were Japanese, 12 had two or more consecutive admissions, which adds up to a total of 63 admissions. However, considering a potential bias toward a correlation, analyses were repeated using only 37 independent patients.

Collection of patient information

Electronic medical records of eligible participants were retrospectively reviewed. As outcome indicators, the following two measures were used: the extent of the decrease in serum phosphorus levels from admission to the nadir phosphorus level during the first 2 weeks after admission and the development of refeeding hypophosphatemia (< 2.5 mg/dl serum phosphorus). Explanatory variables included data at admission, i.e., age, sex, body mass index, anorexia nervosa subtype (restrictive or binge-purge), data obtained from laboratory tests (BUN/Cr ratio, serum phosphorus and potassium levels, hemoglobin, and albumin), and indicators involving treatment, i.e., the rate of weight gain during the first 7 days, caloric intake, and amount of intravenous phosphate administered. Classification of anorexia nervosa subtype, restrictive or binge-purge (bulimic-type), was carried out because binge-purge behavior often influences serum electrolytes levels through repeated vomiting, in particular, serum potassium level [7]. Body mass index was calculated as the weight of the individual (in kilograms) divided by the square of the height of the individual (in meters). To calculate the rate of weight gain during the first 7 days, we divided the kilograms gained during the first 7 days by the initial weight. Total caloric intake (kilocalories) refers to the average total caloric intake from day 1 through day 7 [4], including both oral intake and intravenous infusion therapy. If the patient ate only half the provided 1200-kcal meal, the actual amount of total caloric intake was reduced to 600 kcal. To accurately investigate the effect of energy intake on an individual patient depending on his or her weight, an indicator of total caloric intake per body weight was used for this analysis (total caloric intake divided by body weight), which is widely used for diet therapy for diabetes mellitus [8]. Intravenous phosphorus administration, which was not measured in previous studies of predictors for refeeding hypophosphatemia, was included in this study and was defined as the average total intravenous phosphorus administration (millimoles) from day 1 through day 7. In our unit, phosphorus administration is done intravenously, not orally, during the first 7 days. To better calculate the effect of intravenous phosphorus supplementation on refeeding syndrome, the amount of intravenous phosphorus administered was divided by total caloric intake, and this value was used in the statistical analysis. This is because intracellular movement of serum phosphorus is dependent on reintroduction of nutrients, which is mediated by surges in insulin [9].

A laboratory panel, including serum phosphorus, was carried out on admission. From the second examination onwards, each blood test was conducted at 7:30 in the morning before breakfast. To precisely identify the nadir serum phosphorus level, the patients underwent serial laboratory tests; 47 admissions (74.6%) had the test again on the second hospital day, 45 (71.4%) on the third hospital day, 45 (71.4%) on the fourth hospital day, 29 (46.0%) on the fifth hospital day, and 34 (53.6%) on the sixth day, and they continued to have blood tests until the serum phosphorus level went up again. We note that 59 of 63 admissions (93.7%) had the second laboratory test within 48 h of the first.

Protocol for refeeding and intravenous phosphorus administration

The initial caloric prescription for each patient was decided by individual physicians on admission, based on their assessment of the degree of malnutrition, caloric intake preceding admission, and his or her weight. In addition to oral food, intravenous infusion therapy was often used and, less frequently, nasogastric feeding was also carried out. Normally, the total initial caloric prescription consisted of ~ 600–1400 kcal/day and was usually increased by ~ 200 kcal every day. Intravenous phosphorus administration was not routinely carried out but was prescribed when hypophosphatemia was found in the laboratory test at admission or consecutive tests and when hypophosphatemia was expected to occur [10]. More precisely, when phosphorus levels were below 2.5 mg/dl or within the lower half (2.5 to 3.5 mg/dl) of the standard value of serum phosphorus (2.5 to 4.6 mg/dl) [11], intravenous phosphorus administration was carried out. The amount of phosphorus administration was generally started with 10 or 20 mmol/day, which was adjusted depending on levels of serum phosphorus on serial laboratory tests. This procedure was similarly applied for hypokalemia and hypomagnesemia [10].

Statistical analysis

The development of refeeding hypophosphatemia and the extent of the decrease in the serum phosphorus level were investigated for these 63 admissions. Explanatory variables for these two object variables included demographics (age, sex, anorexia nervosa subtype), data obtained at admission (body mass index, BUN/Cr ratio, serum phosphorus and potassium levels, hemoglobin, and albumin), indicators involving treatment (the rate of weight gain, caloric intake, and amount of intravenous phosphate administered). The correlation matrix for the measured variables is shown in Table 1. No single variable had a correlation of > 0.6 with other variables, indicating that all variables were relatively independent, such that all variables were included in the following analyses. Regarding the serum potassium levels, we compared them between the restrictive and binge-purge types using Student's t-test.

A linear discriminant regression analysis was performed for the development of refeeding hypophosphatemia (< 2.5 mg/dl serum phosphorus). Ten admissions which already had a serum phosphorus level of < 2.5 mg/dl at admission were also included; thus, all 63 admissions were included in this linear discriminant regression

Table 1 Correlation matrix among characteristics of patients with severe malnutrition with respect to development of refeeding hypophosphatemia

	Age	Sex	Restrictive subtype	Body Mass Index	Hemoglobin	Albumin	Serum potassium level	BUN/Cr ratio	Serum phosphorus level at admission	Total energy/kg	Rate of weight gain	Intravenous phosphorus administration
Age	1											
Sex	−0.32	1.00										
Restrictive subtype	0.26	0.11	1.00									
Body Mass Index	−0.01	0.03	0.46	1.00								
Hemoglobin	−0.23	−0.14	−0.18	0.03	1.00							
Albumin	−0.21	0.04	0.07	0.17	0.43	1.00						
Serum potassium level	0.18	0.16	0.50	0.27	0.03	0.25	1.00					
BUN/Cr ratio	0.29	0.21	0.23	−0.22	−0.04	−0.14	0.23	1.00				
Serum phosphorus level at admission	−0.01	−0.03	− 0.23	−0.14	0.36	0.05	0.07	0.13	1.00			
Total energy/kg	0.02	−0.16	−0.16	−0.35	− 0.11	0.01	0.00	0.04	−0.26	1.00		
Rate of weight gain	−0.25	−0.12	− 0.42	−0.08	0.19	0.07	−0.32	−0.29	− 0.11	0.11	1.00	
Intravenous phosphorus administration	0.16	−0.06	0.17	0.04	0.02	−0.23	−0.10	0.18	0.08	−0.58	0.02	1.00

analysis. In addition, a multivariable linear regression analysis was used for the decrease in serum phosphorus levels from admission to nadir hypophosphatemia. Considering potential heterogeneity of patients, i.e., inclusion of 2 male patients, patients with bulimia nervosa, and consecutive admissions, the above-mentioned analyses were also repeated using the three additional cohorts: the female group, the restrictive group, and the independent patient group. For the independent patient group, we used only the data of their first admission. Given low statistical power for the last two groups (n = 45, 37, respectively), explanatory variables for these groups were limited to those having p-values of < 0.1 in the former analyses using all 63 admissions. Regarding outliers, we defined an outlier as a value (residual error for the multiple linear regression analysis or the discriminant score for the linear discriminant regression analysis) that is three standard deviations from the mean in this article. Excel 2010 (Microsoft, Reymond, USA) with add-on Statcel 3 (OMS Ltd., Tokyo, Japan) was used for all statistical analyses. Two-tailed p-values are reported, and p-values of <.05 were considered statistically significant.

Results

Table 2 demonstrates the demographic factors, laboratory data at admission, and treatment indicators for the study group. Of 63 admissions, only 2 (3.2%) were male participants and the remaining 61 (96.8%) were female participants. Regarding the anorexia nervosa subtype, 45 admissions (71.4%) involved the restrictive type, whereas 18 (28.6%) involved the binge-purge type. The average body mass index was extremely low at 11.5 ± 1.6. Although the average serum potassium level at admission was 3.5 ± 0.9 mmol/l, it differed depending on the subtype (Student's t-test, $p < .01$). The average serum potassium level of admissions with the binge-purge type was 2.8 ± 0.8 mmol/l, whereas that with the restrictive type was 3.8 ± 0.8 mmol/l. The average total caloric intake during the first 7 days was 1233 ± 590 kcal/day. The average intravenous phosphorus administration during the first 7 days was 9.2 ± 6.2 mmol/day. The initial serum

Table 2 Demographic factors, laboratory data at admission, and treatment indicators of admissions with severe malnutrition ($N = 63$)

Characteristic	Value	Normal range for Japanese women in their 30s [a]
Age	37.2 ± 10.4 years (range: 14 to 59 years)	
Sex (female participants)	96.8%	
Anorexia nervosa subtype (restrictive subtype)	45 (71.4%)	
Weight at admission (kg)	29.1 ± 4.5	
Body mass index at admission	11.5 ± 1.6	14.1–28.9
Hemoglobin (g/dl)	12.0 ± 2.8 (7.45 ± 0.99 mmol/l)	11.4–14.6 (7.07–9.06 mmol/l)
Albumin (g/dl)	3.7 ± 0.7	4.1–5.0
Serum potassium level (mmol/l)	3.5 ± 0.9	3.6–4.7
Blood urea nitrogen (mg/dl)	27.7 ± 24.5 (9.89 ± 8.75 mmol/l)	7.7–17.7 (2.75–6.32 mmol/l)
Creatinine (mg/dl)	0.86 ± 0.56 (0.08 ± 0.05 mmol/l)	0.49–0.76 (0.04–0.04 mmol/l)
Blood urea nitrogen/creatinine ratio at admission	33.6 ± 19.8	
Serum phosphorus level at admission (mg/dl)	3.9 ± 1.4 (1.23 ± 0.45 mmol/l)	3.0–4.5 (0.97–1.45 mmol/l)
Nadir serum phosphorus level (mg/dl)	2.6 ± 0.8 (0.84 ± 0.26 mmol/l)	3.0–4.5 (0.97–1.45 mmol/l)
Total caloric intake during the first 7 days (kcal/day)	1233 ± 590	
Weight gain during the first 7 days (kg)	1.1 ± 1.8	
Weight gain during hospitalization (kg)	2.9 ± 2.5	
Intravenous phosphorus administration during the first 7 days (mmol/day)	9.2 ± 6.2	
Interval between admission and the hospital day of nadir hypophosphatemia (days)	3.9 ± 4.0	
Duration of hospitalization (days)	43.3 ± 32.4	

[a]https://www.mhlw.go.jp/toukei/kouhyo/data-kou18/data12/junkan-h12-5.pdf and https://www.jslm.org/books/guideline/2018/03.pdf

phosphorus level was 3.9 ± 1.4 mg/dl, which decreased by 1.3 mg/dl to 2.6 ± 0.8 mg/dl at nadir hypophosphatemia, which was recorded at 3.9 ± 4.0 days after their admission, that is, on hospital day 4.9 ± 4.0.

Development of refeeding hypophosphatemia

Of 63 patients, 29 experienced hypophosphatemia. For the female group (n = 61), the restrictive group (n = 45), and the independent patient group (n = 37), the numbers of patients experienced hypophosphatemia are 28, 24, 16, respectively. Each analysis that evaluates predictors of hypophosphatemia included all participants in each group. The linear discriminant regression analysis for development of refeeding hypophosphatemia using all 63 participants was related to severity of BUN/Cr ratio (p = .004), body mass index (p = .007), and restrictive subtype (p = .0499) (Table 3). The results for this model produced Mahalanobis distances of 3.44 (error rate, 0.18). When repeated using only 61 female admissions, it again showed similar results, in which only BUN/Cr ratio (p = .005) and body mass index (p = .007) significantly contributed to development of refeeding hypophosphatemia (Mahalanobis distances of 3.42, error rate of 0.18). When only 45 admissions of restrictive anorexia type were included, the results were similar with severity of BUN/Cr ratio (p = .006), body mass index (p = .01), and serum phosphorus level at admission (p = .047) influencing development of refeeding hypophosphatemia (Mahalanobis distances, 2.58; error rate, 0.21). When repeated with 37 independent participants, BUN/Cr ratio (P = .003) significantly contributed to development of refeeding hypophosphatemia (Mahalanobis distances, 3.20; error rate, 0.19). In this analysis, influence of body mass index did not reach statistical significance with p-Value of 0.13. All the discriminant scores of our linear discriminant regression analysis are normally distributed (normality test, p > 0.05) and there are no outliers in the discriminant scores.

Decrease in serum phosphorus level

Regarding the decrease in serum phosphorus level, the multiple linear regression model explained as much as 80.9% of the observed variance with a p-value of <.01 and an F-value of 22.9. It shows that serum phosphorus level at admission (p < .001), body mass index (p = .02), and BUN/Cr ratio (p = .046) predicted the amount of decrease in the serum phosphorus level (Table 4). When repeated using only 61 female admissions, it again showed similar results, in which only serum phosphorus level at admission (p < .001) and body mass index (p = .02) predicted the amount of decrease in the serum phosphorus level (P < .001, F = 24.6). When only 45 admissions of restrictive anorexia type were included, serum phosphorus level at admission (p < .001) and elevated BUN/Cr ratio (p = .04) influenced development of refeeding hypophosphatemia (P < .001, F = 31.2). Similarly, serum phosphorus level at admission (p < .001) and elevated BUN/Cr ratio (P = .03) significantly contributed to the amount of decrease in the serum phosphorus level (P < .001, F = 22.3) when repeated with 37 independent participants. All the residual errors of the multiple linear regression analysis are normally distributed (normality test, p > 0.05) and there are no outliers in the residual errors.

The fact that the decrease in serum phosphorus levels was predicted by the serum phosphorus levels at admission reflects our intravenous phosphorus administration method, in which phosphorus administration was not routinely carried out but was prescribed when hypophosphatemia was found in the laboratory test and when hypophosphatemia was expected to occur. Accordingly, the extent of decrease in serum phosphorus levels

Table 3 Linear discriminant regression analysis for development of refeeding hypophosphatemia among patients with severe malnutrition

Variable	p-Value	F-value	D2(−i)	Discrimination coefficient
Blood urea nitrogen to creatinine ratio	0.0044	8.9242	2.5175	0.0743
Body mass index	0.0065	8.0656	2.6124	−0.9153
Restrict subtype	0.0499	4.0380	3.0976	2.5952
Serum phosphorus level at admission	0.0605	3.6891	3.1430	−0.6530
Serum potassium level	0.0956	2.8856	3.2500	0.9395
Rate of weight gain	0.1260	2.4217	3.3133	0.1108
Albumin	0.1408	2.2396	3.3384	−1.0653
Total energy intake/kg	0.2831	1.1771	3.4886	−0.0302
Sex	0.2931	1.1290	3.4956	−2.8982
Intravenous phosphorus administration/total energy intake	0.8191	0.0528	3.6545	15.4027
Age	0.8491	0.0366	3.6570	−0.0089
Hemoglobin	0.8768	0.0243	3.6588	0.0283

Table 4 Multiple linear regression analysis for the decrease in serum phosphorus level among patients with severe malnutrition

Variable	p-Value	Standard beta	Regression coefficient	Standard error	Lower 95% confidence limit	Upper 95% confidence limit
Serum phosphorus level at admission	1.886×10^{-15}	0.7877	0.9071	0.0799	0.7466	1.0675
Body mass index	0.0195	−0.1808	−0.1828	0.0757	−0.3349	− 0.0306
Blood urea nitrogen/creatinine ratio	0.0455	0.1452	0.0120	0.0058	0.0002	0.0237
Albumin	0.0514	−0.1363	−0.3339	0.1673	−0.6699	0.0021
Serum potassium level	0.0535	0.1418	0.2571	0.1300	−0.0040	0.5181
Rate of weight gain	0.0645	0.1288	0.0316	0.0167	−0.0020	0.0652
Total energy intake/kg	0.1068	−0.1426	−0.0108	0.0065	−0.0239	0.0024
Hemoglobin	0.2860	0.0777	0.0460	0.0427	−0.0397	0.1318
Restrictive subtype	0.3049	0.0876	0.3146	0.3035	−0.2950	0.9241
Age	0.3582	0.0648	0.0102	0.0110	−0.0119	0.0323
Sex	0.4567	−0.0520	−0.4808	0.6410	−1.7682	0.8066
Intravenous phosphorus administration/total energy intake	0.7604	−0.0247	−4.8280	15.7467	−36.4561	26.8001

tended to be large if a patient had a preserved level of serum phosphorus at admission because patients with higher phosphorus levels at admission did not receive intravenous phosphorus administration until their serum phosphorus levels decreased. However, it is notable that body mass index and BUN/Cr ratio significantly contributed to the decrease in serum phosphorus levels even after the variable of serum phosphorus levels at admission was controlled.

Discussion

Our study showed that development of refeeding hypophosphatemia and a greater decrease in serum phosphorus levels during refeeding period of patient with severe malnutrition was predicted by lower body mass index and elevated BUN/Cr ratio. Although influence of body mass index on development of refeeding hypophosphatemia did not reach statistical significance in the independent patient group, this is probably because of low statistical power and this variable might reach statistical significance in a large-scale study. These findings suggest that body mass index and BUN/Cr ratio are useful when predicting refeeding hypophosphatemia for patients with severe malnutrition. In a previous report on refeeding hypophosphatemia [4], BUN/Cr ratio was used as an indicator for levels of dehydration. Although elevated BUN/Cr ratio is surely influenced by dehydration, causes of elevated BUN/Cr ratio is not specific for dehydration. It is also influenced by other backgrounds, such as protein-energy malnutrition, catabolic state due to starvation, elevated corticosteroid levels, and renal functions, all of which can occur in this cohort. To clarify severity of dehydration, other indicators such as urine specific gravity or orthostatic hypotension are needed. More severe BUN/Cr ratio [4] and lower body mass index [1–3] have already been found to be associated with a greater likelihood of developing refeeding hypophosphatemia, and our study replicated the importance of using BUN/Cr ratio and body mass index as predictors even for patients with severe malnutrition. In fact, The average body mass index for 63 admissions was 11.5 ± 1.6, suggesting that this study group was consistent with the anorexia nervosa with most severe type of malnutrition as classified among other studies that used multivariable regression analysis, in which the body mass indexes ranged from 12.7 to 16.2 [1–4]. The interval between admission and nadir hypophosphatemia was 3.9 days, which is also similar to previous findings of 4.8 days [4] and within the first week of hospitalization [12] for patients with anorexia nervosa. Similarly, patients who are hospitalized with severe burns also show nadir hypophosphatemia between their third and fifth day of hospitalization [13]. The most important finding of the present study is that we found a predictor for the amount of decrease in serum phosphorus levels during the refeeding period, information that might be used to manage refeeding hypophosphatemia in patients with severe malnutrition using electrolyte repletion. Although a lower body mass index led to a substantial decrease in the serum phosphorus level, energy intake was not correlated with the development of refeeding hypophosphatemia or the decrease in the serum phosphorus level. This finding is consistent with recent reports [1, 14–18] that recommend a higher-calorie diet, starting at 1440–2400 kcal/day. The initial serum phosphorus level did not correlate with development of refeeding hypophosphatemia in the present study and in Brown et al.'s study (2015) [1], both of which are the only studies of patients with anorexia nervosa that used the initial serum phosphorus level as a variable.

Why are body mass index and BUN/Cr ratio predictors for refeeding hypophosphatemia? In addition, why doesn't the initial serum phosphorus level correlate with development of refeeding hypophosphatemia? A relevant clue may lie in the very mechanism behind electrolyte imbalances under prolonged starvation and the syndrome associated with subsequent refeeding. According to Mehanna et al. 2008 [10], phosphorus is severely depleted during the period of starvation, although serum phosphorus concentrations can remain normal because most of phosphorus is stored in the intracellular compartment [19], which contracts during starvation. In addition, renal excretion of phosphorus is reduced during prolonged fasting. Accordingly, although extracellular serum phosphorus levels are seemingly normal, phosphorus might have already been depleted within the whole body at admission, which might explain the reason why the initial serum phosphorus level did not correlate with development of refeeding hypophosphatemia. Rather, lower body mass index and probable co-existing dehydration might represent the amount of phosphorus depletion during the period of starvation. With the change to anabolism on refeeding, the insulin surge due to glycemia causes substantial intracellular uptake of phosphorus for all intracellular processes and for the structural integrity of cell membranes that are associated with the synthesis of glycogen, fat, and protein [10]. In addition, phosphorus is used for activation of many enzymes and second messengers as well as energy storage in the form of adenosine triphosphate (ATP). Thus, the combined effects of notable phosphorus consumption during the refeeding period together with depletion of total body stores during starvation causes extracellular hypophosphatemia [18]. Given these mechanisms, it might be impractical to estimate amount of phosphorus storage by using the initial serum phosphate levels. In contrast, a lower body mass index and BUN/Cr ratio might reflect the depleted amount of phosphorus during the period of starvation. In fact, severe malnutrition and probable dehydration often co-exist in patients with anorexia nervosa [4, 20].

Limitations

Our study has several limitations that should be considered. First, absence of a standardized protocol for intravenous phosphorus administration appears to represent a substantial limitation in study design and interpretation of data analyses although amount of intravenous phosphate supplementation was controlled for our statistical analyses. Second, the study population was not large with only 63 admissions. Even with this sample size, however, it was remarkable that the prediction of a decrease in the serum phosphorus level could be explained with an adjusted R-squared of 0.81.Third, this study population might have had a selection bias because we recruited only patients with severe malnutrition. Despite this potential bias, our results are generally compatible with previous research indicating that body mass index and BUN/Cr ratio can predict the severity of refeeding hypophosphatemia among patients with anorexia nervosa [1–4]. Fourth, 4 of 63 admissions (6.3%) did not have the second laboratory tests within 48 h. The average interval between admission and the nadir hypophosphatemia, however, was 93.6 h (3.9 days), which was longer than the 72-h time point at which the four admissions had had the second blood test. Lastly, not all biochemical data were covered, e.g., the serum magnesium level that might have influenced the nadir serum level. This should be addressed in future studies.

Conclusions

Despite the aforementioned limitations, our study demonstrates that body mass index and raised BUN/Cr ratio might predict development of refeeding hypophosphatemia and a change in serum phosphorus levels in patients with severe malnutrition.

Acknowledgements

We wish to thank the patients who participated in these studies. The authors report that there were no sources of funding.

Authors' contributions

MF initiated and coordinated the study. MF, YM, TT, AK, SO, and SK collected the data. MF wrote the first draft of the manuscript. MF and YM interpreted the data and prepared the final manuscript. The author(s) read and approved the final manuscript.

Competing interests

The authors report that there were no conflicts of interest.

Author details

[1]Department of Neuropsychiatry, Ashikaga Red Cross Hospital, 284-1 Yobe, Ashikaga-city, Tochigi 326-0843, Japan. [2]Department of Neuropsychiatry, Keio University School of Medicine, Shinjuku, Tokyo, Japan. [3]Department of Neuropsychiatry, National Hospital Organization Shimofusa Psychiatric Medical Center, Chiba, Japan. [4]Department of Trauma and Critical Care Medicine, Kyorin University School of Medicine, Mitaka, Tokyo, Japan.

References

1. Golden NH, Keane-Miller C, Sainani K, Kapphahn CJ. Higher caloric intake in hospitalized adolescents with anorexia nervosa is associated with reduced length of stay and no increased rate of refeeding syndrome. J Adolesc Health. 2013;53:573–8. https://doi.org/10.1016/j.jadohealth.2013.05.014 Epub 2013 Jul 3.
2. Redgrave GW, Coughlin JW, Schreyer CC, Martin LM, Leonpacher AK, Seide M, Verdi AM, Pletch A, Guarda AS. Refeeding and weight restoration outcomes in anorexia nervosa: challenging current guidelines. Int J Eat Disord. 2015;48:866–73. https://doi.org/10.1002/eat.22390 Epub 2015 Jan 27.
3. Brown CA, Sabel AL, Gaudiani JL, Mehler PS. Predictors of hypophosphatemia during refeeding of patients with severe anorexia nervosa. Int J Eat Disord. 2015;48:898–904. https://doi.org/10.1002/eat.22406 Epub 2015 Apr 2.
4. Kameoka N, Iga J, Tamura M, Tominaga T, Kubo H, Watanabe Y, Sumitani S, Tomotake M, Omori T. Risk factors for refeeding hypophosphatemia in Japanese inpatients with anorexia nervosa. Int J Eat Disord. 2016;49:402–6. https://doi.org/10.1002/eat.22472 Epub 2015 Oct 8.
5. Meczekalski B, Podfigurna-Stopa A, Katulski K. Long-term consequences of anorexia nervosa. Maturitas. 2013;75:215–20. https://doi.org/10.1016/j.maturitas.2013.04.014.
6. Harrington BC, Jimerson M. Initial evaluation, diagnosis, and treatment of anorexia nervosa and bulimia nervosa. Am Fam Physician. 2015;91:46–52.

7. Sato Y, Fukudo S. Gastrointestinal symptoms and disorders in patients with eating disorders. Clin J Gastroenterol. 2015;8:255–63. https://doi.org/10.1007/s12328-015-0611-x Epub 2015 Oct 26.
8. Morino K, Kondo K, Tanaka S, Nishida Y, Nakae S, Yamada Y, Ugi S, Fuse K, Miyazawa I, Ohi A, Nishida K, Kurihara M, Sasaki M, Ebine N, Sasaki S, Katsukawa F, Maegawa H. Total energy expenditure is comparable between patients with and without diabetes mellitus: Clinical Evaluation of Energy Requirements in Patients with Diabetes Mellitus (CLEVER-DM) Study. BMJ Open Diabetes Res Care. 2019;7:e000648. https://doi.org/10.1136/bmjdrc-2019-000648 eCollection 2019.
9. Garber AK, Sawyer SM, Golden NH, Guarda AS, Katzman DK, Kohn MR, Le Grange D, Madden S, Whitelaw M, Redgrave GW. A systematic review of approaches to refeeding hospitalized patients with anorexia nervosa. Int J Eat Disord. 2016;49:293–310. https://doi.org/10.1002/eat.22482.
10. Mehanna HM, Moledina J, Travis J. Refeeding syndrome: what it is, and how to prevent and treat it. BMJ. 2008;336:1495–8. https://doi.org/10.1136/bmj.a301.
11. Nakamura Y, Anayama M, Makino Y, Tamura K, Nagawasa M. Use of lanthanum carbonate for patients with chronic kidney disease at prdialysis stage 4 and 5. Therapeutic Res. 2016;27:485–94 (in Japanese).
12. Ornstein RM, Golden NH, Jacobson MS, Shenker IR. Hypophosphatemia during nutritional rehabilitation in anorexia nervosa: implications for refeeding and monitoring. J Adolesc Health. 2003;32:83–8.
13. Rimaz S, Moghadam AD, Mobayen M, Mohammadi N, Rimaz S, Aghebati R, Jafary Parvar Z, Rad EH. Changes in serum phosphorus level in patients with severe burns: a prospective study. Burns. 2019;45:1864–70. https://doi.org/10.1016/j.burns.2019.03.015 Epub 2019 Nov 2.
14. Whitelaw M, Gilbertson H, Lam PY, Sawyer SM. Does aggressive refeeding in hospitalized adolescents with anorexia nervosa result in increased hypophosphatemia? J Adolesc Health. 2010;46:577–82. https://doi.org/10.1016/j.jadohealth.2009.11.207 Epub 2010 Jan 25.
15. Garber AK, Michihata N, Hetnal K, Shafer MA, Moscicke AB. A prospective examination of weight gain in hospitalized adolescents with anorexia nervosa on a recommended refeeding protocol. J Adolesc Health. 2012;50:24–9. https://doi.org/10.1016/j.jadohealth.2011.06.011 Epub 2011 Aug 26.
16. O'Connor G, Nicholls D. Refeeding hypophosphatemia in adolescents with anorexia nervosa: a systematic review. Nutr Clin Pract. 2013;28:358–64. https://doi.org/10.1177/0884533613476892.
17. Garber AK, Mauldin K, Michihata N, Buckelew SM, Shafer MA, Moscicki AB. Higher calorie diets increase rate of weight gain and shorten hospital stay in hospitalized adolescents with anorexia nervosa. J Adolesc Health. 2013;53:579–84. https://doi.org/10.1016/j.jadohealth.2013.07.014 Epub 2013 Sep 17.
18. Katzman DK, Garber AK, Kohn M, Golden NH. Refeeding hypophosphatemia in hospitalized adolescents with anorexia nervosa. J Adolesc Health. 2014;55:455–7. https://doi.org/10.1016/j.jadohealth.2014.06.010.
19. Bansal VK. Serum inorganic phosphorus. In: Walker HK, Hall WD, Hurst JW, editors. Clinical methods: The History, Physical, and Laboratory Examinations. 3rd edition. Boston: Butterworths; 1990. Chapter 198.
20. Stheneur C, Bergeron S, Lapeyraque AL. Renal complications in anorexia nervosa. Eat Weight Disord. 2014;19:455–60. https://doi.org/10.1007/s40519-014-0138-z.

13

Abnormal bone mineral density and content in girls with early-onset anorexia nervosa

Julia Clarke[1,2*], Hugo Peyre[1,3], Marianne Alison[4], Anne Bargiacchi[1], Coline Stordeur[1], Priscilla Boizeau[5], Grégor Mamou[1], Sophie Guilmin Crépon[4,6,7], Corinne Alberti[7], Juliane Léger[3,6] and Richard Delorme[1]

Abstract

Background: Early-onset anorexia nervosa (EO-AN) represents a significant clinical burden to paediatric and mental health services. The impact of EO-AN on bone mineral abnormalities has not been thoroughly investigated due to inadequate control for pubertal status. In this study, we investigated bone mineral abnormalities in girls with EO-AN regardless of pubertal development stage.

Method: We conducted a cross-sectional study of 67 girls with EO-AN (median age = 12.4 [10.9–13.7 years]) after a median duration of disease of 1.3 [0.6–2.0] years, and 67 healthy age-, sex-, pubertal status- matched control subjects. We compared relevant bone mineral parameters between groups: the total body bone mineral density [TB-BMD], the lumbar spine BMD [LS-BMD], the total body bone mineral content [TB-BMC] and the ratio of the TB-BMC to lean body mass [TB-BMC/LBM].

Results: TB-BMD, TB-BMC, LS-BMD and TB-BMC/LBM were all significantly lower in patients with AN compared to controls. In the EO-AN group, older age, later pubertal stages and higher lean body mass were associated with higher TB-BMC, TB-BMD, and LS-BMD values.

Discussion: Girls with EO-AN displayed deficits in bone mineral content and density after adjustment for pubertal maturation. Age, higher pubertal stage and lean body mass were identified as determinants of bone maturation in the clinical population of patients with EO-AN. Bone health should be promoted in patients, specifically in those with an onset of disorder before 14 years old and with a delayed puberty.

Keywords: Anorexia nervosa, Early onset, Bone mineral density, Bone mineral content, Pubertal maturation

Plain ENGLISH summary

Early-onset anorexia nervosa (EO-AN) – beginning before the age of 14 years and before menarche – represents a significant clinical burden to paediatric and mental health services, with serious medical, psychiatric and psychosocial consequences. The impact of EO-AN on bone mineral abnormalities has not been thoroughly investigated due to inadequate control for pubertal status. In this study, we investigated bone mineral abnormalities in girls with EO-AN regardless of pubertal development stage. We compared bone mineral parameters in 67 girls with EO-AN and 67 healthy age-, sex-, pubertal status-matched control subjects. In our study, all parameters of bone quality were significantly lower in patients with AN compared to controls, showing that girls with EO-AN displayed deficits in bone quality even though the duration of illness was short in these young patients.

* Correspondence: julia.c.clarke@gmail.com
[1]Child and Adolescent Psychiatry Department, Assistance Publique-Hôpitaux de Paris, Robert Debré University Hospital, Paris, France
[2]Université de Paris, Institute of Psychiatry and Neuroscience of Paris, INSERM U1266, Paris, France
Full list of author information is available at the end of the article

Bone health should be promoted in patients, specifically in those with an onset of disorder before 14 years old and with a delayed puberty.

Background

Anorexia nervosa (AN) is characterised by the persistent restriction of energy intake relative to requirements, leading to significantly low body weight, and an intense fear of gaining weight or becoming fat [1]. AN, which has a prevalence of 1% in the general population, has the highest mortality rate of all psychiatric disorders, and serious medical, psychiatric and psychosocial consequences [2, 3]. In most patients AN begins during adolescence or early adulthood, but recent studies have reported an increase in the incidence of early-onset AN (EO-AN), beginning before the age of 14 years [4] and before menarche [5]. EO-AN is a single entity in the broad spectrum of eating disorders, with a significant and specific clinical burden on paediatric and mental health services [6, 7]. The epidemiological and clinical profile of EO-AN display some differences from AN with an onset during adolescence or early adulthood, such as a different sex ratio less unbalanced in favor of women, greater severity of symptoms and specific neurocognitive features [8, 9].

Low spine and whole-body bone mineral density (BMD) and bone mineral content (BMC) have been reported to be associated with AN [10, 11]. These deficits result in a higher risk of spontaneous compression fractures of the vertebrae [12], even in adolescents [13]. More than 50% of adolescents with AN have a BMD more than one standard deviation lower than the mean for age, and approximately 10% of these adolescents have BMD values more than two standard deviations below the mean [14]. This negative effect of the disease on bone health has been found to persist 5 to 10 years after recovery from a severely low BMI at adolescence [15]. In adolescents and adults with AN, the lowest body mass index (BMI) reached during the illness and the total duration of illness (from early symptoms to remission) have consistently been identified as the main factors underlying low BMD [13, 16]. For example, mean bone density loss has been estimated at 2.5% per year in young women with active AN [16]. However, recent findings suggest that the inappropriately low bone densities of patients with AN are driven more by a deficit of bone metabolism in a critical period of development rather than by bone loss (13, [17]. By the age of 18 years, 95% of peak bone mass is achieved, and trabecular bone density increases by about 20% during pubertal growth [18, 19]. Poor bone accrual and a lower peak bone mass in late childhood and early adolescence were therefore thought to have a significant effect on trabecular bone morphology and skeletal strength [20]. Bone acquisition in late childhood is influenced mostly by pubertal stage and growth-related changes in body and skeleton size (including age, height and weight) [21]. During puberty, both nutritional and hormonal factors play major roles in the process of bone development. Increases in bone mineralisation are related to nutritional status (assessed by measuring weight and height) and growth hormone and sex steroid concentrations [22]. Oestrogens are thought to play a key role in increasing and maintaining bone mass in adolescent girls and boys [23]. In girls, peak bone mass gain generally occurs in late puberty, with BMD values increasing up to Tanner stage 4 [22].

The impact of EO-AN on BMD and BMC has not been fully investigated. Previous studies were conducted in subjects with AN beginning during or after the last stages of puberty, i.e. a heterogeneous mixture of children and adolescents in terms of chronological age at AN onset, with inadequate control for pubertal status. In comparisons of patients with pubertal delay with controls (matched only for chronological age and not for Tanner stage), sampling bias may artificially increase the estimated impact of AN on BMC and BMD. We hypothesise that undernutrition has an impact in EO-AN regardless of pubertal development stage (early or late puberty), and that this effect may be greater in patients with severe pubertal delay. In this study, we aimed to fill some of these gaps in our knowledge by assessing the difference in dual-energy X-ray absorptiometry parameters between a unique cohort of girls with restrictive AN beginning before the age of 14 years and a healthy control group matched on the basis of gender, chronological age, but also pubertal status.

Methods

Populations

This study included all consecutive female patients with AN hospitalised over a period of 5 years from 2010 to 2015 at the Child and Adolescent Psychiatry Department of Robert Debré Paediatric Hospital (Paris, France). Patients were enrolled at the time of DXA acquisition, during hospitalisation in a dedicated unit for the treatment of eating disorders. Girls with a retrospective diagnosis of EO-AN were included in the study. The criteria for EO-AN diagnosis were: restrictive AN based on the DSM 5 (we retroactively reassigned the DSM-5 diagnoses for participants recruited before 2013) [24], with an age at onset of the disorder of less than 14 years and onset before menarche. Both pre-14 and pre-menarche age requirements were met. All patients were of European descent. At the time of data acquisition, pubertal development and amenorrhoea status were rated by experienced paediatric endocrinologists (all patients had a diagnosis of EO-AN, and they were at various stages of pubertal development at the time of the inclusion in the study). The Tanner staging was the Tanner of breast development. The final diagnosis of AN was reached by summing the information from the Schedule for Affective Disorders and Schizophrenia for School-Age Children, Present and Lifetime Version (K-SADS-PL) [25] and data from clinical reports from experts in the field. We also used the K-SADS-PL to screen for comorbid psychiatric conditions.

The control individuals for this study were from a large group of healthy female children and adolescents from the general population (n=319). They were aged 6–20 years and were also all of European descent. These individuals were enrolled in a study aiming to establish control values for bone mineral content and body composition [26]. At inclusion, they had no lifetime history of any chronic medical disorder, impaired growth or axis I psychiatric disorders (investigated by a questionnaire completed by the parents) and none of the controls was under any drug treatment at the time of study. Children with height, weight or body mass values more than two standard deviations on either side of the mean were excluded from the control group. None of the study participants was using hormonal contraception. Given the developmental variability of bone mineral content and body composition, all participants with EO-AN from our study were matched with control individuals for Tanner stage. We split Tanner stages into two distinct subgroups, one corresponding to Tanner stage 1 or 2 (early pubertal stages) and the other to Tanner stages 3 to 5 (late stages of puberty), to prevent a lack of power and the biases introduced by multiple testing.

Height and weight were expressed as standard deviation scores (SDS) for age and sex [27]. We also calculated body mass index (BMI) (kg/m^2) as a SDS for age and sex [28]. Pubertal development was assessed according to Tanner stage [29].

Ethics statement

The local ethics committee approved the protocol (Comité de l'Evaluation des Projets de Recherche Biomédicale de Robert Debré).

Dual-energy X-ray absorptiometry

We estimated the BMC and BMD (corresponding to BMC divided by total bone area) for the total body (TB) and for the lumbar spine (LS), L2–L4, by dual-energy X-ray absorptiometry (DXA, GE Lunar Prodigy Corp., Madison. WI). Bone mineral measurements were expressed as standard deviation scores (SDS) for chronological age. TB DXA provided an estimate of body composition: lean body mass (LBM) and body fat mass (BFM), expressed as a percentage. Given the complex relationship between BMC, LBM, age and growth during puberty, we also calculated the TB-BMC/LBM ratio [30, 31].

Statistical analysis

The clinical characteristics of patients with AN and control individuals were compared in appropriate tests. Comparisons of quantitative measures between the patient and control individual groups are made using type III chronological age-adjusted tests from mixed models with a random effect on the pair. We compared relevant bone mineral (TB-BMD and LS-BMD, TB-BMC, TB-BMC/LBM) and body composition (BFM and LBM) measurements between individuals with EO-AN and controls, with adjustment for chronological age. Sensitivity analyses were also conducted separately on subjects in the early (Tanner stages 1 or 2) and late (Tanner stages 3 to 5) stages of puberty. Holms correction for multiple testing was applied to control for type 1 error. The p-values indicated in the tables are the corrected p-values. We used a linear regression model to identify the clinical characteristics (chronological age (years)), BMI (SDS), Tanner status (early vs. later stages), duration of AN, fat mass (kg) and lean mass (kg) associated with our four bone mineral parameters (TB-BMD and LS-BMD, TB-BMC, TB-BMC/LBM). All tests were two-tailed. Statistical analyses were performed with SAS 8.2 software (SAS Institute Inc., Cary, North Carolina).

Results

Clinical characteristics

We enrolled 134 girls in the study: 67 patients with EO-AN and 67 female control children and adolescents matched for Tanner stage (Table 1). At inclusion, the median duration of the illness was 1.3 (0.6; 2.0) years, 19% of the patients (n=13) had secondary amenorrhoea, and 57% (n=38) were at Tanner stage 1 or 2. As expected, current BMI was lower for the patients with EO-AN than for the controls. For a given Tanner stage, patients with AN were older than the controls, consistent with the widely reported puberty delay in patients with EO-AN (Fig. 1).

Bone mineral content and body composition

As expected, patients with EO-AN had a lower BFM and a higher LBM, expressed as percentages, than the controls ($p< 0.01$). As shown Table 2, TB-BMD ($p< 0.01$), TB-BMC ($p< 0.01$), LS-BMD ($p< 0.01$) and TB-BMC/LBM (p=0.02) were all significantly lower in patients with AN compared to control girls (Table 2, Fig. 2).

Predictors of bone parameters in EO-AN patients

In our generalised linear regression model higher TB-BMC, TB-BMC/LBM, TB-BMD, and LS-BMD values were associated with a higher chronological age at the

Table 1 Clinical characteristics of the study population

	EO-AN patients *N*=67 median (25th percentile;75th percentile)	Control individuals *N*=67 median (25th percentile;75th percentile)	Patients vs. control individuals *p*-value
Chronological age (yrs)	12.4 (10.9; 13.7)	11.6 (9.9; 12.4)	$p< 0.01$
Tanner pubertal stage			
1 and 2	38 (57%)	38 (57%)	
3 to 5	29 (43%)	29 (43%)	
Height (SDS)	−0.13 (− 0.86; 1.03)	0.76 (− 0.21; 1.45)	$p< 0.01$
Weight (SDS)	−1.46 (−2.01; − 0.83)	0.80 (0.22; 1.45)	$p< 0.01$
BMI (kg/m^2)	14.0 (12.7; 15.2)	18.1 (16.5; 20.1)	$p< 0.01$
BMI (SDS)	−2.20 (−3.25; − 1.24)	0.53 (− 0.29; 1.16)	$p< 0.01$
Secondary amenorrhoea	13 (19%)		
Age at EO-AN onset (yrs)	11.0 (9.5; 12.5)		
Disease duration (yrs)	1.3 (0.6; 2.0)		

In bold: *p*-value < 0.01
BMI Body Mass Index, *EO-AN* Early Onset Anorexia Nervosa

time of inclusion ($p< 0.001$ in all 4 models), regardless of body mass index. We also found that higher pubertal stage (Tanner 1 or 2 versus 3, 4 or 5; $p=0.004$ for TB-BMC, $p=0.02$ for TB-BMD and $p=0.001$ for LS-BMD) and higher lean body mass ($p< 0.001$ in all 4 models) were positively associated with higher TB-BMC, TB-BMD, and LS-BMD ($p< 0.001$ in all 4 models), regardless of body mass index and age (Table 3). Among EO-AN patients, girls at later pubertal stages had higher TB-BMC, TB-BMD, and LS-BMD values. Age, later pubertal stage and higher lean body mass were determinants of total body and lumbar spine bone mineral content and bone mineral density in the clinical population of EO-AN patients.

Discussion

This observational study provided extensive data for the assessment of bone mineral density and content in a well-characterised cohort of girls with severe restrictive AN beginning before the age of 14 years. Our findings highlight the abnormal bone mineral composition of these patients, affecting bone mineral content and, to a

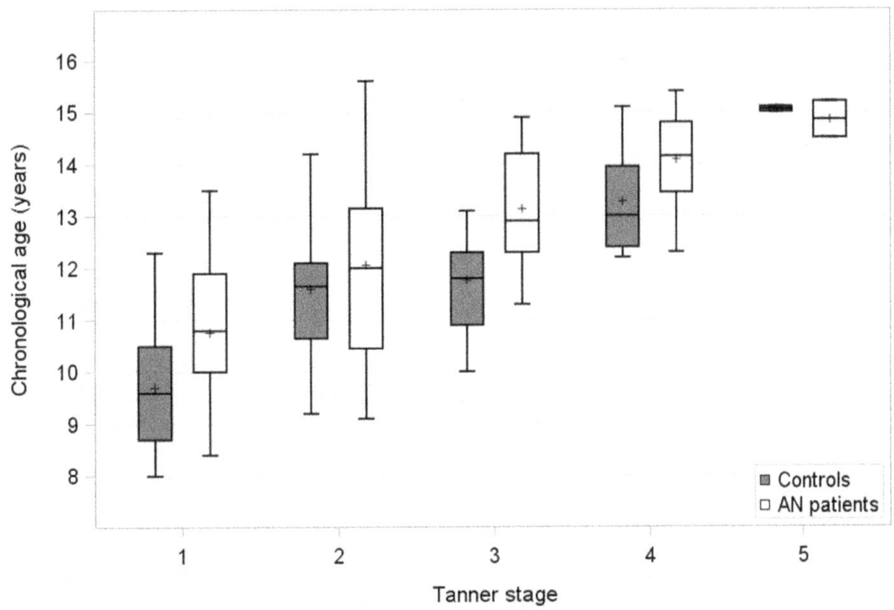

Fig. 1 Box plots of Tanner stages in patients vs. controls individuals (n=134) and distribution by age

Table 2 Comparison of bone mineral characteristics and body composition in 134 children: 67 with EO-AN vs 67 Tanner stage matched control individuals, adjusted for chronological age

	EO-AN patients *N=67* *median (25th percentile;75th percentile)*	*Control individuals* *N=67* *median (25th percentile;75th percentile)*	*Patients vs. control individuals p-value*
BFM (% total weight)	10.9 (6.6; 16.2)	23.0 (18.0; 27.3)	< 0.01
LBM (% total weight)	84.9 (78.1; 89.2)	71.3 (67.0; 76.3)	< 0.01
TB LBM/height	171 (156; 187)	187 (169; 210)	< 0.01
TB BMC (SDS)	−0.82 (−1.55; − 0.23)	− 0.02 (− 0.64; 0.38)	< 0.01
TB BMC/LBM	0.21 (− 0.53; 1.04)	−0.32 (− 0.78; 0.46)	0.02
TB BMD (SDS)	− 0.30 (− 1.17; 0.24)	−0.06 (− 0.74; 0.60)	< 0.01
LS BMD (SDS)	− 0.75 (− 1.70; − 0.09)	− 0.20 (− 0.79; 0.75)	< 0.01

BFM Body Fat Mass, *EO-AN* Early Onset Anorexia Nervosa, *LBM* Lean Body Mass, *TB-BMC* Total Body Bone Mineral Content, *TB-BMC/LBM (SDS)* Ratio of the TB-BMC to Lean Body Mass (LBM), *TB-BMD (SDS)* Total Body Bone Mineral Density, *LS-BMD (SDS)* Lumbar Spine Bone Mineral Density

lesser extent, bone mineral density. Moreover, lumbar spine density was more affected than total body density. The findings of our study are consistent with those of previous studies. Previous studies on prepubertal children and children in the *early stages of puberty* have reported that bone mineral content is a more accurate measurement of bone acquisition than bone mineral density [21]. Moreover, the trabecular bone (lumbar spine) has been shown to be more severely affected than cortical bone in girls with EO-AN [8, 9]. Women with AN beginning during adolescence are known to have a lower bone density than women developing this condition during adulthood, despite similar durations of amenorrhoea [32]. In our study, the decrease in bone mineral content and spinal bone mineral density were very significant (about − 0.8 SDS) despite the short duration of disease. Age, later pubertal stage and higher lean body mass were determinants of bone mineral density and content in our study. Duration of illness has been previously shown to be a negative predictor of LS BMD [13]. The duration of illness was not related with BMD and BMC probably due to the narrow range of the duration of the illness in our cohort (median of 1.3 years).

Adolescence is a time window during which bone accrual must be maximal to attain an optimal peak bone mass. Any deficits occurring during this period may be

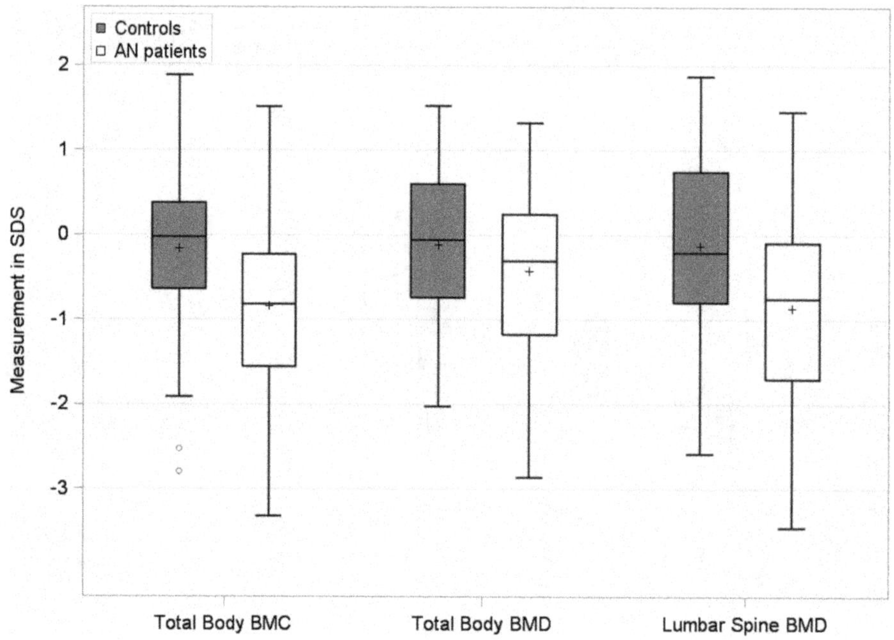

Fig. 2 Box plots of total body bone mineral content (BMC), total body bone mineral density (BMD) and lumbar spine BMD in patients vs. controls (*n*=134)

Table 3 Linear regression model of clinical characteristics (chronological age, BMI, Tanner status, duration of AN, amenorrhea, body fat mass and lean body mass) associated with the four bone mineral parameters (TB-BMD and LS-BMD, TB-BMC, TB-BMC/LBM)

	TB BMC (SDS)			TB BMC/LBM (%)			TB BMD (SDS)			LS BMD (SDS)		
	N=67			N=67			N=67			N=67		
	β	IC-95%	p-value	β	IC-95%	p-value	β	IC-95%	p-value	β	IC-95%	p-value
Chronological age (yrs)	166.2	[133.92; 198.49]	< 0.01	0.13	[0.06; 0.20]	< 0.01	0.03	[0.02; 0.04]	< 0.01	0.06	[0.04; 0.07]	< 0.01
Pubertal stage			< 0.01			0.55			0.02			< 0.01
1 and 2	ref.	ref.		ref.	ref.		ref.	ref.		ref.	ref.	
3 to 5	217.25	[71.32; 363.17]		0.10	[−0.24; 0.44]		0.04	[0.01; 0.08]		0.09	[0.04; 0.15]	
BMI (SDS)	15.45	[−33.00; 63.90]	0.53	−0.13	[− 0.24; − 0.02]	0.07	0.01	[0.00; 0.02]	0.16	0.02	[0.00; 0.04]	0.02
FBM (kg)	−25.10	[−66.67; 16.47]	0.23	0.02	[−0.07; 0.11]	0.61	0.01	[−0.01; 0.00]	0.32	−0.01	[− 0.02; 0.01]	0.45
LBM (kg)	65.11	[53.86; 76.35]	< 0.01	0.04	[−0.01; 0.08]	0.10	0.01	[0.01; 0.01]	< 0.01	0.02	[0.01; 0.02]	< 0.01
Disease duration (yrs)	−60.79	[− 129.85; 8.27]	0.08	−0.03	[− 0.19; 0.12]	0.67	− 0.01	[− 0.02; 0.01]	0.31	−0.03	[− 0.05; 0.00]	0.06

BMI Body mass index, *BFM* Body Fat Mass, *LBM* Lean Body Mass, *TB-BMC* Total Body Bone Mineral Content, *TB-BMC/LBM (SDS)* Ratio of the TB-BMC to Lean Body Mass (LBM), *TB-BMD (SDS)* Total Body Bone Mineral Density, *LS-BMD (SDS)* Lumbar Spine Bone Mineral Density

permanent [17, 33]. EO-AN is a severe disease that affects bone mineralisation before puberty and is associated with a high risk of altered bone mineralisation if symptoms persist during puberty. EO-AN had an impact regardless of pubertal development stage, and this effect was strongest in those with the most severe pubertal delay (suffering from both oestrogen deficiency and undernutrition). An inadequate skeletal mass results in fragile bones and a higher risk of fractures, both in childhood and later in life, as adults [34, 35]. Early diagnosis and intervention are required to prevent such complications in this specific population.

One of the strengths of this study is that the pubertal delay in patients with early AN was considered by matching patients and controls for pubertal stage rather than chronological age. Indeed, the hormonal changes occurring during puberty are known to play a crucial role in bone mineralisation [22, 23]. We found differences in bone mineral parameters between EO-AN patients and control individuals at both early (Tanner 1 or 2) and late (Tanner 3, 4 or 5) stages of puberty. Furthermore, pubertal delay was associated with a greater deficit in bone maturation. In populations of adults with chronic AN, it has been suggested that hormonal adaptations to nutrient deficiency (including hypogonadotropic hypogonadism and growth hormone resistance) mediate a loss of bone mass [17, 36]. However, our study set-up was not appropriate for the testing of this hypothesis. Our results must be interpreted in the light of several limitations. First, AN was particularly severe in our sample of patients, who required hospitalisation in a highly specialised eating disorders unit, with the nationwide recruitment of patients particularly resistant to ambulatory care. Our sample may not, therefore, be entirely representative of the population of girls with EO-AN (with an onset before the age of 14 and primary amenorrhea). Second, although our sample is the largest sample from this clinical population ever studied, it nevertheless remains small. Our study may therefore lack power (i) to detect subtle differences in bone mineral composition (type 2 error) and (ii) to identify some of the clinical characteristics associated with bone mineral content and density in girls with AN. Finally, it was not possible to use our data to further assess the contribution of biological mechanisms to bone deficits in anorexia nervosa. We did not assess calcium intake or physical activity, although both these factors are known to be major determinants of bone mineralisation. Further studies are required to increase our understanding of the factors affecting bone mineral content and density before the completion of pubertal development in women with early-onset AN.

Conclusions

Even after a short duration of disease, girls with early-onset anorexia nervosa display bone loss, with severe effects on bone mineral content and lumbar spine density. These results highlight the need for careful and appropriate monitoring of bone mineral characteristics in these patients and the importance of nutrition rehabilitation to allow pubertal development to occur, given the importance of this process for bone mineral acquisition. Girls with EO-AN may have a high risk of fracture throughout life. Bone health should, therefore, be promoted through nutritional and other interventions (e.g. avoidance of toxic substances, physical activity under medical supervision etc.). Future studies should compare prospective bone mineral content and density in young adults with EO-AN and those with later onset of the disease, taking into account the duration of undernutrition, the pubertal delay (including age at menarche and catch-up growth), and the clinical characteristics of AN (recovery versus relapse and chronicity).

Abbreviations

BFM: Body Fat Mass; BMI: Body Mass Index; DXA: Dual-Energy X-ray Absorptiometry; EO-AN: Early-Onset Anorexia Nervosa; LBM: Lean Body Mass; LS-BMD: Lumbar Spine Bone Mineral Density; SDS: Standard Deviation Scores; TB-BMC/LBM: Ratio of the Total Body Bone Mineral Content to Lean Body Mass; TB-BMC: Total Body Bone Mineral Content; TB-BMD: Total Body Bone Mineral Density

Acknowledgements

The authors gratefully acknowledge the families who accepted to participate in this study. This work was supported by AP-HP and Paris University.

Authors' contributions

JC designed of the work and was a major contributor in writing the manuscript; HP contributed to the interpretation of the data and was a contributor in writing the manuscript; MA allowed for the acquisition of imaging data and was a contributor in writing the manuscript; AB, CS, GM have completed the acquisition of clinical data; PB carried out the statistical analyses; SGC carried out the statistical analyses and contributed to the interpretation of the data; CA participated in the design of the study; JL have drafted the work and substantively revised it; RD was a major contributor in writing the manuscript and substantively revised it. All authors read and approved the final manuscript.

Competing interests

The authors declare that they have no competing interests.

Author details

[1]Child and Adolescent Psychiatry Department, Assistance Publique-Hôpitaux de Paris, Robert Debré University Hospital, Paris, France. [2]Université de Paris, Institute of Psychiatry and Neuroscience of Paris, INSERM U1266, Paris, France. [3]Université de Paris, INSERM UMR 1141, Paris, France. [4]Radiology Department, Assistance Publique-Hôpitaux de Paris, Robert Debré University Hospital, Pediatric, Paris, France. [5]Unit of Clinical Epidemiology, Assistance Publique-Hôpitaux de Paris, Robert Debré University Hospital, Paris, France. [6]Department of Pediatric Endocrinology and Diabetology & Reference centre for Growth and Development Endocrine diseases, Assistance Publique-Hôpitaux de Paris, Robert Debré University Hospital, Paris, France. [7]INSERM UMR-S 1123 ECEVE and CIC-EC 1426, Paris, France.

References

1. American Psychiatric Association. Diagnostic and Statistical Manual of Mental Disorders: American Psychiatric Association; 2013. [cité 1 mai 2015]. 1. (DSM Library). Disponible sur: http://dsm.psychiatryonline.org/doi/book/10.1176/appi.books.9780890425596.
2. Arcelus J, Mitchell AJ, Wales J, Nielsen S. Mortality rates in patients with anorexia nervosa and other eating disorders. A meta-analysis of 36 studies. Arch Gen Psychiatry. 2011;68(7):724–31.
3. Excess mortality, causes of death and prognostic factors in anorexia nervosa. - PubMed - NCBI [Internet]. [cité 14 nov 2018]. Disponible sur: https://www.ncbi.nlm.nih.gov/pubmed/19118319.
4. Lask B, Bryant-Waugh R. Eating disorders. Br J Hosp Med. 1993;49(8):531–3.
5. Russell GF. Premenarchal anorexia nervosa and its sequelae. J Psychiatr Res. 1985;19(2–3):363–9.
6. Nicholls DE, Lynn R, Viner RM. Childhood eating disorders: British national surveillance study. Br J Psychiatry J Ment Sci. 2011;198(4):295–301.
7. Pinhas L, Morris A, Crosby RD, Katzman DK. Incidence and age-specific presentation of restrictive eating disorders in children: a Canadian Paediatric Surveillance Program study. Arch Pediatr Adolesc Med. 2011;165(10):895–9.
8. Mouren-Simeoni MC, Bouvard MP. Anorexie mentale chez l'enfant prépubère: particularités cliniques et évolutives. In: Neuropsychiatrie de l'enfance et de l'adolescence: Elsevier; 1993. p. 291–5. [cité 29 avr 2015]. Disponible sur: http://cat.inist.fr/?aModele=afficheN&cpsidt=4815691.
9. van Noort BM, Lohmar SK, Pfeiffer E, Lehmkuhl U, Winter SM, Kappel V. Clinical characteristics of early onset anorexia nervosa. Eur Eat Disord Rev J Eat Disord Assoc. 2018;26(5):519–25.
10. Robinson L, Aldridge V, Clark EM, Misra M, Micali N. A systematic review and meta-analysis of the association between eating disorders and bone density. Osteoporos Int J Establ Result Coop Eur Found Osteoporos Natl Osteoporos Found USA. 2016;27(6):1953–66.
11. Schorr M, Thomas JJ, Eddy KT, Dichtel LE, Lawson EA. Meenaghan E, et al. Bone density, body composition, and psychopathology of anorexia nervosa spectrum disorders in DSM-IV vs DSM-5. Int J Eat Disord. 2017;50(4):343–51.
12. Lucas AR, Melton LJ, Crowson CS, O'Fallon WM. Long-term fracture risk among women with anorexia nervosa: a population-based cohort study. Mayo Clin Proc. 1999;74(10):972–7.
13. Shepherd S, Kyriakou A, Shaikh MG, McDevitt H, Oakley C, Thrower M, et al. Longitudinal changes in bone parameters in young girls with anorexia nervosa. Bone. 2018;116:22–7.
14. Misra M, Aggarwal A, Miller KK, Almazan C, Worley M, Soyka LA, et al. Effects of anorexia nervosa on clinical, hematologic, biochemical, and bone density parameters in community-dwelling adolescent girls. Pediatrics. 2004;114(6): 1574–83.
15. Mumford J, Kohn M, Briody J, Miskovic-Wheatley J, Madden S, Clarke S, et al. Long-term Outcomes of Adolescent Anorexia Nervosa on Bone. J Adolesc Health Off Publ Soc Adolesc Med. 2019;64(3):305–10.
16. Miller KK, Lee EE, Lawson EA, Misra M, Minihan J, Grinspoon SK, et al. Determinants of skeletal loss and recovery in anorexia nervosa. J Clin Endocrinol Metab. 2006;91(8):2931–7.
17. Fazeli PK, Klibanski A. Effects of Anorexia Nervosa on Bone Metabolism. Endocr Rev. 2018;39(6):895–910.
18. ADG B-J, Faulkner RA, Forwood MR, Mirwald RL, Bailey DA. Bone mineral accrual from 8 to 30 years of age: an estimation of peak bone mass. J Bone Miner Res Off J Am Soc Bone Miner Res. 2011;26(8):1729–39.
19. Gabel L, Macdonald HM, HA MK. Reply to: Challenges in the Acquisition and Analysis of Bone Microstructure During Growth. J Bone Miner Res Off J Am Soc Bone Miner Res. 2016;31(12):2242–3.
20. Mitchell DM, Caksa S, Yuan A, Bouxsein ML, Misra M, SAM BB. Trabecular Bone Morphology Correlates With Skeletal Maturity and Body Composition in Healthy Adolescent Girls. J Clin Endocrinol Metab. 2018; 103(1):336–45.
21. TAL W, Liu X, Pitukcheewanont P, Gilsanz V. Bone acquisition in healthy children and adolescents: comparisons of dual-energy x-ray absorptiometry and computed tomography measures. J Clin Endocrinol Metab. 2005;90(4):1925–8.
22. Yilmaz D, Ersoy B, Bilgin E, Gümüşer G, Onur E, Pinar ED. Bone mineral density in girls and boys at different pubertal stages: relation with gonadal steroids, bone formation markers, and growth parameters. J Bone Miner Metab. 2005;23(6):476–82.
23. Singh D, Sanyal S, Chattopadhyay N. The role of estrogen in bone growth and formation: changes at puberty. Cell Health and Cytoskeleton. 2011;3:1–12.
24. American Psychiatric Association. Diagnostic and statistical manual of mental disorders. 5th ed. Washington: American Psychiatric Association; 2013.
25. Kaufman J, Birmaher B, Brent D, Rao U, Flynn C, Moreci P, et al. Schedule for Affective Disorders and Schizophrenia for School-Age Children-Present and Lifetime Version (K-SADS-PL): initial reliability and validity data. J Am Acad Child Adolesc Psychiatry. 1997;36(7):980–8.
26. Léger J, Marinovic D, Alberti C, Dorgeret S, Chevenne D, Marchal CL, et al. Lower bone mineral content in children with type 1 diabetes mellitus is linked to female sex, low insulin-like growth factor type I levels, and high insulin requirement. J Clin Endocrinol Metab. 2006;91(10):3947–53.
27. Sempé (M). Auxologie, méthode et séquences. Bull Mém Société Anthropol Paris. 1980;7(1):77.
28. Rolland-Cachera MF, Cole TJ, Sempé M, Tichet J, Rossignol C, Charraud A. Body Mass Index variations: centiles from birth to 87 years. Eur J Clin Nutr. 1991;45(1):13–21.
29. Tanner JM, Whitehouse RH. Clinical longitudinal standards for height, weight, height velocity, weight velocity, and stages of puberty. Arch Dis Child. 1976;51(3):170–9.
30. Courteix D, Lespessailles E, Loiseau-Peres S, Obert P, Ferry B, Benhamou CL. Lean tissue mass is a better predictor of bone mineral content and density than body weight in prepubertal girls. Rev Rhum Engl Ed. 1998;65(5):328–36.

31. Högler W, Briody J, Woodhead HJ, Chan A, Cowell CT. Importance of lean mass in the interpretation of total body densitometry in children and adolescents. J Pediatr. 2003;143(1):81–8.
32. Biller BM, Saxe V, Herzog DB, Rosenthal DI, Holzman S, Klibanski A. Mechanisms of osteoporosis in adult and adolescent women with anorexia nervosa. J Clin Endocrinol Metab. 1989;68(3):548–54.
33. Misra M, Klibanski A. Anorexia nervosa and bone. J Endocrinol. 2014;221(3): R163–76.
34. Drabkin A, Rothman MS, Wassenaar E, Mascolo M, Mehler PS. Assessment and clinical management of bone disease in adults with eating disorders: a review. J Eat Disord. 2017;5:42.
35. Faje AT, Fazeli PK, Miller KK, Katzman DK, Ebrahimi S, Lee H, et al. Fracture risk and areal bone mineral density in adolescent females with anorexia nervosa. Int J Eat Disord. 2014;47(5):458–66.
36. Schorr M, Miller KK. The endocrine manifestations of anorexia nervosa: mechanisms and management. Nat Rev Endocrinol. 2017;13(3):174–86.

14

Facilitators and barriers in anorexia nervosa treatment initiation: a qualitative study on the perspectives of patients, carers and professionals

Denise Kästner[1*], Angelika Weigel[1], Ines Buchholz[1], Ulrich Voderholzer[2,3,4], Bernd Löwe[1†] and Antje Gumz[1†]

Abstract

Background: An early psychotherapeutic treatment of anorexia nervosa (AN) is crucial for a good prognosis. In order to improve treatment initiation, knowledge about facilitators and barriers to treatment is needed.

Objective: Against this background, we aimed to identify facilitators and barriers from the perspectives of patients, carers and professionals using a qualitative approach.

Method: To this end, semi-structured interviews were conducted in triads of female patients with AN aged 14 years and older at the beginning of their first psychotherapeutic treatment, their carers, and referring health care professionals. A modified Grounded Theory approach was used for analysis.

Results: In total, 22 interviews were conducted ($n = 6$ adults, $n = 4$ adolescents, 4 full triads). The duration of untreated AN ranged between 30 days and 25.85 years ($M = 3.06 \pm 8.01$ years). A wide spectrum of facilitators and barriers within the patient, the social environment, the health care system and the society were identified. Most prominent factors were 'recognizing and addressing' by close others, 'waiting times and availability' and 'recommendations and referrals' by health care professionals. 'Positive role models for treatment' were perceived as a specific facilitative social influence. Facilitators were more frequently mentioned than barriers and most of the factors seem to hold potential for modifiability.

Conclusion: Overall, the findings suggest that early intervention approaches for AN should not only address patients and the health care system, but may also involve carers and successfully treated former patients.

Keywords: Anorexia nervosa, Early intervention, Facilitators and barriers, Psychotherapy, Qualitative study

* Correspondence: d.kaestner@uke.de
Bernd Löwe and Antje Gumz Shared last authorship
[1]Department of Psychosomatic Medicine and Psychotherapy, University Medical Centre, Hamburg-Eppendorf, Martinistr. 52, W37, 20246 Hamburg, Germany
Full list of author information is available at the end of the article

Plain English summary

An early treatment of Anorexia nervosa (AN) can improve the prognosis and avoid a chronic and severe course of illness. In order to decrease the duration of untreated AN, solid knowledge about the existing facilitators and barriers to treatment is essential. This study aimed to identify facilitators and barriers to psychotherapeutic treatment for AN from different perspectives. To this end, we conducted and analyzed $n = 22$ interviews with ($n = 4$) adolescent and ($n = 6$) adult patients at the beginning of their first treatment, their carers ($n = 7$), and referring health care professionals (n = 4). Our findings confirm previous study results on the importance of the social environment during the process of treatment initiation and on relevant barriers within the health care system like long waiting times and negative previous experiences with health care professionals. Facilitating influences not previously considered resulted from successfully treated former patients acting as 'positive role models for treatment'. If future studies support our findings, successfully treated former patients and carers may be involved more strongly in early intervention approaches for AN.

Introduction

Anorexia nervosa (AN) is a serious illness characterized by self-induced underweight, body image distortions and fear of weight gain [1]. The long-term outcome of AN is highly variable, but it was estimated that about 20% of all individuals with AN remain chronically ill [2, 3]. Moreover, the mortality rate of AN is higher than in any other mental disorder [4, 5]. The prognosis of patients with AN depends highly on how early specialized AN-treatment starts [6, 7]. Over time, eating disorder pathology can become a learned self-perpetuating rewarding process [8] and various medical complications may emerge [9]. In order to avoid hospital admissions, poor treatment outcomes and chronic courses, it is crucial to treat AN at early illness stages [6, 7].

Compared to other mental disorders (especially schizophrenia), research on early diagnosis and treatment in AN is still relatively scarce [10, 11]. Existing evidence suggests that the first 3 years of AN are the critical time window for intervention [12]. However, the mean duration of untreated AN (DUAN) was found to be approximately two to 3 years [13–16]. The DUAN range is usually wide and some patients do receive their first AN treatment only decades after the illness onset. For a closer look, the DUAN can be further divided into 1) the time span without health care contacts and 2) the time from the first AN-related health care contact to the beginning of the specialized treatment. The first interval was found to be about one to two and a half years, the second interval 10 months to 1 year [13, 17, 18]. Consequently, both close others [15] and general practitioners [17] play a decisive role in early treatment initiation. However, studies investigating their perspectives on the process of treatment initiation are missing [19, 20].

So far, widespread early intervention approaches for patients with AN have yet to be developed and implemented [11]. A single novel service for young adults with eating disorders named "First Episode and Rapid Early Intervention for Eating Disorders" showed highly promising results with respect to a reduction of the DUAN (on average 4 months shorter compared to treatment as usual), reduced treatment disengagement and improved patient satisfaction [21–23]. In order to inform the development and the improvement of such services and other approaches to early diagnosis and treatment, knowledge about existing facilitators and barriers to treatment is crucial. Two recent reviews summarized the current evidence on this topic. Accordingly, feelings of shame and stigma, personal beliefs related to the eating disorder (e.g. failure to perceive the severity of the illness), problems associated with the health care system (lack of availability, cost of treatment), and the lack of encouragement from others were identified as important barriers to treatment. Health-related concerns, other mental health problems and/or emotional distress, and social support were relevant facilitators. However, several weaknesses of the current evidence base were outlined. Firstly, most studies did not focus on specific eating disorders but rather aggregate samples of patients with various diagnoses [20]. Secondly, most studies on facilitators and barriers did not include adolescent patients and thereby potentially ignore age-group specific factors [19]. Finally, the perspectives of professionals or close others were not considered in any study despite their important role in the process of treatment initiation [19, 20].

Against this background, we aim to identify facilitators and barriers to specialized AN treatment from the perspective of adolescent and adult patients, carers and referring professionals. Knowledge about the spectrum of facilitators and barriers from multiple perspectives is crucial for improvements. Furthermore, as the first part of a mixed-methods study (Facilitators And Barriers In Anorexia NervosA treatment initiation - FABIANA-study) the present results will also directly contribute to the development of an instrument to assess facilitators and barriers (FABIANA sub-study II) and subsequently test their influence on the DUAN quantitatively (FABIANA sub-study III). In the long-term, the findings of the FABIANA-study will help to inform early intervention approaches and avoid chronic courses of AN.

Method

Study design

The FABIANA-study is a mixed-methods multi-center study with three consecutive sub-studies. The present manuscript reports sub-study I. A detailed overall description can be found within the study protocol [24]. In brief, sub-study I is a qualitative multi-informant study exploring the perspectives of triads of female patients with AN, their carers and referring professionals on facilitators and barriers to treatment initiation using semi-structured interviews. The qualitative approach is useful, common and effective for obtaining rich data on opinions, attitudes, motives, behaviors, and expectations. As part of a mixed-methods design it is a very common first step to develop and inform the quantitative measurement of complex constructs [25]. Data collection and analysis were conducted in line with the Consolidated criteria for reporting qualitative research (COREQ) criteria [26]. Ethical approval was obtained prior to recruitment (PV5108). This manuscript was prepared using the Standards for Reporting Qualitative Research (SRQR) [27].

Participants

Recruitment involved five cooperating partners who offer specialized psychotherapeutic AN treatment (four inpatient clinics, one psychotherapy training center).

Eligible for study participation were female patients with AN aged 14 years and older, who were at the beginning of their first psychotherapeutic AN treatment (i.e., a) start no longer than 3 months ago; b) at least 7 days of inpatient care or 5 sessions outpatient care completed; c) since illness onset no AN treatment). The eligibility criteria were chosen to guarantee a sufficiently consolidated development of cognitive functions such as abstract thinking and reasoning (minimum age), to minimize the risk of recall biases and response shifts (beginning of the first treatment no longer than 3 months ago) and to exclude early treatment dropouts (minimum number of completed inpatient days or outpatient sessions). AN diagnosis was validated in the context of SCID-interviews. Study participants were non-randomly selected using mixed purposeful sampling. In order to select adolescent and adult AN patients and to achieve variance with respect to the DUAN (< vs. ≥ 1 year) stratified purposeful sampling was used; their carers and professionals were included in the study by network (snowball) sampling [28]. The aim was to include complete triads. Recruitment was terminated with theoretical saturation (i.e. new material could be fully described with existing categories).

Data collection

All participants and, in case of minor participants, legal guardians gave written informed consent. To assess basic sample characteristics, participants filled out a short questionnaire prior to the interview. The treating psychotherapist provided information on patients' weight, height and the date of treatment initiation.

Qualitative interviews were based on semi-structured guidelines designed for each perspective. The guidelines were developed by the research team. They were tested in a group consisting of physicians and psychologists and refined accordingly. Interviews were conducted by two female PhD-level psychologists with patients being interviewed face-to-face, and carers and professionals by phone. Interviewers and study participants did not know each other prior to undertaking the study. Prior to data collection, the study team reflected on and noted any a priori assumptions on emerging topics.

Patient interviews were divided into two parts. The first part sought to check inclusion and exclusion criteria and to retrospectively determine the month of AN onset. The procedure is described in detail within the study protocol [24]. The second part of the patient interviews and the interviews with the carers and professionals were concerned with facilitators and barriers for the treatment initiation. At first, all participants were asked to describe the process from the beginning of the first symptoms to the beginning of the treatment with their own words. Afterwards, the interviews focused on factors facilitating or hindering treatment initiation (e.g. "What made it easier/harder for you/ your daughter/your friend/your patient to start treatment?") and became increasingly more specific. All interviews were audio-taped and transcribed using prespecified transcription rules [29].

Data analysis

In line with the applied Grounded Theory approach [30, 31], data analysis was carried out simultaneously to the data collection. By that, the already analyzed material influenced the subsequent data collection (e.g. specifically recruit cases that may provide so far missing information). Each interview was analyzed independently by two members of the study team using MAXQDA (software package for Qualitative Data Analysis named after the sociologist MAX Weber) [32]. Analysis started with open coding of the interviews. Memos were written for each interview and as needed for specific codes. Subsequently, the code tree was gradually developed and repeatedly refined in order to reach the best possible fit with the interview material. In total, four female researchers developed and discussed the categories and coded the interviews (three PhD-level psychologists and one professor for psychosomatic medicine and psychotherapy). In order to measure the influence of specific, well-defined facilitators and barriers in the following FABIANA-sub-studies, rather broad aggregations were avoided within the qualitative analysis.

Subsequently, the developed category system (1. main categories, 2. factors, i.e. F = facilitators and B = barriers sorted by the frequency they were mentioned) is presented. Code names (i.e. categories) are indicated by single quotation marks, exemplary quotes by double quotation marks. Exemplary quotes are selected to further illustrate less self-explanatory factors and to substantiate the findings [27]. Quotes are identified by perspective and a study code linking the triad (P = patient, C = carer, Pr = professional). They are edited for legibility and explanations are added in square brackets were necessary.

Results

Sample characteristics

In total, 22 interviews were conducted with 10 patients, 7 carers, 4 professionals and one study participant, who was both carer (of an adolescent patient) and professional (4 complete triads: 3 with adult patients, 1 with an adolescent patient). The interviews took on average 1 h and 2 min (SD = 14:33 min).

Among the patients were six adults (mean age = 23.33 years, SD = 7.47, range: 20–38 years; mean BMI = 15.9 kg/m^2, SD = 2.25) and four adolescents (mean age = 15.75 years, SD = 1.50, range: 14–17 years; mean BMI = 15.6 kg/m^2, SD = 1.43; mean % expected body weight = 73.41, SD = 4.47). One of the adolescent patients and three of the adult patients had at least one comorbid SCID-I diagnosis. No participant was diagnosed with a personality disorder. Mean DUAN within the sample was 3.06 years (SD = 8.01; median = 0.58 years) with a range between 30 days and 25.85 years. The interviewed carers were four mothers, two fathers and one (female) friend (mean age = 52.00 years, SD = 3.79). The professionals were four general practitioners and one psychotherapist ($n = 4$ female, $n = 1$ male; mean age = 53.40 years, SD = 7.02). Two of the general practitioners were specialized in the treatment of eating disorders.

Overview of the qualitative results

In total, 1.200 codings were assigned. Nearly two third ($n = 772$, 63.28%) of the codings represented a facilitator, and slightly more than one third ($n = 448$, 36.72%) a barrier. The following framework to group facilitators and barriers into broader main categories emerged (s. Figure 1): 'patient' (P), 'social environment' (SE), 'health care system' (HCS) and 'societal factors' (SF). Furthermore, the interactions between these categories had to be differentiated. Four codings could not be mapped and belong to a remaining category.

The next level of the developed code tree gives a more detailed description of the facilitators and barriers. Table 1 lists the 20 most frequently mentioned factors (mean rank based on the number of interview partners mentioning the factor and the number of single codings belonging to the factor). Table S1 gives the top 20 list separated by perspectives and age groups (adolescent vs. adult patients). Accordingly, interview partners generally emphasized factors related to their perspective (e.g., professionals mentioning factors within the 'health care system'). More minor factors are presented in Table S2.

The patient

The most frequently mentioned factors on the part of the patient were 'somatic symptoms' (F) and the occurrence of a (symptom) 'exacerbation or breaking point' (F). As a reason for seeking help, both adolescent and adult patients mentioned a wide variety of somatic

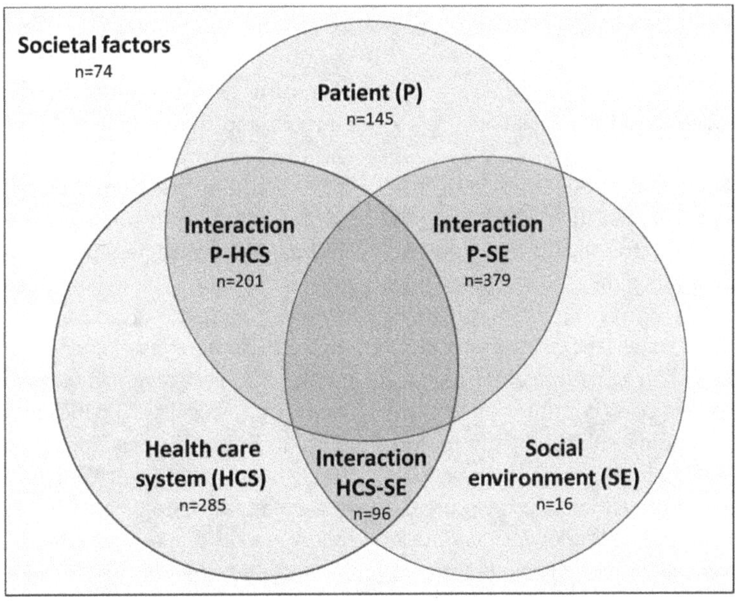

Fig. 1 Framework to group facilitators and barriers including the respective number of codings from 22 qualitative interviews

Table 1 Top 20 facilitators and barriers in AN treatment initiation

Factor	Main category	Rank[a]	Interview partners n (%)	Single codings n (%)
F + B - (Not) recognizing and addressing	SE-P	1	18 (81.8)	83 (6.9)
F + B – Waiting time and availability	HCS	2	16 (72.7)	82 (6.8)
F+ B – (No/wrong) recommendation and referral	HCS-P	3	20 (90.9)	54 (4.5)
F + B – Competence, specialization, training	HCS	3	13 (59.1)	97 (8.1)
B – Non-understanding of AN as illness or the need for treatment	SE-P	5	12 (54.5)	57 (4.8)
F – Health education and de-stigmatization of AN and psychotherapy	SF	6	14 (63.6)	42 (3.5)
F – Exchange, support, concern, understanding	SE-P	6	13 (59.1)	51 (4.3)
F – Positive role models for treatment	SE-P	8	9 (40.9)	57 (4.8)
F+ B – (No) reminding of, making of or accompanying to appointments	SE-P	9	10 (45.5)	40 (3.3)
F – Suggesting or encouraging to seek treatment	SE-P	10	13 (59.1)	24 (2.0)
F – Somatic symptoms	P	10	10 (45.5)	37 (3.1)
F – Good personal connections	SE-HCS	12	11 (50.0)	33 (2.8)
F + B – Networking, cooperation	HCS	13	7 (31.8)	47 (3.9)
F+ B – (No/vaguely) diagnosing or communicating diagnosis	HCS-P	14	8 (36.4)	34 (2.8)
F+ B – (Not) living, being, eating alone	P-SE	15	10 (45.5)	20 (1.7)
F – Exacerbation and personal breaking point reached	P	16	9 (40.9)	20 (1.7)
B – Trivializing and neglected assistance	HCS--P	17	[b]6 (27.3)	34 (2.8)
F + B – Fit between individual patient and service settings	HCS	18	7 (31.8)	[b]16 (1.3)
F + B – (Reducing) comparisons with media ideals	SF	19	[b]6 (27.3)	30 (2.5)
F – Continuity (of care) and regular control examinations	HCS-P	20	[b]6 (27.3)	20 (1.7)
Total			**22**	**1.200**

Note. F facilitator, *B* barrier, *SE* social environment, *HCS* health care system, *P* patient, *SF* societal factors, *AN* anorexia nervosa, [a] Mean rank based on the rank on the level of interview partners (number of interview partners mentioning the factor) and on the level of codings (number of single text passages mentioning the factor). [b] Not among the top 20 within the ranking on the level of interview partners or the level of codings, respectively

symptoms reaching from brittle nails to pericardial effusion. Regarding the facilitator 'exacerbation and breaking point', interview partners stated for example that they were only ready to start treatment when the "limit was reached" (C-771), "it was already so acute" (P-142), they collapsed or had "no real life anymore" (P-765).

Interactions between the patient and the social environment

In general, most of the statements of our interview partners concerned 'interactions between the patient and the social environment' (s. Table 2 for illustrative quotes). First, 'recognizing and addressing' (F + B) the changing or worrying eating behaviors, body weight, or physical activities by close others was experienced as important. In some cases, the early detection and confrontation was found to be essential, in other cases continuity and persistence in making AN-symptoms subject of discussion emerged as crucial. A barrier for treatment initiation, which seemed especially relevant to adolescent patients (s. Tab. S1), was the 'non-understanding of AN as illness and/or of the need for treatment' (B) within the social environment. Besides an underestimation of the seriousness at early illness stages or in general (e.g., "she will deal with that on her own") and simplistic or stigmatizing beliefs (e.g., "just eat normal again"), interview partners also pointed to eating disorders of close others as one reason for non-understanding reactions (e.g., formerly anorectic grandmother who strongly supported the thin body ideal). In contrast, the facilitating influence of positive relationships involving 'exchange, support, concern and understanding' (F) was mentioned. Support without pressure, open, understanding and calm conversations and expressions of concern were perceived as helpful. In addition to such general social support, interactions with other persons, who already found their way into treatment and experienced improvement or even recovery, were described as a specific facilitative influence on so far untreated persons. Such 'positive role models for treatment' (F) were found within the personal lives (e.g., stepsister, colleague) or via (social) media (e.g., Instagram, television documentary). Interview partners stated that positive role models could motivate treatment initiation, answer specific questions about treatments and take fears about treatment. Further facilitative influences relevant for adolescents and adults were seen in practical support by 'reminding of, making of or accompanying to appointments' (F + B) and in

Table 2 Illustrating quotes for facilitators and barriers at the interaction of individuals with AN and their social environment

F + B	(Not) recognizing and addressing	**"I think it really helped me that somebody saw it and then said to me that this is really a disorder." (P-709)** **"My friends reflected on these things and said, "[Patients name], this is not normal!". Then my mind had to admit that this could be true. I think about it. Reluctantly, but I will." (P-249)**
B	**Non-understanding of AN as an illness or of the need for treatment**	"It was that they all [patient's family] thought I had chosen this disorder [...] and I can turn it off and then it's gone. But it does not work that way. It came gradually and it does not go away simply like pushing a button. And they did not understood this." (P-765)
F	**Exchange, support, concern, understanding**	"And I talked a lot about eating, about these issues with my mother and [...] I could basically tell her everything about that and also my worries and my concerns. And I do think that this was not so easy for my mother to hear all this [...]. But at least she tried to stay calm and to deal with that in a good way [...]. This is what helped me."(P-989)
F	**Positive role models for treatment**	*Interviewer*: "Well, my very last question. If you look back on the whole interview and on all the topics we touched, what would you say, makes it easier for people with anorexia to start treatment?" *Patient*: "I think, well, I would say talking to others and I would say talking a lot to other persons, who went already through this process, I believe. Because they [...] can encourage you and they can tell, that it wasn't that bad, or well how they experienced it." (P-771)
F + B	**(No) reminding of, making of or accompanying to appointments**	"... and if you don't have this sturdiness. This never ending "I will call again" [...]. They were already annoyed with me, but it was useful. She then got the place from 1 day to the other." (C-194) "For sure, I would say if it were not for my family, I would not have been there. I would not have managed it to do the steps on my own. My husband organized everything. It was clear to me, that I needed it, but ... calling, driving there, I would not have done that." (P-966)
F	**Suggesting or encouraging to seek treatment**	"We just told her, that she really needs help and professional help, because we are stuck." (C-142) „ ... I have also motivated her that she keeps going through with her idea [...] to go [...] in this clinic. And I really motivated her to actually do that, because I thought it was so right." (C-194)
F + B	**(Not) living, being, eating alone**	"... basically only if you are all the time together with her, you could see that it is really nothing she is eating." (C-249)

Note. F facilitator, *B* barrier, *P* patient, *AN* anorexia nervosa, *C* carer

'suggestions and encouragement to seek treatment' (F). The latter meant for some patients to get an highly important initial external impulse, for others hearing pleas or continuous persuasive efforts, and, usually later in the process, encouraging and motivating words (e.g., "Only way that it will get better.", P-765). Finally, participants noted the relevance of social resources in general or nearby ('(Not) living, eating or being alone' – F + B).

The health care system

One of the most prominent causes for treatment delays were considered to be long 'waiting times and limited availability' (F + B, e.g., "I have said, she is starving to death. You can't tell me [to wait] three months.", C-194). The interview partners, especially carers, called for more treatment places and better availability of outpatient psychotherapists in general and in rural areas in particular. An important concern was that the tediously build treatment motivation decreases during waiting times. To better address this problem, it was recommended that referring professionals should point out the potentially long waiting times as early as possible. Furthermore, patients often stated to choose the service with the shortest waiting time.

Different statements were concerned with 'the competence, the specialization and the training' (F + B) of the referring professionals.. Even though the main tasks of the professionals were merely detection and referral, solid knowledge of the disorder, somatic consequences, and necessary diagnostic procedures (e.g. laboratory parameters), as well as soft skills such as the ability to establish a good patient-physician relationship or communication skills were considered essential. Finding a professional who is competent in dealing with somatic and mental problems was often experienced as a challenge. Two specific suggestions for improvement were mentioned: establishment of a psychosomatic general practitioner and expansion of low-threshold outpatient services located at specialized inpatient facilities. The latter were seen as the best way to assess the need for treatment in a timely manner and to make direct referrals if needed.

Another key factor highlighted by professionals was found to be 'networking and cooperation' (F + B). This primarily concerned collaboration between general practitioners and psychotherapists, and secondarily other professions like gynecologists, school psychologists, counselors, and psychiatrists. Physicians experienced the lack of financial compensation for networking and interdisciplinary collaboration to be a hindrance.

The factor 'fit between patient and service settings' (F + B) subsumes various, mostly non-modifiable circumstances. Positive influences were, for example, if the clinic was close to home or if fellow patients were expected to be in the same age group. Strongly limited phone times of psychotherapists or time slots for appointments during school or working hours constituted a barrier.

Interactions between the patient and the health care system

The most important and obvious factor regarding 'interactions between patient and health care system' was whether and when the consulted professional referred into specialized treatment ('(No/wrong) recommendation and referral' – F + B). Referrals or recommendations which were binding (e.g., "Not only saying 'think about it'.", P-966), timely (e.g., with "notification of urgency", P-249, avoiding prolonged treatments in non-specialized contexts, Pr-709), clear (e.g., "you should, not you could", C-194) and concrete (i.e., specific provider, C-709, C/Pr-547) were described as facilitative. Additionally, a joint decision making involving carers was described as helpful (Pr-771, C-771).

Prior to the referral, the detection of the disorder and the communication about the diagnosis was indicated to be crucial ('(No/vaguely) diagnosing or communicating diagnosis' – F + B). The interview partners described that persons with AN sometimes consult physicians for related reasons or single symptoms (e.g., check for nutritional deficiency or food intolerance, Pr-249; amenorrhea, other mental symptoms, Pr 709). According to various interview partners, especially adult patients, professionals frequently failed to recognize AN in such situations, and an isolated treatment of single symptoms or mental comorbidities was described to prolong treatment initiation. When communicating the diagnosis, patients and carers wished for an unambiguous and clear position of the professional. One adult patient stated receiving her diagnosis in a written form was highly helpful ("copy of the physician's letter", P-966). Another option mentioned was to go through each single diagnostic criterion (Pr-709).

A previous experience of 'trivializing or neglected assistance' (B) emerged as a clear barrier to treatment. Some patients described that professionals normalized the pathology of the eating disorder (e.g., "And then we went to a general practitioner, but she didn't take me seriously. She said, well, that it is normal for adolescents, that it is just a phase in my life, and that we will manage it somehow on our own.", P-989). Others reported situations in which professionals failed to provide adequate care despite the fact some were severely underweight (e.g., sick leave without follow-up appointment, several emergency room admissions without a correct diagnosis or referral, P-966). After such experiences, it often took time for the individuals to seek help again.

In contrast, 'continuity (of treatment) and regular control examinations' (F) performed by the general practitioners were perceived to facilitate a subsequent psychotherapeutic treatment.

Interactions between social environment and health care system

Sometimes, treatment initiation was also influenced by interactions between carers and professionals. Specifically, existing 'good personal connections' (F) between a carer and a professional proved beneficial (e.g., "My grandmother knows this general practitioner and it just so happens the general practitioner is specialized in this field [eating disorders].", P-142).

Societal factors

Societal factors affected the female patients, their social environment and professionals. 'Health education and destigmatization of AN and psychotherapy' (F) was named as a major societal factor. The interview partners were most likely to associate health education with school, but also mentioned fitness studios. Health education should inform and educate about eating disorders in general and the somatic consequences, the importance of early treatment, and the treatment options in particular. According to the interview partners, it should convey a feeling that there is no need to feel guilt or shame because of the disorder or because of seeking treatment (P-989). The interview partners particularly wished for greater awareness among key persons (e.g., pediatricians, general practitioners, teachers, fitness trainers).

A relevant barrier to treatment was 'comparisons with media ideals' (F + B, e.g., "I have to say social media is a big factor [...] where you are influenced by the body sizes of models and then you think, maybe I look similar to them now, but then why should I be sick?", P-142). In this context, participants mentioned the removal of pro-Ana content as an important measure.

Discussion

The main objective of the present study was to identify facilitators and barriers to an early AN treatment using a multi-informant approach involving female adolescent and adult patients, their carers, and referring healthcare professionals. In comparison, facilitating influences were mentioned more frequently than hindering influences. The various interview partners (female patients, carers, professionals) generally focused on facilitators and barriers related to their perspective.

'Positive role models for treatment' was a facilitator that specifically stood out in comparison to the existing evidence base. The factor describes a specific positive influence of successfully treated individuals on so far untreated individuals with AN. To our knowledge, this factor has not been mentioned in any previous study. In line with this finding, it was pointed out that there is little research on the sharing of lived experience despite its relevance in the consumer community [33]. In general, positive and negative effects of these 'interventions' are to be expected [34, 35], but research has long focused almost exclusively on the negative consequences associated with pro-Ana websites [34–36]. An increase in eating disorder pathology from the use of such websites has been demonstrated [34]. However, it has also been shown that critical and recovery-oriented comments ('anti-Ana', 'pro-recovery') clearly dominate on social media platforms [37]. Their effects in terms of earlier treatment initiation have not been studied, but the potential active ingredients of recovery-oriented narratives reported in the literature overlap strongly with the statements of our interview partners. These include increases in treatment motivation, hope, knowledge (insider information), and decreases in fear and stigma [33, 38, 39]. Potential risks could include overestimation of treatment effects [39] and maladaptive social comparisons (peer contagion effect) [40, 41]. Nonetheless, based on the present results, it seems highly promising to further investigate the influences of successfully treated former patients ('positive role models for treatment') on the treatment initiation of so far untreated individuals with AN.

In addition to the specific facilitative social influence of 'positive role models', interactions with family and friends play a crucial role, especially during the period without any contact with health care. The present and previous studies have shown consistently that close others fulfill tasks similar to those of professionals in early stages of illness (e.g. recognition, motivation) and that their recognition (F + B - '(not) recognizing and addressing") [42], understanding (B - 'non-understanding of AN as illness and/or of the need for treatment') [19, 43], emotional and practical support (F - 'exchange, support, concern, understanding', F + B - '(no) reminding of, making of or accompanying to appointments') [20], and encouragement to seek treatment (F - 'suggesting or encouraging to seek treatment') [19, 20], or the lack thereof, may be decisive for treatment initiation. Social problems and isolation (F + B - '(not) living, eating, being alone') can prolong the DUAN [42]. However, the role of close others is also highly challenging. Very little is known about the needs and burden of close others (e.g., need for information, emotional stress, financial strain, impaired social life) specifically in the period before AN treatment starts. It has been suggested that the needs and burden of carers vary depending on the stage of illness [44], but most studies investigated the issue only among carers of AN patients in treatment (e.g. [44, 45]). In early stages, it is essential to recognize the illness, which is often described as a process of gradual realization [46]. According to the present results, adolescents may particularly benefit if carers perceive the difficulties soon in terms of an illness and subsequently recognize the need for professional help (B - 'non-understanding of AN as illness and/or of the need for treatment'). To achieve such understanding, carers need sound information about AN [46]. Counseling services and support programs for carers can provide such information. Additionally, with regard to their own negative emotions (e.g. guilt, helplessness), maladaptive beliefs and behaviors (e.g. over-involvement, criticism) and possible eating problems of their own, they can provide support and counseling to achieve a better coping with the illness [47]. It seems important that such services are open to close others, even if the person with AN is not yet in treatment. Such an early support of carers may indirectly exhibit a positive influence on the treatment initiation of the individual with AN.

However, considerable delays in treatment also occur within the health care system [13, 17, 18]. In particular, we were able to confirm several findings on the relevance of long waiting times or limited availability (F + B – 'waiting time and availability') [13, 19, 20, 48, 49] and past negative experiences with health care professionals (B – 'trivializing and neglected assistance') [19, 20, 43, 48, 49]. Both factors strongly indicate weaknesses within the health care system. Especially, the trivialization of symptoms by professionals obviously counteracted early diagnosis and treatment. Thereby, professionals seem to reinforce maladaptive thoughts of individuals with AN that the problem might be "not serious enough" [48] or that there must be a symptom exacerbation (F – 'exacerbation or breaking point') [50] and/or (severe) 'somatic symptoms' (F) [19, 50] before treatment is initiated. In other instances, and more frequently, professionals failed to make a diagnosis or refer to specialized treatment (F + B – '(no/wrong) recommendation and referral', F + B – '(no/vague) diagnosing or communicating diagnosis') [49, 51]. Thiswas often attributed to a lack of 'competence, specialization, or training' (F + B) regarding eating disorders, especially in primary care [49]. In addition to more intensive training, screening and decision support tools are often recommended [49, 52]. However, the presently interviewed professionals also emphasized the importance of 'networking and collaboration' (F + B) at the interface between primary and secondary healthcare.

Finally, the improvement of mental health literacy [19, 48] can be an important societal factor. Health education and awareness programs (F – 'health education and destigmatization of AN and psychotherapy') can reduce stigma and negative attitudes related to the disorder and the treatment, which are often cited as a barrier to early treatment [19, 20, 43, 48, 50].

Strengths and limitations

The present findings have to be viewed in light of the strengths and weaknesses of our study. To our knowledge, this is the first study to investigate facilitators and barriers to AN treatment initiation using a multi-informant approach. Therefore, we could shed light on factors relevant to female adolescent and adult patients, carers and professionals. Prior studies often focused solely on the perspective of adult patients. It can be argued that the present sample size within each group (e.g., adolescent patients) is relatively small. However, the overall sample size of our study is well within the recommended range [28]. Furthermore, the correct and careful selection of study participants in order to reach theoretical and data saturation is often higher valued in qualitative research than the mere number of study participants [28, 53]. Accordingly, we applied rigorous eligibility criteria (e.g., minimum age, beginning of the first treatment no longer than 3 months ago) and followed a pre-defined sampling scheme. As one consequence of this sampling scheme, we could achieve a wide range of the DUAN within our study sample. However, regarding our sampling, it is also important to note that male patients as well as individuals who never entered specialized treatment were not included in the present analysis. Additionally, two of the general practitioners interviewed had a specialty in eating disorders, which seems atypical. In general, we could gain insights on the spectrum of factors relevant to AN treatment initiation, but we cannot make conclusions about the relative importance of certain facilitators or barriers. Additional quantitative evidence especially on modifiable facilitators and barriers is needed for this purpose. In order to subsequently develop an instrument for the assessment of facilitators and barriers and to gain such evidence (FABIANA sub-studies II and III), the present analyses remained relatively specific and concrete. Consequently, we did not consider potential meta-themes within the qualitative material.

Conclusion

In conclusion, our study set out to better understand the spectrum of facilitators and barriers in AN treatment initiation using a multi-informant approach. Most of the presently identified facilitators and barriers seem to hold potential for modifiability and improvements. Our findings suggest that measures to decrease the duration of untreated AN and avoid chronic illness courses might not only address patients and the health care system, but may also involve close others and successfully treated former patients. A newly identified specific measure to improve the treatment initiation of untreated individuals with AN might be the use of treatment narratives from successfully treated former patients.

Abbreviations

AN: Anorexia nervosa; B: Barrier; BMI: Body-Mass-Index; C: Carer or close other; DSM-IV: Diagnostic and Statistical Manual of Mental Disorders – Fourth Edition; DUAN: Duration of untreated Anorexia nervosa; F: Facilitator; HCS: Health care system; P: Patient; Pr: Health care professional; SCID I/II: Structured clinical interview for DSM-IV Axis I/II diagnoses; SE: Social environment; SF: Societal factors

Acknowledgements

We would like to thank all our interview partners and our cooperating partners who were involved in the recruitment of study participants. Alphabetically ordered, these are: Asklepios Clinic Nord-Ochsenzoll (Hamburg), Asklepios Clinic West Hamburg (Hamburg), Clinic Lüneburger Heide (Bad Bevensen), Dipl.-Psych. B. Matz-Knocke (Hamburg), Dipl.-Psych. M. Axhausen (Hamburg), Dipl.-Psych. S. la Roche (Hamburg), Institute for Behavior Therapy Training Hamburg (IVAH, Hamburg), Medical Care Center for Psychotherapy, Psychiatry and Psychosomatics Falkenried (Hamburg), Psychosomatic Clinic of the Evangelic Hospital Ginsterhof (Rosengarten), Schön Clinic Hamburg Eilbek (Hamburg), Schön Clinic Roseneck (Prien am Chiemsee), Training Center for Behavior Therapy Falkenried (VTFAW, Hamburg).

Authors' contributions

The study's principal investigators, BL and AG, designed the study with DK and AW. Funding was obtained by BL and AG. UV was involved in the recruitment of patients. DK and IB conducted data collection. DK, AW, IB and AG analyzed the interview material. DK wrote the first draft of the manuscript. All other authors provided substantial input to the first draft. All authors read and approved the final manuscript.

Competing interests

The authors declare that they have no competing interests.

Author details

[1]Department of Psychosomatic Medicine and Psychotherapy, University Medical Centre, Hamburg-Eppendorf, Martinistr. 52, W37, 20246 Hamburg, Germany. [2]Schön Clinic Roseneck, Prien am Chiemsee, Germany. [3]Department of Psychiatry and Psychotherapy, University Hospital Freiburg, Freiburg, Germany. [4]Department of Psychiatry and Psychotherapy, University of Munich (LMU), Munich, Germany.

References

1. American Psychiatric Association, Diagnostic and statistical manual of mental disorders. DSM-5. 5th ed. Arlington: American Psychiatric Publishing; 2013.
2. Steinhausen HC. The outcome of anorexia nervosa in the 20th century. Am J Psychiatry. 2002;159(8):1284–93.
3. Fichter MM, et al. Long-term outcome of anorexia nervosa: results from a large clinical longitudinal study. Int J Eat Disord. 2017;50(9):1018–30.
4. Arcelus J, et al. Mortality rates in patients with anorexia nervosa and other eating disorders. A meta-analysis of 36 studies. Arch Gen Psychiatry. 2011; 68(7):724–31.
5. Hoang U, Goldacre M, James A. Mortality following hospital discharge with a diagnosis of eating disorder: national record linkage study, England, 2001-2009. Int J Eat Disord. 2014;47(5):507–15.
6. House J, et al. Comparison of specialist and nonspecialist care pathways for adolescents with anorexia nervosa and related eating disorders. Int J Eat Disord. 2012;45(8):949–56.
7. Treasure J, Russell G. The case for early intervention in anorexia nervosa: theoretical exploration of maintaining factors. Br J Psychiatry. 2011;199(1):5–7.
8. O'Hara CB, Campbell IC, Schmidt U. A reward-centred model of anorexia nervosa: a focussed narrative review of the neurological and psychophysiological literature. Neurosci Biobehav Rev. 2015;52:131–52.

9. Zipfel S, et al. Anorexia nervosa: aetiology, assessment, and treatment. Lancet Psychiatry. 2015;2(12):1099–111.
10. MacDonald K, et al. Pathways to mental health services for young people: a systematic review. Soc Psychiatry Psychiatr Epidemiol. 2018;53(10):1005–38.
11. Schmidt U, et al. Will a comprehensive, person-centered, team-based early intervention approach to first episode illness improve outcomes in eating disorders? Int J Eat Disord. 2016;49(4):374–7.
12. Treasure J, Stein D, Maguire S. Has the time come for a staging model to map the course of eating disorders from high risk to severe enduring illness? An examination of the evidence. Early Interv Psychiatry. 2015;9(3): 173–84.
13. Schlegl S, et al. Pathways to Care and Duration of Untreated Illness of Inpatients with Anorexia and Bulimia nervosa. Psychiatr Prax. 2019;46(6): 342–8.
14. Weigel A, et al. Duration of untreated illness and predictors of late treatment initiation in anorexia nervosa. J Public Health. 2014;22:519–27.
15. Neubauer K, et al. Paths to first treatment and duration of untreated illness in anorexia nervosa: are there differences according to age of onset? Eur Eat Disord Rev. 2014;22(4):292–8.
16. Schoemaker C. Does early intervention improve the prognosis in anorexia nervosa? A systematic review of the treatment-outcome literature. Int J Eat Disord. 1997;21(1):1–15.
17. Volpe U, et al. Pathways to specialist care for eating disorders: an Italian multicentre study. Eur Eat Disord Rev. 2019;27(3):274–82.
18. Gumz A, et al. The psychenet public health intervention for anorexia nervosa: a pre-post-evaluation study in a female patient sample. Prim Health Care Res Development. 2018;19(1):42–52.
19. Ali K, et al. Perceived barriers and facilitators towards help-seeking for eating disorders: a systematic review. Int J Eat Disord. 2017;50(1):9–21.
20. Regan P, Cachelin FM, Minnick AM. Initial treatment seeking from professional health care providers for eating disorders: a review and synthesis of potential barriers to and facilitators of "first contact". Int J Eat Disord. 2017;50(3):190–209.
21. Brown A, et al. The FREED project (first episode and rapid early intervention in eating disorders): service model, feasibility and acceptability. Early Interv Psychiatry. 2018;12(2):250–7.
22. Potterton R, et al. "I'm not a teenager, I'm 22. Why can't I snap out of it?": a qualitative exploration of seeking help for a first-episode eating disorder during emerging adulthood. J Eat Disorder. 2020;8(1):46.
23. Flynn M, et al. Assessing the impact of first episode rapid early intervention for eating disorders on duration of untreated eating disorder: a multi-Centre quasi-experimental study. Eur Eat Disord Rev. 2020. Epub ahead of print.
24. Kästner D, et al. Facilitators and barriers in anorexia nervosa treatment initiation (FABIANA): study protocol for a mixed-methods and multicentre study. BJPsych Open. 2019;5(6):e92.
25. Curry LA, et al. Mixed methods in biomedical and health services research. Circ Cardiovasc Qual Outcomes. 2013;6(1):119–23.
26. Tong A, Sainsbury P, Craig J. Consolidated criteria for reporting qualitative research (COREQ): a 32-item checklist for interviews and focus groups. Int J Qual Health Care. 2007;19(6):349–57.
27. O'Brien BC, et al. Standards for reporting qualitative research: a synthesis of recommendations. Acad Med. 2014;89(9):1245–51.
28. Onwuegbuzie AJ, Leech NL. A call for qualitative power analyses. Qual Quant. 2007;41(1):105–21.
29. Dresing T, Pehl T. Praxisbuch Interview, Transkription & Analyse. Anleitungen und Regelssysteme für qualitativ Forschende [Practice book interview, transcription & analysis. Instructions and rules for qualitative research]. 8th ed. Marburg: Eigenverlag; 2018.
30. Strauss, A. and J. Corbin, Grounded theory: Grundlagen qualitativer Sozialforschung. 1996: Psychologie Verlags Union.
31. Strübing J. In: Bohnsack R, et al., editors. Grounded Theory. 2nd ed. qualitative social research. Wiesbaden: VS Verlag; 2008.
32. Software V. MAXQDA. Berlin: VERBI Software; 2018.
33. Dawson L, et al. Are recovery stories helpful for women with eating disorders? A pilot study and commentary on future research. J Eat Disord. 2018;6:21.
34. Rodgers RF, et al. A meta-analysis examining the influence of pro-eating disorder websites on body image and eating pathology. Eur Eat Disord Rev. 2016;24(1):3–8.
35. Smahelova M, et al. Internet usage by women with eating disorders during illness and recovery. Health Commun. 2019;35(5):1–9.
36. Gale L, et al. Experiences of using pro-eating disorder websites: a qualitative study with service users in NHS eating disorder services. Eat Weight Disord. 2016;21(3):427–34.
37. Branley DB, Covey J. Pro-ana versus pro-recovery: a content analytic comparison of social media Users' communication about eating disorders on twitter and Tumblr. Front Psychol. 2017;8:1356.
38. Aardoom JJ, et al. Internet and patient empowerment in individuals with symptoms of an eating disorder: a cross-sectional investigation of a pro-recovery focused e-community. Eat Behav. 2014;15(3):350–6.
39. Ziebland S, Wyke S. Health and illness in a connected world: how might sharing experiences on the internet affect people's health? Milbank Q. 2012; 90(2):219–49.
40. Beveridge J, et al. Peer mentoring for eating disorders: results from the evaluation of a pilot program. J Eat Disord. 2019;7:13.
41. Shaw LK, Homewood J. The effect of eating disorder memoirs in individuals with self-identified eating pathologies. J Nerv Ment Dis. 2015;203(8):591–5.
42. Treasure J, Nazar BP. Interventions for the Carers of patients with eating disorders. Curr Psychiatry Rep. 2016;18(2):16.
43. Griffiths S, et al. Pathways into treatment for eating disorders: a quantitative examination of treatment barriers and treatment attitudes. Eat Disord. 2018; 26(6):556–74.
44. Blondin S, et al. Caregiving experience and expressed emotion among parents of adolescents suffering from anorexia nervosa following illness onset. Eat Disord. 2019;27(5):453–70.
45. Stefanini MC, et al. Living with someone with an eating disorder: factors affecting the caregivers' burden. Eat Weight Disord. 2019;24(6):1209–14.
46. Fox JR, Dean M, Whittlesea A. The experience of caring for or living with an individual with an eating disorder: a meta-synthesis of qualitative studies. Clin Psychol Psychother. 2017;24(1):103–25.
47. Nicholls DE, Yi I. Early intervention in eating disorders: a parent group approach. Early Interv Psychiatry. 2012;6(4):357–67.
48. Innes NT, Clough BA, Casey LM. Assessing treatment barriers in eating disorders: a systematic review. Eat Disord. 2017;25(1):1–21.
49. Johns G, et al. Current eating disorder healthcare services - the perspectives and experiences of individuals with eating disorders, their families and health professionals: systematic review and thematic synthesis. BJPsych Open. 2019;5(4):e59.
50. Schoen EG, et al. A retrospective look at the internal help-seeking process in young women with eating disorders. Eat Disord. 2012;20(1):14–30.
51. Higgins A, Cahn S. Detection of anorexia nervosa in primary care. Eat Disord. 2018;26(3):213–28.
52. Dingemans AE, et al. Development and validation of a decision tool for early identification of adult patients with severe and complex eating disorder psychopathology in need of highly specialized care. Eur Eat Disord Rev. 2017;25(5):366–72.
53. Malterud K, Siersma VD, Guassora AD. Sample size in qualitative interview studies: guided by information power. Qual Health Res. 2016;26(13):1753–60.

15

Critical incidents in anorexia nervosa: perspectives of those with a lived experience

Jenni Leppanen[1,2*], Lara Tosunlar[2], Rachael Blackburn[2], Steven Williams[1], Kate Tchanturia[2,3,4] and Felicity Sedgewick[5]

Abstract

Background: Although social-emotional difficulties are believed play a key role in anorexia nervosa (AN), there is uncertainty regarding what these difficulties might look like. Previous research has largely focused on a "disease model" of social-emotional processing in AN with little attention paid to positive emotions and experiences. Therefore, the aim of the present study was to obtain a fuller picture of critical life events as identified by those with lived AN experience.

Methods: Thirty-four participants aged 16–48 with current or past AN completed an online survey describing self-defined positive and difficult critical events. Thematic analysis was used to assess patterns in participants narrative responses.

Results: Two major themes were identified in the descriptions of positive critical events: *Moments of celebration* and *Unexpected positive outcomes*. These major themes revealed increased external focus and some corrective experiences that challenged the participants pre-existing expectations leading to new positive outcomes. Difficult events clustered into life events that were identified as *Eating disorder (ED) related* and *Non-ED related* and included the dimensions of relational conflict and feeling unsupported.

Discussion: The findings suggest that although negative emotionality was identified in the accounts of those with lived experience of AN capacity for "*big-picture*" thinking with and explicit focus on others was also identified. Moreover, an openness to corrective experiences that worked to challenge negative expectations was evident for some participants. Together these findings have scope as targets for further clinical research and treatment interventions.

Keywords: Anorexia nervosa, Critical events, Positive experiences, Difficult experiences, Information processing bias, Thematic analysis

* Correspondence: jenni.leppanen@kcl.ac.uk
[1]Department of Neuroimaging, Institute of Psychology, Psychiatry and Neuroscience, King's College London, London, UK
[2]Department of Psychological Medicine, Institute of Psychology, Psychiatry and Neuroscience, King's College London, 103 Denmark Hill, London SE5 8AF, UK
Full list of author information is available at the end of the article

Plain English summary

Anorexia nervosa (AN) is a serious, life-threatening illness, and difficulties in emotional processing and social relationships are believed to perpetuate this illness by increasing isolation. However, what these difficulties might look like is uncertain. Furthermore, sole focus on such a "disease model" of AN has recently been challenged as it fails to consider positive emotions and experiences, and thus ignores the full human experience of someone with AN. This online study aimed to address this by asking people with lived experience of AN about both positive and difficult critical events. When describing positive critical events some participants discussed moments of celebration which reflected external focus and "big picture" thinking. Others discussed unexpected positive outcomes which revealed some negative biases that were met with positive actions. Difficult critical life events largely included discussion of relational conflict and loneliness, which for some participants took place against the backdrop of the eating disorder. These findings suggest that although AN may be largely characterised by negative emotions and loneliness, this is not the full picture. Many participants described living rich lives with both difficult and positive experiences and were open to have their negative expectations challenged with positive actions.

Background

Anorexia nervosa (AN) is a complex eating disorder (ED) characterised by malnutrition and very low bodyweight [4]. Theoretical models of AN have suggested that social-emotional difficulties play an important role in perpetuating the illness [28, 73, 80]. Such difficulties are believed to lead to conflict in social relationships, which can in turn lead to increased isolation and create space for the ED to take over the person's life [72, 73]. Although many interventions have been developed targeting various aspects of social-emotional functioning in AN [19], treatment response remains a significant challenge with only around 33% of patients reaching full recovery [1, 51, 66, 67]. Therefore, further investigation of social-emotional processing in AN could help improve understanding of the illness and aid the development of new interventions.

Over the years there has been a great deal of interest in examining social-emotional difficulties in AN using experimental paradigms. Large scale meta-analytic reviews of these studies report that people with AN have difficulties in several areas of social-emotional processing, including emotion recognition, theory of mind, and emotional expression [14, 59, 60, 65]. However, more recent work with larger sample sizes and utilising tasks with greater ecological validity, have found that people with AN have no general difficulties in explicit recognition of emotions or complex theory of mind tasks [2, 24, 82]. It has been suggested that previously reported difficulties in correct attribution of emotional states may be related to negative information processing biases in AN [3, 24], indicating that there is still a great deal of uncertainty regarding social-emotional difficulties in AN. Furthermore, over the past few years there have been calls to examine positive emotions and experiences in AN, highlighting the importance of studying resilience, hope, and optimism rather than focusing solely on difficulties [70]. At a time of uncertainty regarding the types of social-emotional difficulties that people with AN might have, it is valuable to gain further insight by adopting different methods and approaches.

As outlined above, the majority of previous work examining social-emotional processing in AN have been behavioural experiments or self-report questionnaire studies. Such quantitative work lacks the flexibility and ability to capture multiple aspects of behaviour and experiences that people may have. In contrast, a qualitative approach can provide unique insights into a variety of experiences and perspective on social relationships, which can further elucidate what social-emotional difficulties in AN might look like. The few qualitative studies in this area have documented that people with AN report difficulties with emotion expression, blocking or suppressing emotions, and in recognising their own emotions [49, 55]. Many also reported oversensitivity to, or misinterpretation of, others emotions, fixating on events or over-analysing the behaviour of others [46, 55, 79]. However, most of these studies have focused on exploring specific aspects of social-emotional processing, such as friendships or experience of emotions [79], or investigated patients' views in the context of an interventional study [55]. A more implicit approach, examining broader emotional experiences of those with lived experience of AN with participants discussing key life events in their own life, expands the scope of qualitative studies on the topic of social and emotional processing.

To address the gaps in the literature outlined above, the aim of the present study was to shed light on both *positive* and *difficult* emotional experiences in AN by retrospectively exploring critical life events identified by those with a lived experience of AN in the acute phase of illness. We were specifically interested in events involving other people, as this would allow us to gain insight into social relationships and interactions during the acute stage of illness. Using the Critical Incident Technique (CIT [31];), we sought to answer the following research questions:

1) What are the important events participants choose to describe?
2) What emotional responses do participants report as linked to their recollections of positive and negative critical events?

3) What are the social relationships involved and how are they portrayed?

This study was exploratory in nature and therefore we did not seek to test a priori hypotheses.

Method

Participants

Thirty-four participants completed the study. All of the participants were 16 years old or older with current or history of AN. The sample demographic and clinical characteristics are presented in Table 1. Diagnosis was established by asking the participants to report if they had a diagnosis of AN and who diagnosed them (psychiatrist, psychologist, general practitioner, or other). All participants reported having been diagnosed with AN, ten of whom considered themselves to be recovered (REC). Twenty people reported having been diagnosed by a psychiatrist, 12 by their general practitioner, one by a clinical nurse specialist, and one by a clinical psychologist. As shown in Table 1, on average, the participants reported BMI below 18.5 but those who considered themselves recovered reported numerically higher than those with current AN. Additionally, on average our participants reported ED symptomatology, as measured by the Eating Disorder Examination Questionnaire (EDEQ), that was more than double of that reported by healthy individuals in the community [27]. Participants who reported being recovered reported numerically lower levels of ED symptomatology than those with current AN. Still, it is of importance to note that as this study was conducted online, no third person confirmation about the participants' stage of illness or recovery was obtained. Twenty-three people also reported having other diagnoses in addition to AN, the most common of which were depression ($N = 10$, 43.48%), anxiety ($N = 8$, 34.78%) and obsessive compulsive disorder ($N = 7$, 30.43%). For further details please see Supplementary Table 1.

The participants were recruited through online adverts on social media (Twitter, Facebook) and from ED charity (BEAT) website. As the study took place online, all the participants were required to complete an online consent form prior to completing the study. The study was approved by the King's College London Psychiatry, Nursing and Midwifery Research Ethics Subcommittee, United Kingdom (HR-19/20–13,004). All procedures were conducted in accordance with the latest version of the Declaration of Helsinki (2013).

Critical incident technique

Participants were asked to recount critical positive and difficult situations or events they had experienced while acutely ill using the CIT [31]. The CIT is an effective qualitative research technique used to systematically collect observations of significant events of which the person has first-hand experience. CIT has been used in numerous fields, including psychology, medicine, business, employee performance appraisal, and marketing [13, 22, 26, 34, 45, 64]. The CIT allows participants to self-define a critical or important event they wish to discuss further, rather than relying on the researchers' views on what is considered critical. This approach empowers participants and actively includes them in the research process. As part of the CIT process, the participants are then asked variety of open-ended questions about the background of the event, the event itself,

Table 1 Clinical and demographic sample characteristics

	Whole sample ($N = 34$)	Current AN ($N = 24$)	Recovered AN (N = 10)
Age M (SD)	26.43 (8.48)	27.11 (8.22)	24.81 (9.31)
Age at diagnosis M (SD)	16.97 (5.50)	17.88 (5.80)	14.80 (4.16)
BMI M (SD)	18.31 (3.13)	17.58 (3.17)	20.58 (1.05)
EDEQ Total M (SD)	3.25 (1.72)	3.93 (1.34)	1.48 (0.94)
Gender N (%)	Female 28 (82.4%) Male 4 (11.8%) non-binary 1 (2.9%)	Female 18 (75.0%) Male 4 (16.7%) Non-binary 1 (4.2%)	Female 10 (100%)
Marital status N (%)	Single 29 (85.3%) Domestic partnership 2 (5.9%) Married 1 (2.9%) Civil partnership 1 (2.9%) Separated 1 (2.9%)	Single 20 (83.3%) Domestic partnership 1 (4.2%) Married 1 (4.2%) Civil partnership 1 (4.2%) Separated 1 (4.2%)	Single 9 (90.0%) Domestic partnership 1 (10.0%)
Ethnicity N (%)	White 32 (94.1%) Mixed 1 (2.9%) Other/non-specified 1 (2.9%)	White 22 (91.7%) Mixed 1 (4.2%) Other/non-specified 1 (4.2%)	White 10 (100%)

AN anorexia nervosa, *BMI* body mass index, *EDEQ* eating disorders examination questionnaire, *M* mean, *SD* standard deviation, *N* number and the consequences of the event to gather as much information about the participants' direct observations as possible. The use of such in-depth questions makes the CIT a particularly useful technique for research involving participants recalling important past events. Furthermore, the CIT technique places the focus of the analysis on the context of the event in addition to the event itself, enabling the researchers to explore the emotions, cognitions, and motivations surrounding it. Therefore, we used the CIT in the present study to enable us to reach our aims and answer our research questions.

The CIT is typically used as a semi-structured interview, but here it was adapted to questionnaire format (for original CIT and adapted version used in this study see Supplementary materials) to make the study more accessible and enable wider recruitment of participants. We created two CIT style questionnaires asking participants about critical positive and difficult life event. At the beginning of each questionnaire, participants were first asked to identify an event which included a social element, that is it involved some other people. Whether these other people were friends, family members, a partner, or someone else, was up to the participants. They were then asked for further details about the event as outlined above. Additionally, participants were asked how they felt about their own and the other people's actions, whether they felt that the consequences were what they had hoped for, and how they thought the other people involved felt about the situation. All of the participants completed the CIT questionnaires.

Qualitative data analysis

Participants' responses to the CIT were subject to thematic analysis [9]. The thematic analysis was conducted by two authors, JL and FS. An inductive thematic analysis approach was chosen because it is primarily used to identify reoccurring similarities and differences in the narratives. In other words, this approach allowed data from multiple participants to be examined simultaneously, which in turn enabled us to meet the main aim of the present study. Additionally, inductive thematic analysis offers a flexible approach to data that enabled us to examine key positive and difficult social incidents in the lives of people with lived experience of AN and to explore other concepts such as different types of social-emotional difficulties, including information processing biases, emotion processing problems, and maladaptive emotion regulation styles.

Thematic analysis has been proposed to either involve inductive process whereby themes are identified from the data without prior expectations or theoretically driven analysis where the researcher's prior knowledge of the phenomenon studied shapes the process [9, 10]. In the present study we used an inductive approach. CIT questions were used to probe participants to provide further detail about the event in question and the context surrounding it. Participants' narrative responses to questions about positive and difficult events, were then analysed separately to identify commonly occurring themes and subthemes within each event category. We paid particular attention to: what were the social interactions that participants chose to discuss, how the participants described their own and others' behaviour, what emotions were discussed or emerged from the narratives, and how satisfied the participants were with the outcome. Within each event category themes were identified without reference to previous work, thus representing inductive themes.

Before starting thematic analysis, all CIT responses were divided according to event category, descriptions of positive and difficult events were examined independently. We adopted a six-step approach to thematic analysis. We began with (1) data familiarisation, during which the narrative responses were read thoroughly. After this (2) initial codes were generated to identify content features, which represented commonalities and differences between the narratives. The feature codes were then grouped and (3) broader themes were identified. Following standard practice, during this stage, certain content feature codes were discarded if they were identified in fewer than 3 participants' narratives or if they did not fit in any of the other broader themes already generated. Next the themes generated by grouping the feature codes were (4) reviewed to ensure clear relationship between themes and subthemes and avoid duplication. After review, (5) themes and subthemes were defined according to the concepts they represented and the (6) final report was produced. The codes and themes were agreed upon independently by the two authors. Any disagreement or uncertainty regarding the codes and themes were brought to the whole team for further discussion.

Results

Positive critical events

When the participants were asked to reflect on positive critical events, some discussed events that were positive throughout and left them feeling good about themselves. However, most participants chose to discuss events that had at least some negative components, either reflecting their own negatively biased expectations or focusing on negative events in a perceived absence of positive experiences. Thus, three major themes reflecting different emotional valences were identified in participants' narrative responses to the CIT questions about positive critical events: (1) Unexpected positive outcomes, (2) Moments of celebration, (3) Nothing positive to report

(Fig. 1). Each theme and their corresponding subthemes are presented in Fig. 1 and discussed further below.

Unexpected positive outcomes

The *Unexpected positive outcomes* theme was identified in several narrative descriptions of events where the participants described feeling low and alluded to having negative expectations of themselves, the event itself, or the other people involved. Instead of having these expectations met, the participants talked about how they were pleasantly surprised by the actions of others: *"My sister found my food that I was hiding behind my bed. It was positive because [she] wasn't rude and horrible about it" (AN-05).* This theme suggests that although many participants recognised having negative information processing biases, assuming they were worthless and unloved, or the people around them did not care or understand them, they were open to having these biases challenged. Despite such negative context surrounding the events, it was clear from participants' descriptions of the outcomes that these were critical positive experiences.

The *Unexpected positive outcomes* theme comprised of two subthemes: (a) *positive reminders* and (b) *understanding and acceptance.* Several participants discussed receiving *positive reminders* from their loved ones during times when they were feeling low or going through hard times. In all these narratives, our participants briefly alluded to their low self-esteem and low mood, which they assumed their loved ones knew about. This knowledge was discussed as the catalyst that led their loved ones to show the participants through actions that they were indeed loved and worthy. *"My chest infection had been worsening in the few days preceding this incident, and in turn my mood had dropped quite a bit, so my self-esteem had been particularly low...Two of the day staff volunteered to take me [to the Emergency department] ... them going above and beyond made me feel cared for and worthy" (AN-07).* A few participants also mentioned that although the positive reminders made them feel loved and gave them motivation to work hard on their recovery, they also triggered feelings of guilt: *"I was in hospital on Christmas day and my father visited. He brought with him a big jar of notes that my friends had written as well as small gifts from them, all [the] memories from the past and things they liked about me ... I felt very emotional, but also guilty" (REC-05).* This further indicates that some people with AN may battle with a deep sense of worthlessness such that even positive exchanges can give rise to negative emotions, which in turn can make it difficult to cope with or accept these positive interactions. This illustrates the complexity of emotional experiences among people with AN.

Another subtheme was *understanding and acceptance,* which included discussion of significant stages of illness. These included having other people find out about ED related behaviours and needing hospital treatment. Hiding the illness is common in AN, often fuelled by feelings of embarrassment, shame, or desire to protect the illness, which can be seen as something valuable and positive. This, in turn, often leads to avoidance and further social isolation, creating barriers to help-seeking. Although all the participants talked about how other people discovering their ED was a daunting prospect, they also discussed their desire for support and acceptance: *"[I] wanted no one to find out. But it was good that they found out ... I felt supported and less alone with*

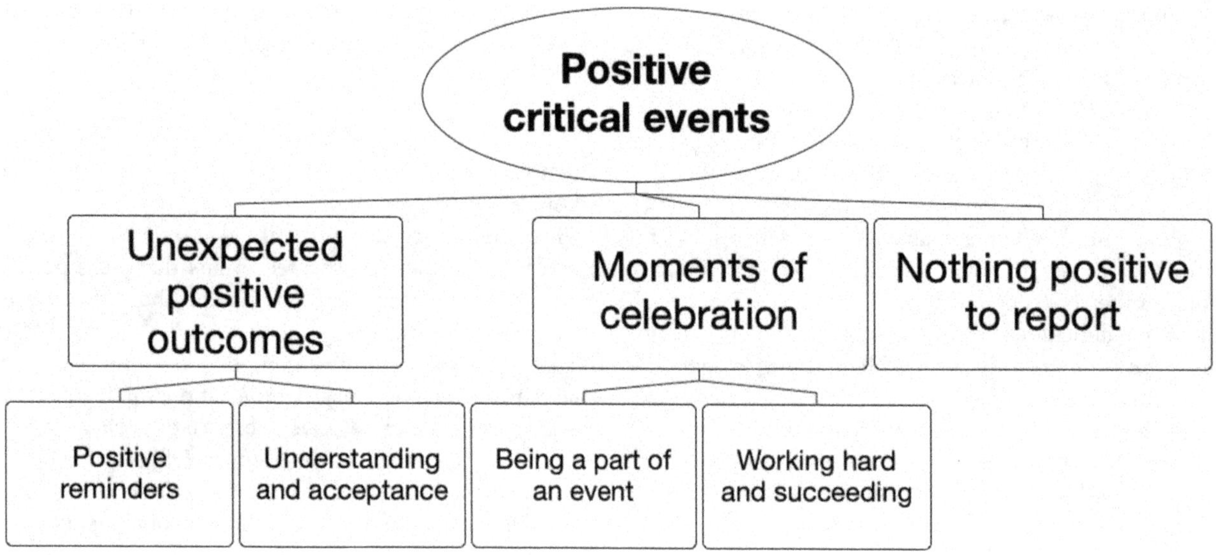

Fig. 1 Positive critical events. The map shows themes that were identified in participants' narrative descriptions of positive important events

what I was doing" (AN-05). Being met with compassion and understanding also served as an opportunity for more open discussion and learning in the context of treatment: *"I have a tendency in these [confusing and upsetting] situations to withdraw from conversations and this was noticed by the therapist ... Our sessions individually had initially focused on her gaining an understanding of my personality and thought patterns ... "[It] planted the seed around navigating through negative emotions, rather than around them, and the skills I developed during this time enabled me to communicate this better to the people around me" (REC-02).* It was clear in the narratives that understanding and acceptance from loved ones and professionals was instrumental to enable the participants to communicate without judgement, and direct compassion towards themselves and allow themselves to engage with treatment.

Moments of celebration

The theme *Moments of celebration* included written accounts of being part of a fun event, such as a wedding or a birthday celebration, and achieving goals, such as getting accepted into university. The participants described the events using language that suggested they felt the events were positive throughout. Interestingly, this theme was generally characterised by an external focus of attention, with the participants primarily describing the event and the other people involved. This could reflect an attempt to reduce self-focused attention to lower social anxiety. Indeed, a few participants discussed how focusing on activities and their loved ones enabled them to see the *"big picture"*, *"get out of [their] own head" (REC-01)* and enjoy the moment. This theme comprised of two subthemes, (a) *Being a part of an event* and (b) *Working hard and succeeding,* which are discussed further below.

The first subtheme, *Being part of an event,* included recollections of both significant occasions such as a wedding or birth of a relative, as well as smaller get-togethers, including birthday celebrations and days out. All narratives within this subtheme were characterised by reduced self-focused attention and active involvement, and the participants discussed how being part of the event and focusing on the activities made them feel more hopeful and connected to their loved ones: *"By saying 'yes' to one thing, and seeing I was still okay after it, I was more likely to say 'yes' to the next. As I engaged in more things, I enjoyed myself more as had more confidence that the consequences would be okay." (REC-07).* It was clear this sense of belonging and shared experiences made participants feel like they were able to function competently as part of their community, which for some participants served as motivation to strive towards recovery form AN: *"His [nephew's] birth gave me the determination to work hard on my recovery so that I could watch him grow into a bright young boy and spend valuable time with him" (AN-08).*

Another subtheme was *Working hard and succeeding* which was characterised by the participants discussing how they worked hard to reach their goals. Although some participants mentioned how receiving support and encouragement from their loved ones during this time was important in keeping them focused and calm, the primary focus was on their own work and efforts: *"I worked hard to get where I wanted to go [University of choice] ... [my family offered] Lots of support and encouragement which helped" (AN-14).* This sense of accomplishment made people feel proud and competent: *"Having been so unwell that I had previously been unable to undertake barely any physical activity ... [I] felt a huge sense of achievement in being able to take my young daughter onto the ice rink" (AN-09).* It was clear that the feeling of achievement allowed individuals to view themselves in a more positive light and feel more capable, which in turned strengthened their self-compassion and sense of self-acceptance.

Nothing positive to report

Unexpectedly, three people recounted negative experiences with no clear positive themes as their positive critical events. These included accidental death of a loved one and being victimised. One person also talked about missing out on an otherwise important, positive family event: *"My brother asked his girlfriend to marry him ... I missed him asking her ... I felt like a failure and a let down to the family ... [The others] never spoke to me about it. They just left me. It was just my brother that said I'd upset him by not coming." (AN-09).* Although it was clear from the quote that celebrating and being part of this important event would have aligned with their values, the narrative description of the memory was very different compared to those in 5.1.2. Their focus was largely on letting others down and feeling guilty about doing so, rather than on celebrating a positive experience with loved ones. A tendency to associate the self with negative experiences is common in AN [61], and these narratives could be a reflection of an extreme case of negative bias whereby these participants felt that they had nothing positive to discuss or that nothing positive had happened to them. Alternatively, these narratives may reflect the number of significant negative life events our participants have experienced. Indeed, people with AN have been found to report more negative and stressful experiences than a healthy comparison group [20], as well as other psychiatric inpatients including people with depression and anxiety [44, 76].

Difficult critical events

When asked to recount difficult critical events in their lives, twenty participants discussed situations that were in some way related to their ED. It became clear that for these individuals, the AN was often at the centre of important negative social experiences. This is to be expected as the illness and associated symptoms often serve as both the cause and consequence of shame and distress. Interestingly, the other 14 participants discussed difficult events that were not necessarily directly tied to AN, but were to do with other distressing life events that happened to occur when they were ill. Thus, the following themes were identified in the narratives: (1) ED-related difficult events and (2) non-ED difficult events. The themes and their corresponding subthemes are presented in Fig. 2 and discussed further below.

ED-related difficult events

The *ED-related difficult events* theme was identified in narratives where people wrote about interactions with their loved ones or ED services that revolved around the illness and which resulted in conflict and personal distress. The participants primarily wrote how other people's reactions to the illness or associated behaviours made them feel pressured or ashamed. This theme suggests that people with AN have many complex emotions tied to their illness, which can be difficult to navigate during stressful events, causing them to react in ways contrary to their values of belonging and care for the people around them. Indeed, people wrote how these difficult interactions left them feeling alone and unsupported, but also how the illness made them feel like the odd one out and isolated them from their loved ones. It was clear that these social events formed a significant step in their illness journey. The *ED-related difficult events* theme comprised of two subthemes: (a) *Losing self* and (b) *Breaking through denial,* all of which are discussed in more detail below.

As part of the first subtheme, *Losing self,* people wrote about a particularly turbulent time in their lives when AN was dominant, disrupted their daily lives, and prevented them from engaging with activities in line with their values and desires. Several participants implied that they felt unable to stop themselves from engaging in ED behaviours and cognitions, which frequently led to personal distress and relational conflict. Social eating especially made participants feel pressured to challenge their ED thinking style and behaviours, which they felt unable to do, resulting in negative outcomes: *"Family dinner and [I] had to choose what to eat and how much [I] wanted from each part. [It was] difficult because it was hard to know if eating too much or too little and difficult because my family saw me hide it in my sleeves and it was embarrassing … my sister shouted at me" (AN-05).* Individuals also wrote about how they wanted to join in and be part of activities but the illness made them feel it all impossible, *"Went out for dinner and ended up crying because I ate" (AN-01),* which led to further feelings of guilt and shame: *"I upset my family and ruined the evening. Also embarrassed myself … I didn't want to react*

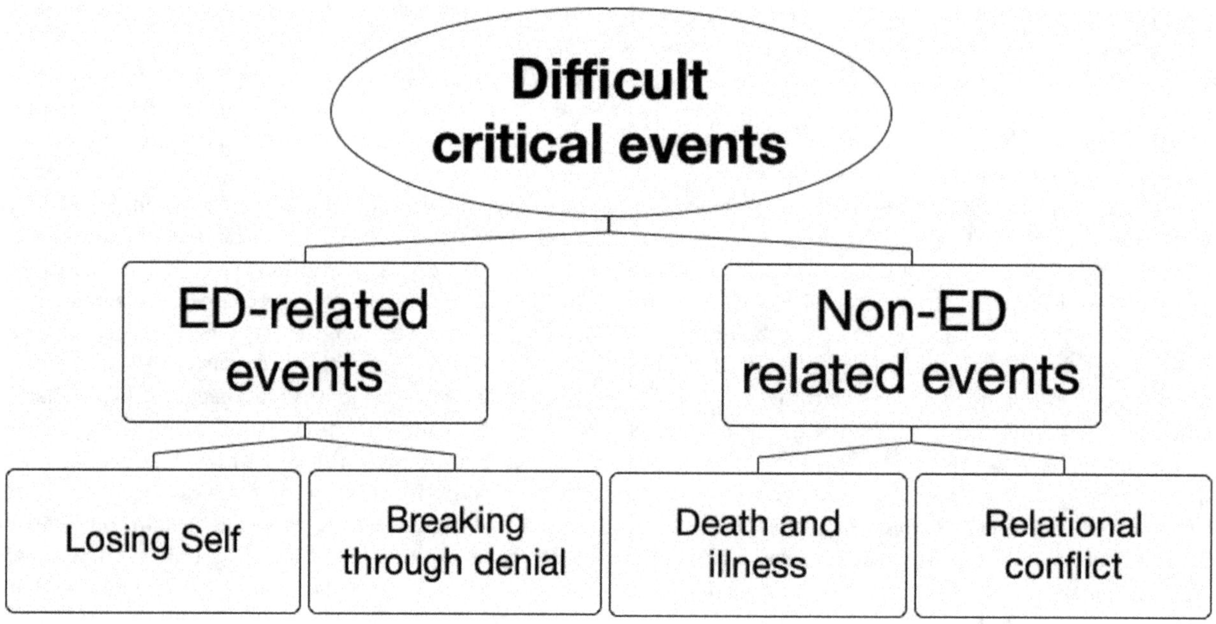

Fig. 2 Difficult critical events. The map shows themes that were identified in participants' narrative descriptions of difficult important events. ED = eating disorder

that way but at the time it helped me cope." (REC-01). These recollections convey a feeling that losing oneself to AN is very isolating experience.

Other participants found that being under pressure frequently resulted in conflict and made them feel misunderstood or ignored when they tried to explain or express their feelings and thoughts. In these narratives people wrote about engaging in behaviours and thinking styles that could be interpreted as protecting the illness identity. Indeed, several participants talked about relational conflict in a manner that suggested a *me*-versus-*them* mentality: *"As my mum and I exited the ward that Friday night, my care-coordinator handed a meal plan for that weekend to my mum. It wasn't the one we had discussed ... My anorexia was talking for half of the conversation, trying to get my mum to change the meal plan ... I felt extremely betrayed both by my care-coordinator (who I got on with and thought I could trust) and my mum (who I felt was taking the hospital's side and not her own daughter's)" (REC-07).* Frequently, people also reported that these difficult interactions solidified their impressions that their loved ones were not there to support them when they were overwhelmed by the illness, so could not reach out and ask for help when they needed it: *"I felt belittled, like she [a friend] didn't really care. I felt scared that others felt the same as her, and that I shouldn't talk to others about how I felt because they would start resenting me" (AN-19).* Interestingly, in all these narratives, the participants conveyed a feeling that things could have turned out better if they had been heard instead of being dismissed and rejected.

Breaking through denial was another clear subtheme, including discussions of situations where individuals were suddenly made aware of the extent of their illness and how it impacted other people around them. Denial of the illness or its impact on the person's health is common in AN. This thinking style can be thought of as a coping mechanism, which can help the person feel strong and in control whilst simultaneously becoming increasingly isolated and being at the mercy of AN. Thus, unsurprisingly some participants seemed shocked to receive diagnosis of AN when they were going to see their doctor for other reasons: *"I was diagnosed with anorexia nervosa and was about to be hospitalized ... I did not believe this was happening. I did not think there is anything wrong with me. I have heard about anorexia, but I did not think I am the one having it." (REC-10).* These participants also alluded to often being unaware of the impact AN had on their loved ones, which made having to suddenly face the reality of the illness an even more difficult experience: *"I passed out at the GP and it made my mum very upset ... I did not want to upset or worry my mum." (REC-03).* In this recollection the participant was concerned about how she was consumed by the illness to the extent that it made her blind to the impact it was having on not only on herself but her loved one. In the end, despite the difficulties, some participants also wrote about positive outcomes and relief associated with having to face their illness: *"I was almost relieved to be diagnosed, it felt like I could finally speak to somebody about it." (AN-10).*

Non-ED related difficult events

The narratives that formed the *Non-ED related difficult events* theme involved negative life experiences that were not directly related to the ED, but rather happened to occur while the participants were ill. These primarily included recollections of very difficult experiences, which the participants struggled to cope often resulting in feelings of loneliness and shame. Other people's and their own reactions often compounded these feelings later on, further deepening their experience of social isolation. This theme comprised of two subthemes: (a) *Death and illness*, and (b) *Relational conflict.*

Under the *Death and illness* subtheme, our participants discussed grieving the loss of a loved one or dealing with a family members illness. When discussing losing a loved one, the participants described going through common stages of grief, but appeared to react in one of two ways: some felt upset and overwhelmed to the point that they either did not want, or know how, to reach out for help: *"I was on the way to a party on the bus and got a message from a friend that our friend had died. I continued to the party and didn't mention it to anyone there ... I felt very dissociated and didn't know what to do. I got quite upset and no one knew why. I felt very alone and distressed when I should've gone home and spoken to someone about it." (REC-05).* Other participants, on the other hand, talked about how the loss made them feel exasperated: *"The death of my godmother/aunt. I was feeling very angry as she was sick and I wanted to swap places with her" (AN-16).* A few participants talked about how their need to stick to their routine at the time of the incident made them feel guilty and ashamed later: *"My mum had a seizure ... I was upset and frustrated as I stressed about how I'd get to work and who would make my lunch. I should've been more upset and caring and stayed at home" (AN-04).* This could reflect cognitive rigidity and resistance to change common in AN, which can prevent a person from behaving and responding in accordance with their value of compassion towards others and themselves causing further distress and shame.

The other subtheme identified in the narratives was *Relational conflict.* This subtheme included discussions of difficult interactions with loved ones which left participants feeling alone and upset, when what they desired was support and encouragement from their loved ones:

"I was in hospital after having a blackout and badly injuring my face, and I texted [my friend] to let her know, but received an abusive reply ... She told me our friendship was over" (AN-18). Interestingly, similar to ED-related relational conflict discussed above, the narratives under this subtheme also included discussions of how these difficult interactions left the participants feeling dismissed, which was often interpreted as an indicator that nobody truly cared and there would be no point in reaching out to others in the future: *"My mum disregarding my feelings made me feel invalidated and added to my belief that I shouldn't open up to people." (AN-22).* Taken together, this could be one of the factors influencing the development or maintenance of negative cognitive biases in AN.

Discussion

The present study aimed to explore positive and difficult events in the lives of people with lived experience of AN. The participants completed two CIT-style questionnaires asking them questions about these critical events and the resulting narratives were subject to thematic analysis. Many of the themes identified in the positive and difficult narratives were presented against the backdrop of the eating disorder, which formed a large part of the participants' lives when they were acutely unwell. Importantly, the findings suggest that individuals with lived experience of AN have the capacity, even in the acute stage of the illness, to engage and recount rich, enjoyable experiences demonstrating optimism and hope.

Over the past few years there have been calls to study positive emotions in AN [70], however, to our knowledge no studies have thus far explored narratives of positive experiences among this group. In the present study, the critical events that were entirely positive under the theme *Moments of celebration* frequently involved discussions of achievements, having something to look forward to, and active engagement in activities. Such focus on other people and future events could reflect reduced self-focused attention. Self-focused attention, sometimes referred to as rumination or dwelling on one's own emotions and internal experiences, has been extensively studied in the field of social anxiety. Reduced self-focused attention been associated with less negative interpretation bias and reduced tendency to exaggerate others' negative feelings towards oneself [5, 8, 56]. Reducing self-focused attention, particularly to negative aspects of the self, has been found beneficial in reducing social anxiety and fear of negative evaluation [8, 25, 43, 48]. This finding suggests that people with AN can shift their focus of attention and have rich, enjoyable experiences, demonstrating optimism and hope even in the acute stage of illness.

Fully engaging in activities and focusing on other people can also be interpreted as increased *"big picture"* oriented thinking and living authentically in accordance with their personal values. Experimental research within the general population has documented that increased *"big picture"* thinking is associated with a tendency to react in a positive manner and increases positive affect [33, 42]. Interventions targeting excessive detail focus in AN, such as cognitive remediation therapy, have been found to improve mood and increase *"big picture"* thinking in experimental tasks [23, 37, 50]. Similarly, authenticity and openly living according to one's own values has been associated with increased positive affect, while inauthenticity has been reported to be associated with negative affect, increased rumination, and lack of clarity about one's own emotions [41, 54]. Furthermore, qualitative research has found that the ability to see the *"big picture"*, and living according to own values of care, may be a key component in supporting recovery from AN [15, 18, 78]. When discussing their recovery journey, people with lived experience of AN have reported that focusing more on their loved ones enabled them to start to questioning the illness and recognise its full impact on their own and others' lives [78]. This was identified as a turning point in the illness journey at which the person felt able to start distancing themselves from the illness and to develop an identity independent of AN. Taken together, these findings suggest that further investigating and building on the strengths and resilience people with AN have may be a useful target for further interventions. Sole focus on a "disease model" of emotional processing in AN often fails to examine the full human experience of someone with AN [70].

In the present study, several participants seemed to demonstrate negative biases when asked to discuss important positive events. This is in line with previous experimental work finding that people with AN show increased attention towards negative stimuli and a tendency to interpret ambiguous scenes in a negative way [3, 16, 17, 74]. Interestingly, our participants found these experiences to be positive because their own negative expectations were met with positive actions from the people around them, particularly when they were met with support, validation, and understanding that they may have felt unable to ask for. These events could be interpreted as so-called corrective experiences, in which a person challenges their own biases and expectations resulting in a new, often more positive way of viewing others and the self [38]. Corrective experiences are argued to play a key role in the transformative processes promoted in psychotherapy and are associate with breakthroughs in a person's willingness to feel previously demonised and feared emotions and adopt new behaviours [21]. Corrective experiences have been reported to provide people with new understanding of previous important experiences through reflection [35, 36, 81]. This in turn leads to improved self-esteem, reduced reliance on defence mechanisms, and greater social support achieved through disclosure and sharing of emotional experiences [35, 36]. Although corrective experiences have not been extensively researched in the field of ED, one study examining the usefulness of psychodrama reported that by creating corrective experiences, the group allowed the participants with ED to re-evaluate their previous emotional, personal, and cognitive experiences [63].

In previous qualitative work, people with AN highlighted the importance of allowing themselves to accept social support and open up to others when recounting their experiences of recovery [29, 47, 78]. These participants engaged in careful expectation management, first gauging others reactions before opening up, which in the end gave them the affiliate support they were seeking, aiding their recovery [29, 78]. Taken together with the present findings, this suggests that people with AN are open to corrective experiences, which highlights need for further research into how these experiences may be facilitated in a therapeutic context. Importantly in the present study, a few participants discussed how the positive actions and gifts from others made them feel loved, but also triggered feelings of guilt. This could be interpreted as evidence of an internalised sense of worthlessness and shame, which makes believing and accepting positive words and actions towards oneself difficult. Indeed, previous work has found that people with AN frequently report feeling worthless, which can interfere with social relationships and recovery [29, 58, 71, 77]. Taken together, these findings suggest that negative cognitive biases can be challenged with corrective experiences in AN, but the actions and reactions of others, and navigating through feelings of worthlessness are key in order to not further alienate the person.

Difficult critical events could be broadly divided into ED-related and non-ED events. When the participants were discussing ED-related difficult events they talked about how losing self to the illness led to personal distress and relational conflict, and how breaking through denial forced to face the consequences of the illness. Our participants mostly talked about how the illness made them feel like the odd one out and how others' behaviours and reactions made them feel pressured, misunderstood, and alone, with some participants talking about how they wanted to escape situations where they felt unable to cope. Previous studies with people with history of AN have reported that feeling alone with the illness and unheard or misunderstood made participants feel less safe and more reluctant to accept changes [29, 32, 52, 53]. This led to increased distrust between the patient and their loved ones, enforcing feelings of loneliness, and negatively impacted the therapeutic alliance [32, 52]. As a result, participants reported that they often fell intentionally silent and did not want to reach out. However, such reduced expressiveness and responsiveness has been found to be associated with reduction in social support offered by others and disrupted communication [11, 12, 40]. Combined, this may create a vicious cycle of reduced social support and isolation, leaving the person at the mercy of the illness.

Interestingly, a few participants who discussed breaking through denial as a critical difficult experience also found that in the end these were key events in their recovery. This could be taken as *"hitting rock bottom"* and suggests that having to finally face the impact the illness had on them and their loved ones was an important source of motivation for these participants. Together with the experience of losing self to the illness, these events enabled the participants to witness how the illness prevented them from living in accordance with their personal values. Indeed, many participants wrote about how they cared for their loved ones and didn't want to upset them, but they felt they weren't strong enough to fight or challenge the illness, which then led to the conflict. This could be taken as a shift in thinking, moving from denial to acknowledging the impact of the illness. Indeed, previous studies have reported that people who have recovered from AN found having to face the personal, health, and social consequences of the illness was a turning point in their illness journey [47, 78]. It enabled them to see the *"bigger picture"* and how their actions impacted others around them, which in turn gave them motivation to work on the their recovery [78]. These findings suggest that by reflecting on difficult life events some people were able to turn them into a positive creating more space for and motivation for change. These findings highlight the importance of examining how AN impacts an individual's ability to live authentically in accordance with their values, which in turn could be an important target for interventions helping the individual distance themselves from AN.

When recounting both ED-related and non-ED difficult life events several participants wrote about relational conflicts as particularly important interactions. Our participants wrote about how others' negative reactions to their attempts to seek support or ED-related coping strategies made them feel alone and rejected, which were in direct contrast with the understanding and supportive reactions described under the theme *Unexpected positive outcomes*. Many participants also mentioned how these interactions served to further enforce their pre-existing notion that other people did not truly care about them and that they were alone with their illness. Such feelings of loneliness and rejection, possibly compounded by past traumatic and painful experiences, could be one of the factors influencing the development and maintenance of negative cognitive biases in AN, similar to those alluded to in the *Unexpected positive outcomes* theme. This could be interpreted as the formation of a maladaptive coping strategy founded in negatively valenced expectation management, whereby the person begins to expect others to respond in a negative fashion based on previous experiences. A tendency to generalise others' negative feelings towards oneself has been associated with increased negative self-focused attention, poor social functioning, and increased rejection sensitivity [5, 6, 8, 56]. Previous experimental studies have reported that people with AN report elevated rejection sensitivity, perceived lower social rank, and reduced social adjustment [15, 18, 62, 69, 75]. When expecting to be rejected by others, people who experience high rejection sensitivity may engage in passive, hostile behaviours including avoidance and withdrawal of love and support [6, 7]. Such strategies then tend to become self-fulfilling prophecies, often leading to more social difficulties, including further social rejection [6, 7]. However, as shown in the present study, people with AN are open to having these maladaptive cognitive biases challenged through positive actions. Further investigation of the development of negative cognitive biases in AN, their role in illness maintenance, and strategies for challenging them, may be of interest.

Research and clinical implications

The present study highlights the importance of studying both positive and negative life experiences in AN which may form the foundation of the behaviours documented in previous experimental work. Future research could benefit from investigating how difficult social interactions and relational conflict shape the perceptions of people with AN and how these interactions may influence illness progression. The present findings suggest that participants' negative interpersonal experiences may influence the development of cognitive biases and possible maladaptive coping strategies. Maladaptive coping styles, including experiential avoidance and unwillingness to share own experiences, have been found to be associated greater illness severity and worse outcome in AN [57, 73]. This finding is relevant for clinical work highlighting the importance of focusing on relationships and trauma in the treatment of individuals with AN. Interventions, such as family therapy, aim to target some of these factors, namely family dynamics, and there is some evidence that family therapy can be effective in promoting remission [30]. It would be of interest to build on these findings and examine the effectiveness of interventions that target social relationships and complex trauma more broadly, reaching outside of the immediate family.

Importantly, the present findings demonstrate that people with lived experience of AN recount rich, enjoyable social experiences, as well as showing optimism and hope, even in the acute stages of illness. These findings highlight that people with AN can and do demonstrate strength and resilience and future research may benefit from further exploring the role of these positive traits in AN. Such an approach would not only allow us to explore the full human experience of someone with AN [70], but also help capitalise on strengths, such as "*big picture*" thinking, which has been found to play a key role in recovery [78], when developing new interventions. Shifting focus from the "disease model" of AN towards building on strengths can help support existing clinical interventions, increase motivation, and help the individual feel more confident in being able to reach recovery.

In the present study many participants alluded to the role of personal values in their recollections of positive and difficult life events. Positive life events were associated with feeling able to live authentically, in accordance with their value system. Difficult life events, on the other hand, especially those related to the illness, were associated with shame and distress caused by failing to live up to one's own values, such as value of caring for others. These findings highlight the importance of knowing oneself and one's identity outside of AN in the recovery journey. Maintaining the illness can contradict things an individual values about themselves, such as caring for family members but knowing that you are upsetting them. Recognising this tension could help an individual to distance themselves from the illness creating opportunities for change and aiding recovery. To our knowledge, previous work exploring personal values in AN have largely focused on examining illness-related values such as the value of thinness [39, 68]. Therefore, further research into personal values that extend beyond AN and investigation of interventions that capitalise on strengths and values outside of the illness would be of interest.

Limitations

The main limitation of the present study was that it was conducted online. This may have limited the extent to which participants felt able to disclose painful negative events and how they interpreted them. Additionally, as the study was conducted online, we were not able to obtain third person confirmation of participants stage of illness or recovery. This limits the conclusions that can be drawn from this study. Future studies are needed to confirm the present findings using methods that make participants feel safe to disclose and discuss difficult life events. Additionally, conducting the study online meant that it was not possible to conduct a full assessment to confirm diagnosis or stage of illness. Additionally, the sample was almost entirely white, British, and female, which limits generalisability. Future studies may benefit from targeting specifically gender- and ethnic minorities as their experiences of AN and related difficulties are likely to be different.

The CIT was adapted into questionnaire format, which allowed us to recruit participants from more widely across the country without placing an additional burden on participants. However, this format limited the responsiveness inherent to an interview setting. For instance, had the study been conducted face-to-face, it would have been possible to ask why participants described negative experiences when asked for positive events. Since only a few participants recounted negative or upsetting memories when asked about positive critical events, it is possible that these participants misunderstood the question.

Conclusions

The present study aimed to investigate positive and difficult critical incidents in AN. Several participants talked about positive events that involved *Moments of celebration*, with focus on reduced self-focused attention, ability to live authentically, and increased *"big-picture"* thinking. Still, the majority of the positive critical events also involved some negative experiences that then ended on a positive note. When discussing these *Unexpected positive outcomes* participants revealed some evidence of openness to corrective experiences to challenge their negative biases. Difficult critical events broadly involved discussion of *ED-related* and *Non-ED life events*. When discussing *ED-related life events* participants wrote about how losing themselves to the illness made them feel like they couldn't join in even when they wanted to and prevented them from behaving in accordance with their personal value system. Some participants also recounted how others around them made them feel under pressure, asking for too much too soon ultimately resulting in relational conflict. Interestingly, relational conflict appeared in both ED-related and Non-ED related life events and discussion of how these conflicts solidified participants pre-existing expectations that other did not truly care about them and convinced them. These findings suggest that negative experiences may play a role in the development of negatives biases and possible maladaptive coping strategies in AN. Importantly, however, it seems that these negative biases could be challenged through corrective experiences, suggesting that it is possible to modify negative biases in AN. Moreover, the present findings highlight the need for further research into personal values in AN that extend beyond the illness such as value of caring for their loved ones.

Abbreviations

AN: Anorexia nervosa; ED: Eating disorder; REC: Recovered; CIT: Critical incident technique; BMI: Body mass index; N: Number; M: Mean; SD: Standard deviation

Acknowledgements

Not applicable.

Authors' contributions

JL, LT, RB, and FS contributed to the conception of the study and designed the online questionnaire. JL, LT, and RB also contributed to the recruited participants and data collection. JL and FS contributed to the data analysis and interpretation of findings with final approval from LT, RB, KT, and SW. All authors contributed to drafting the final paper. All authors read and approved the final manuscript.

Competing interests

The authors declare that they have no competing interests.

Author details

[1]Department of Neuroimaging, Institute of Psychology, Psychiatry and Neuroscience, King's College London, London, UK. [2]Department of Psychological Medicine, Institute of Psychology, Psychiatry and Neuroscience, King's College London, 103 Denmark Hill, London SE5 8AF, UK. [3]South London and Maudsley NHS Foundation Trust National Eating Disorder Service, London, UK. [4]Psychology Department, Illia State University, Tbilisi, Georgia. [5]School of Education, University of Bristol, Bristol, UK.

References

1. Abbate-Daga G, Amianto F, Delsedime N, de-Bacco C, Fassino S. Resistance to treatment in eating disorders: a critical challenge. BMC Psychiatry. 2013; 13(1). https://doi.org/10.1186/1471-244X-13-294.
2. Adenzato M, Todisco P, Ardito R. Social cognition in anorexia nervosa: evidence of preserved theory of mind and impaired emotional functioning. Plos One. 2012;7(8):e44414. https://doi.org/10.1371/journal.pone.0044414.t003.
3. Ambwani S, Berenson KR, Simms L, Li A, Corfield F, Treasure J. Seeing things differently: An experimental investigation of social cognition and interpersonal behavior in anorexia nervosa. Int J Eating Disord. 2016;49(5): 499–506. https://doi.org/10.1002/eat.22498.
4. American Psychiatric Association (2013) Diagnostic and statistical manual of mental disorders (DSM-5®). American Psychiatric Pub, doi: https://doi.org/10.1176/appi.books.9780890425596.
5. Anderson B, Goldin PR, Kurita K, Gross JJ. Self-representation in social anxiety disorder: linguistic analysis of autobiographical narratives. Behav Res Ther. 2008;46(10):1119–25. https://doi.org/10.1016/j.brat.2008.07.001.
6. Ayduk O, Mendoza-Denton R, Mischel W, Downey G, Peake PK, Rodriguez M. Regulating the interpersonal self: strategic self-regulation for coping with rejection sensitivity. J Pers Soc Psychol. 2000;79(5):776–92. https://doi.org/10.1037/0022-3514.79.5.776.
7. Ayduk O, May D, Downey G, Higgins ET. Tactical differences in coping with rejection sensitivity: the role of prevention pride. Pers Soc Psychol Bull. 2003;29(4):435–48. https://doi.org/10.1177/0146167202250911.
8. Bögels SM, Mansell W. Attention processes in the maintenance and treatment of social phobia: Hypervigilance, avoidance and self-focused attention. Clin Psychol Rev. 2004;24(7):827–56. https://doi.org/10.1016/j.cpr.2004.06.005.
9. Braun V, Clarke V. Using thematic analysis in psychology. Qual Res Psychol. 2006;3(2):77–101. https://doi.org/10.1191/1478088706qp063oa.
10. Braun, V. and Clarke, V. (2013) Successful Qualitative Research a practical guide for beginners. Available at: https://books.google.co.uk/books?hl=en&lr=&id=nYMQAgAAQBAJ&oi=fnd&pg=PP2&dq=braun+and+clarke+successful+qualitative+research&ots=SpQxDfGV3v&sig=E8kD3ZP48b2t2Q1UMnSh0-nLuxY. Accessed 23 June 2020
11. Butler EA, Egloff B, Wlhelm FH, Smith NC, Erickson EA, Gross JJ. The social consequences of expressive suppression. Emotion. 2003;3(1):48–67. https://doi.org/10.1037/1528-3542.3.1.48.
12. Butler EA, Lee TL, Gross JJ. Emotion regulation and culture: are the social consequences of emotion suppression culture-specific? Emotion. 2007;7(1): 30–48. https://doi.org/10.1037/1528-3542.7.1.30.

13. Butterfield LD, Borgen WA, Amundson NE, Maglio AST. Fifty years of the critical incident technique: 1954-2004 and beyond. Qual Res. 2005;5(4):475–97. https://doi.org/10.1177/1468794105056924.
14. Caglar-Nazali HP, Corfield F, Cardi V, Ambwani S, Leppanen J, Olabintan O, et al. A systematic review and meta-analysis of "Systems for Social Processes" in eating disorders. Neurosci Biobehav Rev. 2014;42:55–92. https://doi.org/10.1016/j.neubiorev.2013.12.002.
15. Cardi V, Matteo RD, Corfield F, Treasure J. Social reward and rejection sensitivity in eating disorders: an investigation of attentional bias and early experiences. World J Biol Psychiatry. 2013a;14(8):622–33. https://doi.org/10.3109/15622975.2012.665479.
16. Cardi V, Corfield F, Leppanen J, Rhind C, Deriziotis S, Hadjimichalis A, et al. Emotional processing, recognition, empathy and evoked facial expression in eating disorders: an experimental study to map deficits in social cognition. Plos One. 2015;10(8):e0133827. https://doi.org/10.1371/journal.pone.0133827.
17. Cardi V, Turton R, Schifano S, Leppanen J, Hirsch CR, Treasure J. Biased interpretation of ambiguous social scenarios in anorexia nervosa. Eur Eat Disord Rev. 2017;25(1):60–4. https://doi.org/10.1002/erv.2493.
18. Cardi V, Cunha A, Treasure J. The use of guided self-help delivered on mobile technology in anorexia nervosa. Appetite. 2013b;71:471. https://doi.org/10.1016/j.appet.2013.06.013.
19. Cardi V, Tchanturia K, Treasure J. Premorbid and illness-related social difficulties in eating disorders: an overview of the literature and treatment developments. Curr Neuropharmacol. 2018;16(8):1122–30. https://doi.org/10.2174/1570159X16666180118100028.
20. Castellon P, Sudres J, Voltzenlogel V. Self-defining memories in female patients with anorexia nervosa. Eur Eating Disord Rev. 2020;28(5):513–24. https://doi.org/10.1002/erv.2739.
21. Castonguay LG, Hill CE. Transformation in psychotherapy: corrective experiences across cognitive behavioral, humanistic, and psychodynamic approaches. Am Psychol Assoc. 2012. https://doi.org/10.1037/13747-000.
22. Chou, F. *et al.* (2016) Participatory critical incident technique: a participatory action research approach for Counselling psychology technique d'incident critique participative : Une approche de recherche-action participative pour la psychologie du counseling.
23. Dahlgren CL, Lask B, Landrø NI, Rø Ø. Developing and evaluating cognitive remediation therapy (CRT) for adolescents with anorexia nervosa: a feasibility study. Clin Child Psychol Psychiatry. 2014;19(3):476–87. https://doi.org/10.1177/1359104513489980.
24. Dapelo MM, Surguladze S, Morris R, Tchanturia K. Emotion recognition in blended facial expressions in women with anorexia nervosa. Eur Eating Disord Rev. 2015;24(1):34–42. https://doi.org/10.1002/erv.2403.
25. Donald J, Abbott MJ, Smith E. Comparison of attention training and cognitive therapy in the treatment of social phobia: a preliminary investigation. Behav Cogn Psychother. 2014;42(1):74–91. https://doi.org/10.1017/S1352465812001051.
26. Durand M. Employing critical incident technique as one way to display the hidden aspects of post-merger integration. Int Business Rev. 2016;25(1):87–102. https://doi.org/10.1016/j.ibusrev.2015.05.003.
27. Fairburn CG, Beglin SJ. Assessment of eating disorders: interview or self-report questionnaire? Int J Eating Disord. 1994;16(4):363–70.
28. Fairburn CG, Cooper Z, Shafran R. Cognitive behaviour therapy for eating disorders: a "transdiagnostic" theory and treatment. Behav Res Ther. 2003; 41(5):509–28. https://doi.org/10.1016/S0005-7967(02)00088-8.
29. Federici A, Kaplan AS. The patient's account of relapse and recovery in anorexia nervosa: a qualitative study. Eur Eat Disord Rev. 2008;16(1):1–10. https://doi.org/10.1002/erv.813.
30. Fisher CA, Skocic S, Rutherford KA, Hetrick SE, Cochrane Common Mental Disorders Group. Family therapy approaches for anorexia nervosa. Cochrane Database Syst Rev. 2019;2019(5). https://doi.org/10.1002/14651858.CD004780.pub4.
31. Flanagan JC. The critical incident technique. Psychol Bull. 1954;51(4):327–58. https://doi.org/10.1037/h0061470.
32. Fogarty S, Ramjan LM. Factors impacting treatment and recovery in anorexia nervosa: qualitative findings from an online questionnaire. J Eating Disord. 2016;4(1):1–9. https://doi.org/10.1186/s40337-016-0107-1.
33. Fredrickson BL, Joiner T. Positive emotions trigger upward spirals toward emotional well-being. Psychol Sci. 2002;13(2):172–5. https://doi.org/10.1111/1467-9280.00431.
34. Fridlund, B., Henricson, M. and Mårtensson, J. (2017) Critical Incident Technique applied in nursing and healthcare sciences. Available at: www.symbiosisonline.orgwww.symbiosisonlinepublishing.com. Accessed 24 Nov 2019.
35. Friedlander ML, Sutherland O, Sandler S, Kortz L, Bernardi S, Lee HH, et al. Exploring corrective experiences in a successful case of short-term dynamic psychotherapy. Psychother. 2012;49(3):349–63. https://doi.org/10.1037/a0023447.
36. Friedlander ML, Lee H-H, Bernardi S. Corrective experiences in everyday life. Counseling Psychol. 2013;41(3):453–79. https://doi.org/10.1177/0011000012439476.
37. Giombini L, Moynihan J, Turco M, Nesbitt S. Evaluation of individual cognitive remediation therapy (CRT) for the treatment of young people with anorexia nervosa. Eating Weight Disord. 2017;22(4):667–73. https://doi.org/10.1007/s40519-016-0322-4.
38. Goldfried, M. R. (2012) 'The corrective experience: A core principle for therapeutic change.', in Transformation in psychotherapy: Corrective experiences across cognitive behavioral, humanistic, and psychodynamic approaches. American Psychological Association, pp. 13–29. doi: https://doi.org/10.1037/13747-002.
39. Grisso T, Appelbaum PS. Appreciating anorexia: decisional capacity and the role of values. Psychiatry Psychol. 2006;13(4):293–7. https://doi.org/10.1353/ppp.2007.0030.
40. Gross JJ. Emotion regulation: affective, cognitive, and social consequences. Psychophysiology. 2002:281–91. https://doi.org/10.1017/S0048577201393198.
41. Gross JJ, John OP. Individual differences in two emotion regulation processes: implications for affect, relationships, and well-being. J Pers Soc Psychol. 2003;85(2):348–62. https://doi.org/10.1037/0022-3514.85.2.348.
42. Gu L, Yang X, Li LMW, Zhou X, Gao DG. Seeing the big picture: broadening attention relieves sadness and depressed mood. Scand J Psychol. 2017;58(4): 324–32. https://doi.org/10.1111/sjop.12376.
43. Hedman E, Mörtberg E, Hesser H, Clark DM, Lekander M, Andersson E, et al. Mediators in psychological treatment of social anxiety disorder: individual cognitive therapy compared to cognitive behavioral group therapy. Behav Res Ther. 2013;51(10):696–705. https://doi.org/10.1016/j.brat.2013.07.006.
44. Horesh N, Apter A, Lepkifker E, Ratzoni G, Weizmann R, Tyano S. Life events and severe anorexia nervosa in adolescence. Acta Psychiatrica Scand. 1995; 91(1):5–9. https://doi.org/10.1111/j.1600-0447.1995.tb09734.x.
45. Hwang J, Seo S. A critical review of research on customer experience management: theoretical, methodological and cultural perspectives. Int J Contemp Hosp Manage. 2016:2218–46. https://doi.org/10.1108/IJCHM-04-2015-0192.
46. Ison J, Kent S. Social identity in eating disorders. Eur Eat Disord Rev. 2010; 18(6):475–85. https://doi.org/10.1002/erv.1001.
47. Jenkins J, Ogden J. Becoming "whole" again: a qualitative study of women's views of recovering from anorexia nervosa. Eur Eating Disord Rev. 2012; 20(1):e23–31. https://doi.org/10.1002/erv.1085.
48. Junghans-Rutelonis AN, Suorsa KI, Tackett AP, Burkley E, Chaney JM, Mullins LL. Self-esteem, self-focused attention, and the mediating role of fear of negative evaluation in college students with and without asthma. J Am Coll Health. 2015;63(8):554–62. https://doi.org/10.1080/07448481.2015.1057146.
49. Kyriacou O, Easter A, Tchanturia K. Comparing views of patients, parents, and clinicians on emotions in anorexia. J Health Psychol. 2009;14(7):843–54. https://doi.org/10.1177/1359105309340977.
50. Lang K, Treasure J, Tchanturia K. Acceptability and feasibility of self-help cognitive remediation therapy for anorexia nervosa delivered in collaboration with carers: a qualitative preliminary evaluation study. Psychiatry Res. 2015;225(3):387–94. https://doi.org/10.1016/j.psychres.2014.12.008.
51. Legenbauer TM, Meule A. Challenges in the treatment of adolescent anorexia nervosa - is enhanced cognitive behavior therapy the answer? Front Psychiatry. 2015;6. https://doi.org/10.3389/fpsyt.2015.00148.
52. Linville D, Brown T, Sturm K, McDougal T. Eating disorders and social support: perspectives of recovered individuals. Eat Disord. 2012;20(3):216–31. https://doi.org/10.1080/10640266.2012.668480.
53. McNamara N, Parsons H. "Everyone here wants everyone else to get better": the role of social identity in eating disorder recovery. Br J Soc Psychol. 2016; 55(4):662–80. https://doi.org/10.1111/bjso.12161.
54. Mohr JJ, Markell HM, King EB, Jones KP, Peddie CI, Kendra MS. Affective antecedents and consequences of revealing and concealing a lesbian, gay, or bisexual identity. J Appl Psychol. 2019;104(10):1266–82. https://doi.org/10.1037/apl0000399.
55. Money C, Genders R, Treasure J, Schmidt U, Tchanturia K. A brief emotion focused intervention for inpatients with anorexia nervosa: a qualitative

study. J Health Psychol. 2011;16(6):947–58. https://doi.org/10.1177/1359105310396395.
56. Mor N, Winquist J. Self-focused attention and negative affect: A meta-analysis. Psychol Bull. 2002;128(4):638–62. https://doi.org/10.1037/0033-2909.128.4.638.
57. Munro C, Randell L, Lawrie SM. An integrative bio-psycho-social theory of anorexia nervosa. Clin Psychol Psychother. 2017;24(1):1–21. https://doi.org/10.1002/cpp.2047.
58. Offord A, Turner H, Cooper M. Adolescent inpatient treatment for anorexia nervosa: a qualitative study exploring young adults' retrospective views of treatment and discharge. Eur Eat Disord Rev. 2006;14(6):377–87. https://doi.org/10.1002/erv.687.
59. Oldershaw A, Hambrook D, Stahl D, Tchanturia K, Treasure J, Schmidt U. The socio-emotional processing stream in anorexia nervosa. Neurosci Biobehav Rev. 2011;35(3):970–88. https://doi.org/10.1016/j.neubiorev.2010.11.001.
60. Oldershaw A, et al. Emotion generation and regulation in anorexia nervosa: a systematic review and meta-analysis of self-report data. Clin Psychol Rev. 2015:83–95. https://doi.org/10.1016/j.cpr.2015.04.005.
61. Oldershaw A, Startup H, Lavender T. Anorexia nervosa and a lost emotional self: a psychological formulation of the development, maintenance, and treatment of anorexia nervosa. Front Psychol. 2019;10:1–22. https://doi.org/10.3389/fpsyg.2019.00219.
62. De Paoli T, et al. Social rank and rejection sensitivity as mediators of the relationship between insecure attachment and disordered eating. Eur Eating Disord Rev. 2017;25(6):469–78. https://doi.org/10.1002/erv.2537.
63. Prosen S. Psychodrama in the group of patients diagnosed with eating disordersPsychodrama in einer PatientInnengruppe mit Essstörungen. Zeitschrift für Psychodrama und Soziometrie. 2016;15(S1):131–41. https://doi.org/10.1007/s11620-015-0305-x.
64. Santha B, et al. The critical incident technique in dental research: A review'. CHRISMED J Health Res. 2016;3(1):10. https://doi.org/10.4103/2348-3334.172406.
65. Sedgewick F, et al. Similarities and differences in theory of mind responses of patients with anorexia nervosa with and without autistic features. Front Psychiatry. 2019;10. https://doi.org/10.3389/fpsyt.2019.00318.
66. Steinhausen H-C. The outcome of anorexia nervosa in the 20th century. Am J Psychiatry. 2002;159(8):1284–93. https://doi.org/10.1176/appi.ajp.159.8.1284.
67. Steinhausen H-C. Outcome of eating disorders. Child Adolesc Psychiatric Clin North Am. 2009;18(1):225–42. https://doi.org/10.1016/J.CHC.2008.07.013.
68. Tan, D. J. O. A. *et al.* (2006) 'Competence to make treatment decisions in anorexia nervosa: thinking processes and values', Philos Psychiatry Psychol 13(4), p. 267. Available at: /PMC/articles/PMC2121578/?Report=abstract. Accessed 22 Jan 2021.
69. Tchanturia K, Hambrook D, Curtis H, Jones T, Lounes N, Fenn K, et al. Work and social adjustment in patients with anorexia nervosa. Compr Psychiatry. 2013;54(1):41–5. https://doi.org/10.1016/j.comppsych.2012.03.014.
70. Tchanturia K, Dapelo MAM, Harrison A, Hambrook D. Why study positive emotions in the context of eating disorders? Curr Psychiatry Rep. 2015;1(1): 537. https://doi.org/10.1007/s11920-014-0537-x.
71. Tierney S, Fox JRE. Trapped in a toxic relationship: comparing the views of women living with anorexia nervosa to those experiencing domestic violence. J Gender Stud. 2011;20(1):31–41. https://doi.org/10.1080/09589236.2011.542018.
72. Treasure J, Cardi V. Anorexia nervosa, theory and treatment: where are we 35 years on from Hilde Bruch's foundation lecture? Eur Eating Disord Rev. 2017;25(3):139–47. https://doi.org/10.1002/erv.2511.
73. Treasure J, Schmidt U. The cognitive-interpersonal maintenance model of anorexia nervosa revisited: a summary of the evidence for cognitive, socio-emotional and interpersonal predisposing and perpetuating factors. J Eating Disord. 2013;1(1):13. https://doi.org/10.1186/2050-2974-1-13.
74. Turton R, et al. Modifying a negative interpretation bias for ambiguous social scenarios that depict the risk of rejection in women with anorexia nervosa. J Affect Disord. 2018;227:705–12.
75. Via E, Soriano-Mas C, Sánchez I, Forcano L, Harrison BJ, Davey CG, et al. Abnormal social reward responses in anorexia nervosa: an fmri study. Plos One. 2015;10(7):e0133539. https://doi.org/10.1371/journal.pone.0133539.
76. Wade TD, Gillespie N, Martin NG. A comparison of early family life events amongst monozygotic twin women with lifetime anorexia nervosa, bulimia nervosa, or major depression. Int J Eating Disord. 2007;40(8):679–86. https://doi.org/10.1002/eat.20461.
77. Watson MJ, Lydecker JA, Jobe RL, Enright RD, Gartner A, Mazzeo SE, et al. Self-forgiveness in anorexia nervosa and bulimia nervosa. Eating Disord. 2012;20(1):31–41. https://doi.org/10.1080/10640266.2012.635561.
78. Weaver K, Wuest J, Ciliska D. Understanding women's journey of recovering from anorexia nervosa. Qual Health Res. 2005;15(2):188–206. https://doi.org/10.1177/1049732304270819.
79. Westwood H, et al. Exploration of friendship experiences, before and after illness onset in females with anorexia nervosa: a qualitative study'. Plos One. 2016;11(9):e0163528. https://doi.org/10.1371/journal.pone.0163528.
80. Wildes JE, Ringham RM, Marcus MD. Emotion avoidance in patients with anorexia nervosa: initial test of a functional model. Int J Eating Disord. 2010; 43(5):398–404. https://doi.org/10.1002/eat.20730.
81. Wiraszka-Lewandowska K, Sym A, Kokoszka A. The corrective experience of values in psychotherapy: its relations with the change of defense mechanisms and symptom intensity in a course of short-term. Eur Psychother. 2005;6:5–19 Available at: https://www.researchgate.net/profile/Agnieszka_Sym/publication/271199089_The_corrective_experience_of_values_in_psychotherapy_its_relations_with_the_change_of_defense_mechanisms_and_symptom_intensity_in_a_course_of_short-term_psychodynamic_group_psychotherapy/links/54c0ac4b0cf28eae4a696da2.pdf. Accessed 20 Sept 2020.
82. Wyssen A, Lao J, Rodger H, Humbel N, Lennertz J, Schuck K, et al. Facial emotion recognition abilities in women experiencing eating disorders. Psychosomatic Med. 2019;81(2):155–64. https://doi.org/10.1097/PSY.0000000000000664.

16

Changes in brain and behavior during food-based decision-making following treatment of anorexia nervosa

Karin Foerde[1,2], B. Timothy Walsh[1,2], Maya Dalack[1], Nathaniel Daw[3], Daphna Shohamy[4] and Joanna E. Steinglass[1,2*]

Abstract

Background: Anorexia nervosa is a severe illness with a high mortality rate, driven in large part by severe and persistent restriction of food intake. A critical challenge is to identify brain mechanisms associated with maladaptive eating behavior and whether they change with treatment. This study tested whether food choice-related caudate activation in anorexia nervosa changes with treatment.

Methods: Healthy women ($n = 29$) and women hospitalized with anorexia nervosa ($n = 24$), ages 18 to 40 years, completed a Food Choice Task during fMRI scanning at two timepoints. Among patients, procedures occurred upon hospital admission (Time 1) and again after patients had gained to normal weight (Time 2). Healthy controls were tested twice at an interval group-matched to patients. Choice-related caudate activation was assessed at each timepoint, using parametric analyses in an a priori region of interest.

Results: Among patients, the proportion of high-fat foods selected did not change over time (p's > 0.47), but decreased neural activity in the caudate after treatment was associated with increased selection of high-fat foods ($r_{23} = -0.43$, $p = 0.037$). Choice-related caudate activation differed among women with anorexia nervosa vs healthy control women at Time 1 (healthy control: $M = 0.15 \pm 0.87$, anorexia nervosa: $M = 0.70 \pm 1.1$, $t_{51} = -2.05$, $p = 0.045$), but not at Time 2 (healthy control: $M = 0.18 \pm 1.0$, anorexia nervosa: $M = 0.37 \pm 0.99$, $t_{51} = -0.694$, $p = 0.49$).

(Continued on next page)

* Correspondence: js1124@cumc.columbia.edu
[1]New York State Psychiatric Institute, 1051 Riverside Drive, Unit 98, New York, NY 10032, USA
[2]Psychiatry Department, Columbia University Irving Medical Center, 1051 Riverside Drive, Unit 98, New York, NY 10032, USA
Full list of author information is available at the end of the article

(Continued from previous page)
Conclusions: Caudate activity was more strongly associated with decisions about food among individuals with anorexia nervosa relative to healthy comparison individuals prior to treatment, and decreases in caudate engagement among individuals with anorexia nervosa undergoing treatment were associated with increases in high-fat food choices. The findings underscore the need for treatment development that more successfully alters both eating behavior and the neural mechanisms that guide it.

Keywords: Anorexia nervosa, Treatment, fMRI, Neuroscience, Longitudinal, Eating behavior

Plain English summary

Treatment that leads to full weight restoration in anorexia nervosa (AN) is accompanied by improvements in psychological symptoms. Yet, restrictive eating does not improve. Prior studies have shown that different neural circuits are engaged when deciding what to eat for patients with AN, compared with healthy controls. Here, we tested whether there were changes in brain activation associated with eating after weight restoration. Overall, food choices did not change with weight restoration, again showing that restrictive eating is resistant to change. However, changes among patients with AN showed a significant association between increased selection of high-fat foods and decreased activity in the caudate, with treatment. These findings highlight the importance of specific brain systems related to eating in the treatment of AN.

Background

The first step in the treatment of anorexia nervosa (AN) is weight restoration [1]. Behaviorally-based structured programs incentivizing patients with AN to consume adequate calories and normative macronutrient composition (i.e., at least 30% kcal from dietary fat) have high success rates [2]. Yet, relapse and rehospitalization of adults with AN are common, even after full weight restoration [3]. A central behavioral disturbance that contributes to relapse and chronicity of illness is the persistent restriction of food intake [4]. The neural mechanisms that underlie decisions about eating in AN have become a focus of recent research, providing an opportunity to test empirically how such mechanisms are affected by treatment. Increased understanding of the effects of treatment on neural mechanisms underlying the decision of what to eat may be useful in identifying biomarkers and new treatment targets.

In standard treatment programs for AN, renourishment is accomplished by providing appropriate nutrition, supervision around meals, and behavioral and psychological therapy to promote healthy eating and weight restoration [2]. Success rates for inpatient treatment are high in terms of weight normalization, resolution of medical instability, and improvement in associated psychological symptoms including depression and anxiety [5]. In these structured settings, individuals with AN are able to consume the ~4000 kcal per day that are required to gain weight at an appropriate pace. And yet, as soon as treatment incentives are removed after hospital discharge, these same individuals struggle to consume adequate nutrition and often lose weight [6, 7]. In two laboratory meal studies, hospitalized patients with AN showed significant improvement in psychological measures after successful weight restoration, but still consumed significantly fewer calories and less fat than healthy volunteers at both timepoints [8, 9]. The persistence of this maladaptive eating pattern indicates that it is important to understand this behavior.

Decision science has recently yielded advances in understanding the behavioral, computational, and neural mechanisms of choices [10–13]. Much of this research has involved food choices, partly for convenience of experimental design, leading to insights of particular relevance for eating disorders. Choice is a complex phenomenon that incorporates multiple cognitive and neural processes, such as attention, valuation, and action selection [14]. In decisions about what to eat, healthiness and tastiness have repeatedly been shown to be distinguishable values that are integrated into choice selection [12, 15–17]. The neurobiology of food choice has been shown to involve regions associated with value representations ventromedial prefrontal cortex (VMPFC) and self-control dorsolateral prefrontal cortex (DLPFC) [12]. The neural mechanisms of decision-making, and decisions about what foods to eat, have received relatively little attention in AN. Yet understanding the neural bases of maladaptive eating behavior may be important in order to improve treatment.

In two studies from our group, food choices made by adult women with AN were associated with neural activity in the dorsal striatum (specifically, the anterior caudate) [18, 19], which differed from healthy peers. This research used a food choice task that has been demonstrated to capture the maladaptive restrictive choices of patients with AN [20, 21] with both the restricting and the binge-eating/purging subtypes [22]. Task-based choices have been related to actual food intake in a laboratory meal [19], and test-retest reliability of the task has been demonstrated among healthy individuals [23].

However, changes in the neural underpinnings of decision-making about food have not been examined after weight restoration treatment.

Here, we examined whether food choice-related activation in regions of interest identified in previous studies [12, 19, 24], primarily the anterior caudate, VMPFC, and DLPFC changed, with treatment. Patients with AN participated in a Food Choice Task during fMRI scanning twice, once at admission for inpatient weight restoration treatment, and again after treatment. Change with treatment was compared with a group of healthy comparison (HC) women, who were studied twice, at an interval matched to the AN group. We hypothesized that individuals with AN would show greater choice-related activation of the anterior caudate as compared with HC and that this difference between groups would diminish after patients received weight restoration treatment, whereas groups would not differ in choice-related activation in the VMPFC and DLPFC. We additionally explored differences between groups and changes with treatment in choice-related, as well as tastiness and healthiness rating-related, activation in whole-brain analyses.

Methods

Participants

Participants were female HC and female inpatients with AN at the New York State Psychiatric Institute (NYSPI). Eligible patients met DSM-5 [25] criteria for AN at the time of admission assessed via Eating Disorders Assessment for DSM-5 [26]. HC were included if they had no current or lifetime psychiatric illness (including an eating disorder) and had a body mass index (BMI) between 18.5 and 25.0 kg/m^2. In both groups, individuals were excluded if they were taking psychotropic medication, had a known history of a neurological disorder or injury, had any contraindication to MRI, or were pregnant. All participants were right-handed, between the ages 18–40 years, and had an estimated IQ > 80. Participants were enrolled between November 2015 and August 2018.

Procedures occurred twice, once upon admission (Time 1) and once again after weight restoration (Time 2) for individuals with AN, and within 1–2 months for HC, to match the treatment time frame. Inpatient treatment at NYSPI is provided at no cost and consists of a behaviorally-based program aimed at full weight restoration [2] with a BMI goal between 19.5–20.5 kg/m^2. HC were compensated $150 for participation at each timepoint ($300 for both).

Only data from individuals who completed the Choice phase of the Food Choice Task during neuroimaging at both timepoints were analyzed. Time 1 data from these participants were included in one previous publication of food choice, focused on individuals across a spectrum of restrictive eating [18]. Of 31 HC, two were excluded from analyses due to loss of neuroimaging data (1 scanner error, 1 excessive motion) leading to a study sample of 29 HC. Of 26 AN, two were excluded due to a loss of task responses during neuroimaging, leaving a study sample of 24 AN (9 restricting subtype and 15 binge-eating/purging subtype). Two HC were additionally excluded from the Healthiness rating phase (1 due to excessive motion, 1 due to image artifact), and one AN was additionally excluded from the Healthiness and Tastiness rating phase due to excessive motion.

This study was approved by the NYSPI Institutional Review Board and all participants provided written informed consent.

Procedure

Height was measured on a Seca 240 wall-mounted stadiometer. Weight was measured in the morning at each timepoint on a Detecto balance-beam scale.

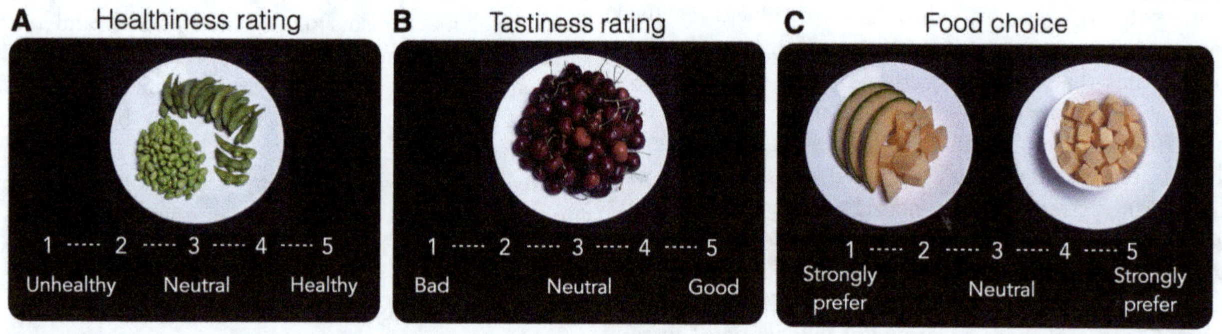

Fig. 1 Food Choice Task. The task consisted of two rating phases and a choice phase. In each phase participants made decisions about 76 food items. On each trial, the food stimulus was presented for 4 s, during which the participant made her response. **a** Healthiness rating phase. Participants rated the healthiness of each food item on five-point Likert scale from Bad to Good (or Good to Bad, counterbalanced across participants). **b** Tastiness rating phase. Participants rated the tastiness of each food item on five-point Likert scale from Unhealthy to Healthy (or Healthy to Unhealthy, counterbalanced across participants). **c** Choice phase. On each trial, participants indicated their preference for a changing food item (shown on the right) relative to a repeated reference item (previously rated neutral on healthiness and tastiness; shown on the left). After task completion, one Choice trial was randomly selected and the participant served a snack-sized portion of the food selected on that trial

Participants were given a standardized lunch (4 oz. turkey breast, 2 slices whole wheat bread, 1 packet mayonnaise, Nutrigrain bar, and 8 oz. water, ~ 500 kcal) at noon. At Time 2, for patients with AN, the post-treatment standardized lunch was increased in calories, such that the percent of the daily caloric prescription was the same at both timepoints. At approximately 2 pm, participants were brought to the NYSPI MR Unit for the Food Choice Task with fMRI scanning. At the end of the task, the participant was served a snack based on one of her choices in the task (see below), observed by staff. Procedures at Time 2 were identical.

Food choice task with fMRI (Fig. 1)

Food Choice Task procedures have been described previously [19]. The task consisted of three phases: Healthiness rating, Tastiness rating, and a Choice block (Fig. 1). In each block, participants rated 76 foods on a 5-point scale. Half of the foods were classified as "high-fat" (> 30% of the calories from fat; images and macronutrient information available at Columbia Academic Commons: https://doi.org/10.7916/d8-497c-2724 [17]. The rating scale appeared at the bottom of the screen for each item and participants were instructed that they could rate it as "neutral" or along the scale. For the Healthiness block, the anchors were "Unhealthy" to "Healthy." For the Tastiness block, the anchors were "Bad" to "Good." For the Tastiness block, participants were additionally instructed to rate it *only* for tastiness. All task parameters (including order of the rating scale) were counterbalanced and randomized across participants. After completion of the rating scales, a "Reference" item was selected for each participant that had been rated by her as "Neutral" on both Healthiness and Tastiness. If no item neutral on both scales was identified, an item was selected that was rated neutral on Healthiness and 1 point in the positive direction on Tastiness, in order to minimize biasing choices based on taste value. In the Choice block, participants made a selection by indicating whether they 'Strongly Preferred' or 'Preferred' the Reference item (which was constant) or the other food (which varied on each trial) using a 5-point scale. To ensure that responses reflected true preferences, participants were told that they would be served one of their choices at the conclusion of the task. One Choice trial was randomly selected, and the participant received a snack-sized portion of the item chosen on that trial.

In all blocks, the food stimulus was presented for 4 s on each trial, during which the participant made her response. Each trial was followed by a fixation cross inter-trial interval (ITI). The duration of ITIs was jittered for optimization of event-related fMRI design. Stimulus presentation sequence and timing were optimized using the optseq2 algorithm (http://surfer.nmr.mgh.harvard.edu/optseq/). Each learning run lasted 480 s. Mean ITI = 2.3 s, median = 2 s, and range = 1–10 s, across all three phases. All task phases were presented using Matlab and the Psychophysics toolbox [27].

Whole-brain imaging data were acquired on a GE 3 T MR750 scanner with a 32-channel phased-array head coil. Structural images were collected using a high-resolution T1-weighted BRAVO pulse sequence (1 × 1 × 1 mm voxel size) for image registration. Functional images were collected using a gradient echo T2*-weighted echoplanar (EPI) sequence with blood oxygenation level-dependent (BOLD) contrast (TR = 2000 ms, TE = 19 ms, flipangle = 77, 3 × 3 × 3 mm voxel size, 45 contiguous axial slices, FOV = 19.2, interleaved acquisition). Each Food Choice Task run consisted of 240 volumes.

Data analysis

Demographic and clinical characteristics were compared using Student's t-tests and chi-square, as appropriate. Repeated measures ANOVA were used to test for significance of change over time within each group. Tests were two-tailed unless otherwise specified. Analyses were conducted in JASP [28] (https://jasp-stats.org), and alpha was set at $p = 0.05$.

Food choice task

Rating and choice data were analyzed using multilevel regression models lme4 linear mixed effects package for R [29]. For the Choice phase, responses on the 5-point scale were converted to binary 'Yes' (1) or 'No' (0) preferences for the trial-unique food versus the Reference item, and neutral responses were omitted from analyses. Binomial choice data were modelled with multilevel logistic regression, in which participant choice (selection of the trial-unique food item over the reference food) was the dependent variable. Continuous outcome rating data from the Healthiness and Tastiness phases were modelled using multilevel linear regression. To assess relationships between ratings and choices, participant choice (selection of the trial-unique food item over the reference food) was the dependent variable and (z-scored) healthiness and tastiness ratings entered as independent variables. The relationship between Healthiness and Tastiness was assessed with Healthiness ratings as the dependent variable and (z-scored) Tastiness ratings as the independent variable. In all analyses, Group (HC/AN, coded as − 1/1), Food type (low-fat/high-fat, coded as − 1/1), and Time (Time 1/Time 2, coded as − 1/1) were entered as independent variables, and models included by-subject random intercepts and slopes and by-item (food images) random intercepts [30, 31].

Correlations between brain, behavior, and demographic measures were assessed using Pearson correlation. Robust regression was implemented as needed due to presence of outlier data points using the rlm function in the MASS package with bisquare weighting [32].

fMRI analyses

Imaging data were converted from DICOM to NIFTI format and preprocessed and analyzed using the FSL (http://fsl.fmrib.ox.ac.uk/fsl/) package version 6 (FMRIB's Software Library; Oxford Centre for Functional Resonance Imaging of the Brain, FMRIB) [33].

Image pre-processing Functional images were aligned using the MCFLIRT tool [34] and the six scan-to-scan head motion parameters estimated during motion correction obtained. The skull was removed from functional images using the brain extraction tool (BET) [35] and from structural images using Freesurfer [36, 37]. Spatial smoothing was applied with a Gaussian kernel of 5 mm (FWHM). Data and design matrix were high-pass filtered with a cutoff period of 100 s. After analysis at the individual level, the results were normalized to a standard template: Functional images were first aligned to the T1-weighted image using a boundary-based registration method implemented in FSL6 (BBR) and then the structural image to the standard MNI152 2-mm template using FLIRT (12 degrees of freedom) and FNIRT (10-mm warp resolution) [34, 38].

Analyses At the level of individual participants, each event was convolved with a canonical hemodynamic response function (except added confound regressors, see below) and entered into a general linear model (GLM). The temporal derivative of each regressor (except added confound regressors) was also included in the model. To account for any residual effects of subject movement, we included the six scan-to-scan head motion parameters estimated during motion correction as well as framewise displacement (FD) and root mean square intensity difference from one volume to the next (DVARS) [39] as confound regressors. In addition, volumes with FD and DVARS exceeding a threshold of 0.5 were modeled out by adding a single time point regressor for each volume to be 'dropped' from analysis [40]. Runs for which more than 25% of volumes were dropped were excluded from analysis: one Tastiness rating run at Time 1 (AN), two Healthiness rating runs at Time 2 (1 HC, 1 AN). The number of dropped volumes did not differ between groups (ps > 0.05, Supplemental Table S1).

Parametric analysis of food choices and ratings were conducted (rating-related results in Supplemental Figure S1) [19]. Each person's choices were normalized to their own response range; analyses were therefore not biased by overall differences in choice preferences. The GLMs for the choice and rating phases included the following regressors: onsets for each trial on which a response was made (i), onsets for each trial on which a response was made parametrically modulated by the (demeaned) rating on that trial (ii) and the (demeaned) response time on that trial (iii), and onsets for missed trials (iv). Regressors i-iii were modeled with duration equal to the response time on each trial, and regressor iv with duration equal to the trial length (4 s). Motion and confound regressors were included as outlined above. Linear contrasts were performed on specific comparisons of interest. These contrasts were used for mixed-effects group analyses using FSL's FLAME 1 (FMRIB's local analysis of mixed effects) tool, using two-sample unpaired *t*-tests to compare groups and paired *t*-tests to compare changes between Time 1 and Time 2.

ROI analyses

Based on a previous study indicating involvement of the right anterior caudate in food choices [19], an anatomical region of interest (ROI) was obtained from the Harvard-Oxford probabilistic atlas included in FSL, thresholded at 25% probability and anterior to y = 0 (Fig. 3a). Additional ROIs were included based on their implication in food choices in healthy individuals, with the VMPFC involved in value-based decisions and the DLPFC implicated in self-control [12]. Moreover, VMPFC regions (e.g., OFC) have been implicated in studies of decision making in AN [41] and DLPFC has been used as a target for neuromodulation (rTMS) intervention in AN [20]. Six-mm spheres were created centered on MNI coordinates taken from a previous study using the Food Choice task [12]: VMPFC (MNI = [3 51 3]; Fig. 3b) and DLPFC (MNI = [− 48 15 24]; Fig. 3c).

Whole-brain analyses

Whole-brain higher-level analyses were thresholded using clusters determined by $Z > 3.1$ and a whole-brain corrected, FWE cluster significance threshold of $p = 0.05$ [42]. For exploratory purposes, we additionally considered analyses thresholded at $Z > 2.3$, FWE cluster significance threshold of $p = 0.05$ [43].

Results are displayed on a study-specific mean anatomical image resulting from averaging all participants' normalized high-resolution structural images.

Results

Clinical characteristics of participants are presented in Table 1. Psychological measures differed between individuals with AN and HC at both timepoints, and the AN group showed improvement in all psychological measures and BMI from Time 1 to Time 2. At Time 2, AN and HC groups were well matched on BMI ($t_{51} = 1.29$, $p = 0.20$). The average time between scans was similar in both groups ($mean_{HC}$: 49 ± 21 days; $mean_{AN}$: 58 ± 21 days, $t_{51} = -1.4$, $p = 0.17$).

Table 1 Demographics and clinical characteristics of participants

	Time 1						Time 2						Time 1 versus Time 2			
	HC (n = 29)		AN (n = 24)				HC		AN				HC		AN	
	M	SD	M	SD	t	*p*	M	SD	M	SD	t	*p*	t	*p*	t	*p*
Age (years)	25.8	5.2	26.9	6.5	−0.7	*0.50*										
Caucasian (n,%)	22	76%	16	67%	0.55[a]	*0.46*										
Estimated IQ	117.3	13.4	112.0	9.5	1.7	*0.11*										
LNS	12.0	3.1	11.7	2.4	0.4	*0.67*										
BMI (kg/m2)	21.0	1.4	16.3	1.9	10.3	*< .001*	21.0	1.6	20.5	0.9	1.4	*0.17*	−0.33	*0.75*	−13.4	*< .001*
Duration of Illness (years)			8.6	6.9												
EDE-Q Global	0.4	0.5	4.3	1.7	− 12.2	*< .001*	0.4	0.4	2.8	1.3	−9.1	*< .001*	−0.54	*0.6*	6.6	*< .001*
TFEQ-Restraint	5.9	4.2	17.4	3.6	−10.6	*< .001*	6.1	4.8	14.2	5.3	−5.9	*< .001*	−0.43	*0.67*	3.9	*< .001*
BDI	2.1	2.3	31.1	13.4	−11.5	*< .001*	3.1	2.5	17.4	14.4	−5.2	*< .001*	−1.94	*0.06*	5.3	*< .001*
STAI(T)	32.6	6.5	62.9	11.4	−12.2	*< .001*	32.9	8.2	56.0	12.2	−8.2	*< .001*	−0.26	*0.8*	3.6	*0.003*

[a]Chi square statistic
Missing data: BDI is missing from 1 individual with AN
AN anorexia Nervosa, *BDI* beck depression index [44], *BMI* body mass index, *EDE-Q* eating disorder examination-questionnaire version [45], *HC* healthy control, *LNS* letter number sequence from the Weschler Adult Intelligence Scale [46], *STAI(T)* Spielberger trait anxiety inventory [47], *TFEQ-Restraint* Three Factor Eating Questionnaire Restraint subscale [48] Estimated IQ was assessed with the Wechsler Abbreviated Scale of Intelligence [49]

Food choice task behavior

All participants were able to respond within the response window, indicated by response rates exceeding 96% in all task phases and in both groups. Response rates did not differ between groups (ps > 0.25).

Choices of high-fat and low-fat foods (proportion of trials chosen over the Reference food) did not change significantly between Time 1 and Time 2 (ps > 0.16) (Fig. 2a). On average, the AN group chose high-fat foods less often than the HC group at both time points (Group X Food type interaction: Est = − 0.42, z = − 4.72, $p < 0.00001$; Supplemental Table S2; significant effect of Group for high-fat foods: Est = − 0.14, z = − 4.61, $p < 0.0001$, but not for low-fat foods: Est = − 0.0008, z = − 0.03, $p = 0.97$).

Healthiness ratings did not change significantly with treatment (ps > 0.05, Fig. 2b, Supplemental Table S3). High-fat foods were rated lower in healthiness than low-fat foods overall (Est: − 0.75, $t_{80.3} = -6.70$, $p = 2.6 \times 10^{-9}$) and significantly more so among individuals with AN (Group X Food type interaction: Est = − 0.05, $t_{50.8} = -2.02$, $p = 0.048$; significant effect of Group for high-fat foods: Est = − 0.15, $t_{51} = -2.84$, $p = 0.006$, but not for low-fat foods: Est = − 0.04, $t_{51} = -1.15$, $p = 0.26$).

Tastiness ratings did not change with treatment (Fig. 2c, Supplemental Table S4). Individuals with AN rated high-fat foods as less tasty than did HC (Food type X Group: Est = − 0.14, t = − 3.23, $p = 0.002$; Group: Est = − 0.13, t = − 2.51, $p = 0.015$; significant effect of Group for high-fat foods: Est = − 0.28, $t_{51} = -3.22$, p = 0.002, but not for low-fat foods: Est = 0.007, $t_{51} = 0.14$, $p = 0.89$), and this pattern did not change over time (all other effects ps > 0.27).

Associations between ratings and choices

Across both timepoints Healthiness influenced Choice more among individuals with AN relative to HC (Est = 0.49, z = 3.94, $p = 8.2 \times 10^{-5}$) and Tastiness influenced Choice more among HC relative to individuals with AN (Est = − 0.46, z = − 3.69, $p = 0.0002$). There was a Time by Tastiness interaction (Est = 0.17, z = 2.08, $p = 0.037$), with Tastiness influencing Choice more at Time 2 in both groups (Fig. 2d, Supplemental Table S5). Healthiness was more strongly associated with Tastiness among AN relative to HC (Est = 0.13, z = 2.19, p = 0.03; Fig. 2e, Supplemental Table S6) and the relationship between Healthiness and Tastiness ratings did not change over time (ps > 0.25).

Neuroimaging

Anterior caudate

During the Choice phase there was no significant interaction between Group and Time in a rmANOVA (F [1, 51]=1.19, $p = 0.28$) nor a main effect of Time (F [1, 51]= 0.87, $p = 0.36$). The main effect of Group approached statistical significance (F [1, 51]=2.997, $p = 0.089$) and groups differed significantly during Choice at Time 1 ($t_{51} = -2.05$, $p = 0.045$). In contrast, group differences at Time 2 were not significant ($t_{51} = -0.694$, $p = 0.49$; Fig. 3a. During Healthiness and Tastiness ratings there were no effects of Group or Time (ps > 0.05; Supplemental Figure S1A).

We next examined whether change in caudate activation over time was related to changes in choice behavior in AN. Among individuals with AN, increased choice of high-fat foods was associated with decreased activation of the caudate during the Choice block ($r_{22} = -0.427$,

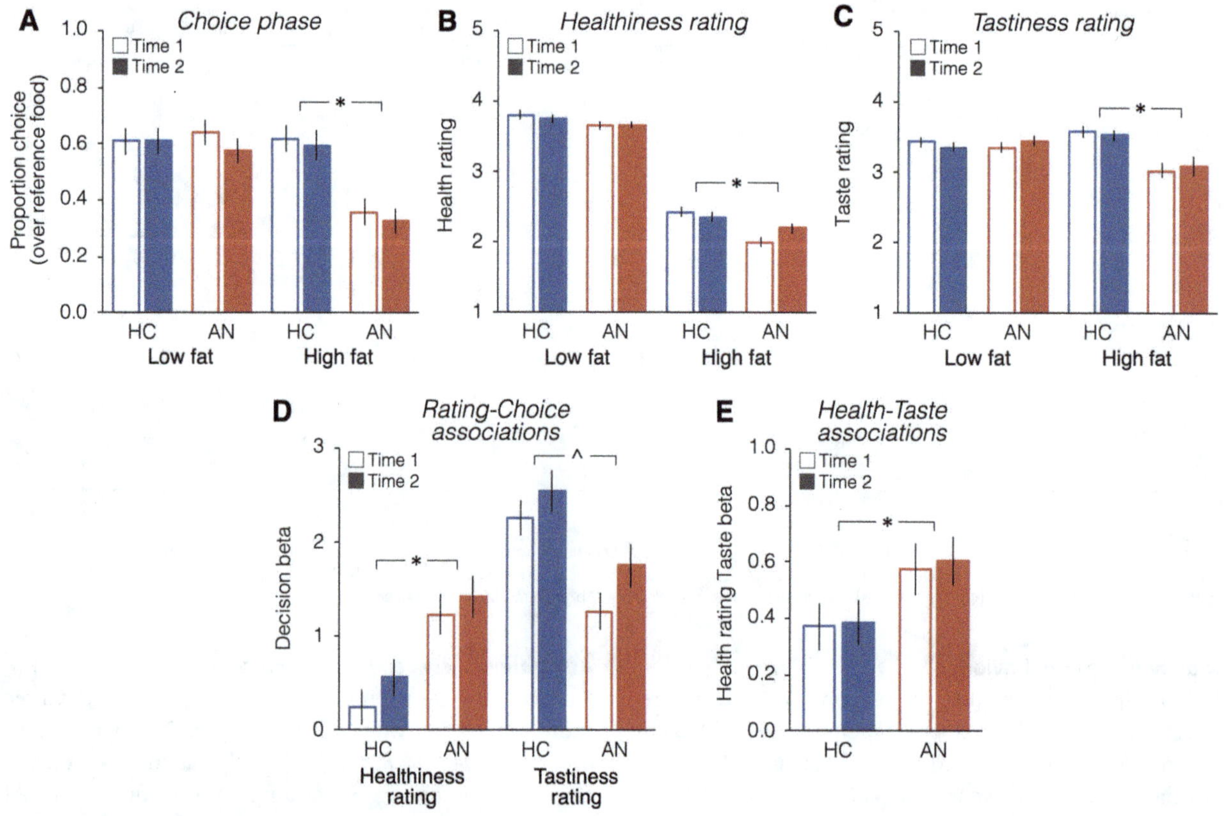

Fig. 2 Food choice task behavior at Time 1 and Time 2. **a** High-fat and low-fat food choices did not change significantly from Time 1 to Time 2 (ps > 0.37). The AN group made fewer high-fat, but not low-fat, food choices before and after treatment (Supplemental Table S2). **b** Overall low-fat items were rated higher on healthiness than high-fat items. High-fat foods were rated as lower in healthiness than low-fat foods overall and the groups differed significantly (Supplemental Table S3). **c** The AN group rated high-fat foods specifically lower in tastiness than did the HC group and this did not change with treatment (Supplemental Table S4). **d** Logistic regression of Healthiness and Tastiness ratings on choice. Choice was influenced more by tastiness among HC than AN, whereas choice was influenced more by healthiness among AN relative to HC (Supplemental Table S5). **e** Regression of Healthiness on Tastiness ratings. Ratings were more strongly associated among AN than HC (Supplemental Table S6). * indicates $p < 0.05$. ^ indicates significant Group difference and significant difference between Time 1 and Time 2 in both groups

$p = 0.037$, robust regression: $p = 0.036$; Fig. 3a). This relationship between neural activation and behavior was not found among the HC ($r_{27} = -0.11$, $p = 0.57$; Fig. 3a). Changes in choices of low-fat foods were not related to caudate engagement in either group (AN: $r_{22} = -0.08$, $p = 0.70$; HC: $r_{27} = -0.02$, $p = 0.90$).

Prefrontal cortex activity and food choice

As in previous studies [12, 19], there was significant choice-related activation in the VMPFC ROI. That activation did not differ between groups (F [1, 51]=0.007, $p = 0.93$) or across time (F [1, 51]=0.57, $p = 0.45$) nor was there a significant interaction (F [1, 51]=0.19, $p = 0.67$; Fig. 3b). We additionally explored whether the DLPFC, previously implicated in the use of self-control for food choices [12], was differentially engaged across groups and time, but found no significant differences (Time: F [1, 51]=0.16, $p = 0.69$; Group: F [1, 51]=1.32, $p = 0.26$; Group x Time: F [1, 51]=1.00, $p = 0.32$; Fig. 3c). There were no effects of Group or Time during Healthiness and Tastiness ratings (ps > 0.05; Supplemental Figure S1BC).

Whole-brain analyses to explore areas outside a priori ROIs revealed a group difference at Time 1 in the superior parietal lobule/precuneus, with greater choice related engagement in the AN than the HC group (Supplemental Figure 2). To examine changes over time in the parietal region, we extracted values at Time 2 from the cluster identified at Time 1. There were no group differences at Time 2 ($t_{51} = -0.15$, $p = 0.88$; Group X Time Interaction: F [1, 51]=6.67, $p = 0.013$; Fig. 3d). For completeness, as for the anterior caudate, we explored the relationship between changes from Time 1 to Time 2 in the parietal region and high-fat food choice changes and found a significant correlation ($r_{22} = -0.476$, $p = 0.019$; robust regression: $p = 0.022$; Fig. 3d). Changes over time in the anterior caudate and parietal lobe were significantly correlated in the AN group ($r = 0.745$, $p < 0.001$)

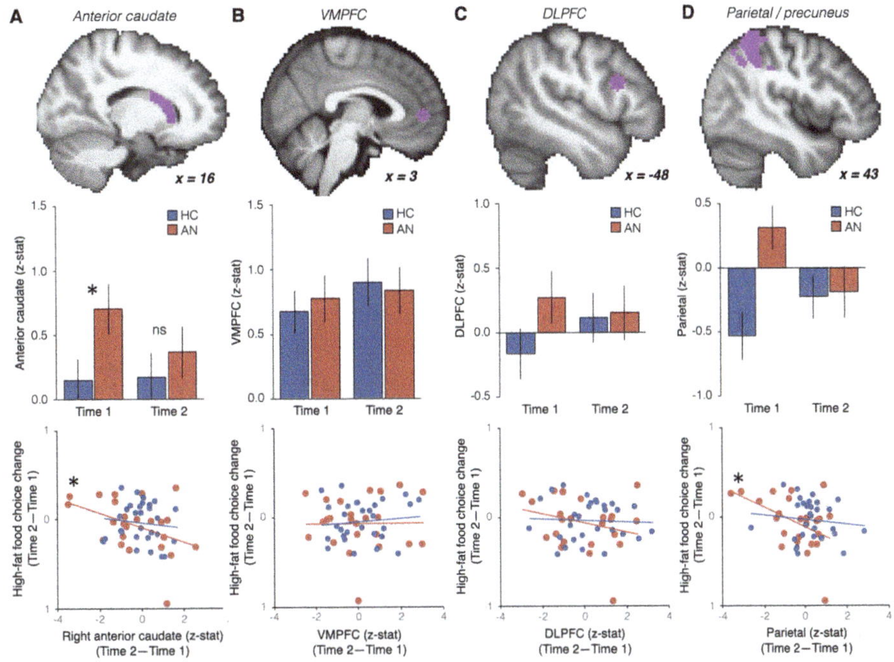

Fig. 3 Choice-related engagement in regions of interest before and after treatment and relationship with eating behavior. **a** Values extracted from the parametric choice analysis in our a priori anatomical ROI in the right anterior caudate (top panel). Choice-related activation in the caudate differed significantly between HC and AN at Time 1, but not at Time 2 (middle panel). Change in activity in the caudate from Time 1 to Time 2 was significantly correlated with the change in proportion high-fat food choices on the food choice task among individuals with AN, but not HC. Robust regression was used due to the presence of outliers. **b** Same analyses as in **a** for the a priori VMPFC ROI (MNI = [3 51 3]; top panel). **c** Same analyses as in **a** for the a priori DLPFC ROI (MNI = [− 48 15 24]; top panel). **d** For illustration purposes the same analyses as in **a** are presented for the parietal region identified in exploratory whole-brain analyses

but not in the HC group ($r = 0.338$, $p = 0.073$); the difference in correlation between groups was significant ($p = 0.038$).

Whole-brain analyses of the Choice phase (Supplemental Figure S2), Healthiness rating phase (Supplemental Figure S3), and Tastiness rating phase (Supplemental Figure S4) did not reveal any other regions that changed between Time 1 and Time 2 or differed between groups.

Discussion

This study tested whether neural mechanisms associated with maladaptive food choice in AN change with acute weight restoration. The fMRI findings during a Food Choice Task immediately following hospital admission were consistent with prior results, with greater choice-related engagement of the anterior caudate among individuals with AN. Increased selection of high-fat foods following weight restoration was associated with decreased choice-related caudate activation. On average, however, patients with AN did not substantially increase their selection of high-fat foods from Time 1 to Time 2, consistent with a prior study demonstrating the persistence of dietary restriction after treatment [9]. Additionally, whole brain analyses identified choice-related activation in a parietal/precuneus region that normalized with weight restoration. Change over time in this region was also associated with food-choice change and with caudate change. These findings underscore the association between restrictive eating and choice-related activation of the caudate in AN and suggest this brain-behavior link may be a target for treatment development.

The lack of change in choice of high-fat foods for a snack after ~ 2.5 months of hospital care is disappointing, though not surprising. The challenge of changing eating behavior, even during inpatient treatment, has been demonstrated in laboratory meal studies [8, 9] and is consistent with the high rate of relapse following hospital discharge. The ability to select a diet higher in energy density at the end of hospital care is associated with better treatment outcomes 1 year later [4, 50], suggesting that interventions that effect change in dietary patterns are likely necessary to decrease relapse. The caudate region implicated here is important for action control and choice, in general [51]. Change in maladaptive behavior in AN may depend on therapeutic techniques that focus directly on the difficult problem of changing food choices. A habit reversal based approach that targeted cues for maladaptive eating routines was successful in changing behavior in AN in a pilot study [52]. Similarly, exposure therapies that emphasize finer-grained focus on maladaptive eating have also shown promise [53]. Neuromodulation of the dorsal frontostriatal system using transcranial magnetic stimulation (TMS) showed some impact in decreasing excessive self-control over food choices among individuals with chronic AN [20]. Targeting the brain systems identified here may amplify the effects of existing treatments for AN.

In addition to the a priori ROI analyses that largely confirmed hypotheses about the caudate in food-based decision making in AN, exploratory whole-brain analyses suggested that the brain-behavior link also includes parietal/precuneus regions. The parietal lobe has been implicated in decision making and choice [54, 55]. In addition, parietal cortex is often considered part of a cognitive control network (fronto-cingulo-parietal system) [56–58], with functions that could be relevant for food choice (e.g., selective attention, response inhibition, etc.). The precuneus has been shown to play a role in a variety of higher cognitive functions, including self-referential processing and episodic memory retrieval [59]. Abnormalities in precuneus activation among individuals with AN have been identified several studies that include food related tasks [60–62] and, notably, is the most highly implicated region associated with the term 'anorexia nervosa' on the Neuroquery meta-analysis tool [63]. While the present study design does not allow for inferences about the specific contribution to decision-making, the findings suggest that further investigation of these cognitive processes is warranted. Although, reverse inference of cognitive processes based on brain activity is of limited utility, one hypothesis potentially worth investigating based on differential engagement of the precuneus among AN and HC, is that individuals with AN rely on memory retrieval differently than do HC; the role of episodic memories in decision making among individuals with AN has not been carefully examined. These cortical regions might also be targets for neuromodulation.

There are limited data about brain systems that contribute to the persistence of AN, especially as few studies have examined neural systems before and after treatment. The mean age and duration of illness in this study is representative of a general sample of treatment seeking adults, and is within the range seen in across neuroimaging research [64]. However, duration of illness has not been systematically considered in neuroimaging studies in AN, and may influence brain findings [65]. Existing longitudinal data, across different imaging modalities, have indicated that renourishment is associated with some brain changes. For example, structural brain abnormalities, such as gray matter volume decreases and cortical thinning, are seen among individuals with AN at low weight and tend to normalize with weight restoration [66–68]. However, studies of white matter abnormalities have not consistently reported normalization with weight restoration [69, 70]. One task-based fMRI study indicated that learning related response abnormalities in the striatum normalized after weight restoration [71]. Two studies of monetary decision-making found increases in neural activity in the striatum [72] and the dorsal anterior cingulate after weight restoration [73]. These studies together indicate that the brain is altered by starvation (and by renourishment) and that fronto-striatal circuits are among regions that undergo change across multiple studies and modalities. The stability of the neural response in the HC group in the present study supports the utility of the longitudinal assessments and strengthens the ability to draw inferences from the changes seen in the AN group. And, unlike prior longitudinal research, the present study directly examined treatment-associated changes in neural mechanisms of restrictive eating - the behavioral disturbance most directly connected to relapse, morbidity, and mortality. These findings highlight the value of explicitly linking brain and behavior by using a task demonstrated to capture maladaptive eating behavior in AN.

Limitations

The current results should be viewed in light of several limitations. First, the sample size was modest, and it is possible that there was insufficient power to detect the full effect of treatment on neural circuits. Small sample size is a common limitation in studies of AN and suggests a need for standardization of methods such that studies can be pooled. Second, patients were studied at the end of acute inpatient treatment, shortly after full weight restoration. While weight restoration is a necessary first step in treatment of AN, it is not associated with full resolution of psychological and behavioral symptoms and may not be the optimal moment to assess brain changes in AN. On the other hand, it has been suggested that neural changes should precede behavioral effects, hopefully permitting understanding of the neural mechanisms of treatment response [74]. Third, examination of brain regions that may become engaged only after weight restoration was limited by a priori regional hypotheses. It may be that the ROIs selected (VMPFC and DLPFC) were not the most relevant or sensitive to change and, in this small study, we were unable to detect other regions of increased activation in a whole brain analysis.

Conclusions

By linking brain and behavior, this study confirmed previous findings that during active decisions about what to eat, acutely ill individuals with AN differed from HC in engagement of the anterior caudate. The change (decrease) in caudate activation after treatment was associated with an increased tendency to choose high-fat foods, and similar activation patterns occurred in the parietal/precuneus region. Additional research is needed to determine whether food choice behavior—and associated neural mechanisms—change with longer-term remission.

Abbreviations

AN: Anorexia nervosa; BMI: Body mass index; BOLD: Blood-oxygen level dependent; DLPFC: Dorsolateral prefrontal cortex; GLM: General linear model; HC: Healthy control volunteer; ITI: Intertrial interval; NYSPI: New York State Psychiatric Institute; VMPFC: Ventromedial prefrontal cortex; IQ: Intelligence quotient; DICOM: Digital Imaging and Communications in Medicine; NIFTI: Neuroimaging Informatics Technology Initiative; FSL: FMRIB Software Library; MNI: Montreal Neurological Institute; FD: Framewise Displacement

Acknowledgments

We would like to thank Akram Bakkour, PhD for technical assistance with the data analyses, and thoughtful contributions to discussions of these data. The authors would like to thank the patients and staff of the New York State Psychiatric Institute for their contributions to this research.

Authors' contributions

JS, DS, KF, and BTW conceptualized and designed the study. KF conducted analyses and DS and ND contributed to analytic design and interpretation. MD contributed to data collection and management, and manuscript review. JS, KF, and BTW wrote and edited the manuscript. All authors reviewed the manuscript. The author(s) read and approved the final manuscript.

Competing interests

Dr. Steinglass receives royalties from UpToDate. Dr. Walsh reports receiving royalties and honoraria from Guilford Press, McGraw-Hill, Oxford University Press, UpToDate, British Medical Journal, Johns Hopkins Press and Guidepoint Global. Drs. Daw, Foerde, and Shohamy and Ms. Dalack report no financial relationships with commercial interests.

Author details

[1]New York State Psychiatric Institute, 1051 Riverside Drive, Unit 98, New York, NY 10032, USA. [2]Psychiatry Department, Columbia University Irving Medical Center, 1051 Riverside Drive, Unit 98, New York, NY 10032, USA. [3]Princeton Neuroscience Institute, Department of Psychology, Princeton University, Princeton, NJ 08540, USA. [4]Psychology Department and Zuckerman Mind Brain and Behavior Institute, Columbia University, 3227 Broadway, New York, NY 10027, USA.

References

1. American Psychiatric Association. Treatment of patients with eating disorders,third edition. Am J Psychiatry. 2006;163(7 Suppl):4–54.
2. Attia E, Walsh BT. Behavioral management for anorexia nervosa. N Engl J Med. 2009;360(5):500–6. https://doi.org/10.1056/NEJMct0805569.
3. Khalsa SS, Portnoff LC, McCurdy-McKinnon D, Feusner JD. What happens after treatment? A systematic review of relapse, remission, and recovery in anorexia nervosa. J Eat Disord. 2017;5(1):20. https://doi.org/10.1186/s40337-017-0145-3.
4. Schebendach J, Mayer LE, Devlin MJ, Attia E, Walsh BT. Dietary energy density and diet variety as risk factors for relapse in anorexia nervosa: a replication. Int J Eat Disord. 2012;45(1):79–84. https://doi.org/10.1002/eat.20922.
5. Attia E, Haiman C, Walsh BT, Flater SR. Does fluoxetine augment the inpatient treatment of anorexia nervosa? Am J Psychiatry. 1998;155(4):548–51. https://doi.org/10.1176/ajp.155.4.548.
6. Kaplan AS, Walsh BT, Olmsted M, Attia E, Carter JC, Devlin MJ, et al. The slippery slope: prediction of successful weight maintenance in anorexia nervosa. Psychol Med. 2009;39(6):1037–45. https://doi.org/10.1017/S003329170800442X.
7. Uniacke B, Wang Y, Biezonski D, Sussman T, Lee S, Posner J, et al. Resting-state connectivity within and across neural circuits in anorexia nervosa. Brain Behav. 2019;9(1):e01205. https://doi.org/10.1002/brb3.1205.
8. Sysko R, Walsh BT, Schebendach J, Wilson GT. Eating behavior among women with anorexia nervosa. Am J Clin Nutr. 2005;82(2):296–301. https://doi.org/10.1093/ajcn/82.2.296.
9. Mayer LE, Schebendach J, Bodell LP, Shingleton RM, Walsh BT. Eating behavior in anorexia nervosa: before and after treatment. Int J Eat Disord. 2012;45(2):290–3. https://doi.org/10.1002/eat.20924.
10. Rangel A, Camerer C, Montague PR. A framework for studying the neurobiology of value-based decision making. Nat Rev Neurosci. 2008;9(7): 545–56. https://doi.org/10.1038/nrn2357.
11. Rangel A. Regulation of dietary choice by the decision-making circuitry. Nat Neurosci. 2013;16(12):1717–24. https://doi.org/10.1038/nn.3561.
12. Hare TA, Camerer CF, Rangel A. Self-control in decision-making involves modulation of the vmPFC valuation system. Science. 2009;324(5927):646–8. https://doi.org/10.1126/science.1168450.
13. Hare TA, Malmaud J, Rangel A. Focusing attention on the health aspects of foods changes value signals in vmPFC and improves dietary choice. J Neurosci. 2011;31(30):11077–87. https://doi.org/10.1523/JNEUROSCI.6383-10.2011.
14. Krajbich I, Armel C, Rangel A. Visual fixations and the computation and comparison of value in simple choice. Nat Neurosci. 2010;13(10):1292–8. https://doi.org/10.1038/nn.2635.
15. Maier SU, Raja Beharelle A, Polania R, Ruff CC, Hare TA. Dissociable mechanisms govern when and how strongly reward attributes affect decisions. Nat Hum Behav. 2020;4(9):949–63. https://doi.org/10.1038/s41562-020-0893-y.
16. Suzuki S, Cross L, O'Doherty JP. Elucidating the underlying components of food valuation in the human orbitofrontal cortex. Nat Neurosci. 2017;20(12): 1780–6. https://doi.org/10.1038/s41593-017-0008-x.
17. Lloyd EC, Shehzad Z, Schebendach J, Bakkour A, Xue AM, Assaf NF, et al. Food Folio by Columbia Center for Eating Disorders: A Freely Available Food Image Database. Front Psychol. 2020;11(3556). https://doi.org/10.3389/fpsyg.2020.585044.
18. Foerde K, Schebendach JE, Davis L, Daw N, Walsh BT, Shohamy D, et al. Restrictive eating across a spectrum from healthy to unhealthy: behavioral and neural mechanisms. Psychol Med. 2020:1–10. https://doi.org/10.1017/S0033291720003542.
19. Foerde K, Steinglass JE, Shohamy D, Walsh BT. Neural mechanisms supporting maladaptive food choices in anorexia nervosa. Nat Neurosci. 2015;18(11):1571–3. https://doi.org/10.1038/nn.4136.
20. Dalton B, Foerde K, Bartholdy S, McClelland J, Kekic M, Grycuk L, et al. The effect of repetitive transcranial magnetic stimulation on food choice-related self-control in patients with severe, enduring anorexia nervosa. Int J Eat Disord. 2020;53(8):1326–36. https://doi.org/10.1002/eat.23267.
21. Steinglass J, Foerde K, Kostro K, Shohamy D, Walsh BT. Restrictive food intake as a choice--a paradigm for study. Int J Eat Disord. 2015;48(1):59–66. https://doi.org/10.1002/eat.22345.
22. Uniacke B, Slattery R, Walsh BT, Shohamy D, Foerde K, Steinglass JE. A comparison of food-based decision making between restricting and binge-eating/purging subtypes of anorexia nervosa. In J Eat Disord. 2020;53(10): 1751–6. https://doi.org/10.1002/eat23359.
23. Foerde K, Gianini L, Wang Y, Wu P, Shohamy D, Walsh BT, et al. Assessment of test-retest reliability of a food choice task among healthy individuals. Appetite. 2018;123:352–6. https://doi.org/10.1016/j.appet.2018.01.010.
24. Bartra O, McGuire JT, Kable JW. The valuation system: a coordinate-based meta-analysis of BOLD fMRI experiments examining neural correlates of subjective value. Neuroimage. 2013;76:412–27. https://doi.org/10.1016/j.neuroimage.2013.02.063.
25. American Psychiatric Association. Diagnostic and statistical manual of mental disorders. 5th ed. Arlington: American Psychiatric Association; 2013. https://doi.org/10.1176/appi.books.9780890425596.
26. Sysko R, Glasofer DR, Hildebrandt T, Klimek P, Mitchell JE, Berg KC, et al. The eating disorder assessment for DSM-5 (EDA-5): development and validation of a structured interview for feeding and eating disorders. Int J Eat Disord. 2015;48(5):452–63. https://doi.org/10.1002/eat.22388.
27. Brainard DH. The psychophysics toolbox. Spat Vis. 1997;10(4):433–6. https://doi.org/10.1163/156856897X00357.
28. JASP Team (2020). JASP (Version 0.14.1)[Computer software].
29. Bates D, Maechler M, Bolker B, Walker S. lme4: linear mixed-effects models using Eigen and S4. R package version. 2014;1(7):1–23.
30. Barr DJ, Levy R, Scheepers C, Tily HJ. Random effects structure for confirmatory hypothesis testing: Keep it maximal. J Mem Lang. 2013;68(3): 255–78. https://doi.org/10.1016/j.jml.2012.11.001.

31. Barr DJ. Random effects structure for testing interactions in linear mixed-effects models. Front Psychol. 2013;4:328. https://doi.org/10.3389/fpsyg.2013.00328.
32. Venables WN, Ripley BD. Modern applied statistics with S. Fourth ed. New York: Springer; 2002. https://doi.org/10.1007/978-0-387-21706-2.
33. Smith SM, Jenkinson M, Woolrich MW, Beckmann CF, Behrens TE, Johansen-Berg H, et al. Advances in functional and structural MR image analysis and implementation as FSL. Neuroimage. 2004;23(Suppl 1):S208–19. https://doi.org/10.1016/j.neuroimage.2004.07.051.
34. Jenkinson M, Bannister P, Brady M, Smith S. Improved optimization for the robust and accurate linear registration and motion correction of brain images. Neuroimage. 2002;17(2):825–41. https://doi.org/10.1006/nimg.2002.1132.
35. Smith SM. Fast robust automated brain extraction. Hum Brain Mapp. 2002; 17(3):143–55. https://doi.org/10.1002/hbm.10062.
36. Fischl B, Sereno MI, Tootell RB, Dale AM. High-resolution intersubject averaging and a coordinate system for the cortical surface. Hum Brain Mapp. 1999;8(4):272–84. https://doi.org/10.1002/(SICI)1097-0193(1999)8:4<272::AID-HBM10>3.0.CO;2-4.
37. Segonne F, Dale AM, Busa E, Glessner M, Salat D, Hahn HK, et al. A hybrid approach to the skull stripping problem in MRI. Neuroimage. 2004;22(3): 1060–75. https://doi.org/10.1016/j.neuroimage.2004.03.032.
38. Andersson JL, Jenkinson M, Smith S. Non-linear registration aka spatial normalisation FMRIB Technial report TR07JA2. Oxford: FMRIB Analysis Group of the University of Oxford; 2007.
39. Power JD, Barnes KA, Snyder AZ, Schlaggar BL, Petersen SE. Spurious but systematic correlations in functional connectivity MRI networks arise from subject motion. Neuroimage. 2012;59(3):2142–54. https://doi.org/10.1016/j.neuroimage.2011.10.018.
40. Siegel JS, Power JD, Dubis JW, Vogel AC, Church JA, Schlaggar BL, et al. Statistical improvements in functional magnetic resonance imaging analyses produced by censoring high-motion data points. Hum Brain Mapp. 2014;35(5):1981–96. https://doi.org/10.1002/hbm.22307.
41. Bodell LP, Keel PK, Brumm MC, Akubuiro A, Caballero J, Tranel D, et al. Longitudinal examination of decision-making performance in anorexia nervosa: before and after weight restoration. J Psychiatr Res. 2014;56:150–7. https://doi.org/10.1016/j.jpsychires.2014.05.015.
42. Eklund A, Nichols TE, Knutsson H. Cluster failure: why fMRI inferences for spatial extent have inflated false-positive rates. Proc Natl Acad Sci U S A. 2016;113(28):7900–5. https://doi.org/10.1073/pnas.1602413113.
43. Bakkour A, Palombo DJ, Zylberberg A, Kang YH, Reid A, Verfaellie M, Shadlen MN, Shohamy D. The hippocampus supports deliberation during value-based decisions. Elife. 2019;8:e46080. https://doi.org/10.7554/eLife.46080.
44. Beck AT, Steer RA. Depression inventory manual. San Antonio: Psychological Corporation, Harcourt, Brace; 1993.
45. Fairburn CG, Beglin SJ. Assessment of eating disorders: interview or self-report questionnaire? Int J Eat Disord. 1994;16(4):363–70.
46. Wechsler D. Wechsler Adult Intelligence Scale - III. San Antonio: The Psychological Corporation; 1997.
47. Spielberger CD, Gorsuch RL, Lushene R, Vagg PR, Jacobs AG. Manual for the state-trait anxiety inventory. Palo Alto: Consulting Psychologists Press, Inc.; 1983.
48. Stunkard AJ, Messick S. The three-factor eating questionnaire to measure dietary restraint, disinhibition and hunger. J Psychosom Res. 1985;29(1):71–83. https://doi.org/10.1016/0022-3999(85)90010-8.
49. Wechsler D. Wechsler abbreviated scale of intelligence manual. San Antonio: The Psychological Corporation; 1999.
50. Schebendach JE, Mayer LE, Devlin MJ, Attia E, Contento IR, Wolf RL, et al. Dietary energy density and diet variety as predictors of outcome in anorexia nervosa. Am J Clin Nutr. 2008;87(4):810–6. https://doi.org/10.1093/ajcn/87.4.810.
51. Liljeholm M, O'Doherty JP. Contributions of the striatum to learning, motivation, and performance: an associative account. Trends Cogn Sci. 2012;16(9):467–75. https://doi.org/10.1016/j.tics.2012.07.007.
52. Steinglass JE, Glasofer DR, Walsh E, Guzman G, Peterson CB, Walsh BT, et al. Targeting habits in anorexia nervosa: a proof-of-concept randomized trial. Psychol Med. 2018;48(15):2584–91. https://doi.org/10.1017/S003329171800020X.
53. Butler RM, Heimberg RG. Exposure therapy for eating disorders: a systematic review. Clin Psychol Rev. 2020;78:101851. https://doi.org/10.1016/j.cpr.2020.101851.
54. Platt ML, Glimcher PW. Neural correlates of decision variables in parietal cortex. Nature. 1999;400(6741):233–8. https://doi.org/10.1038/22268.
55. Pesaran B, Nelson MJ, Andersen RA. Free choice activates a decision circuit between frontal and parietal cortex. Nature. 2008;453(7193):406–9. https://doi.org/10.1038/nature06849.
56. Niendam TA, Laird AR, Ray KL, Dean YM, Glahn DC, Carter CS. Meta-analytic evidence for a superordinate cognitive control network subserving diverse executive functions. Cogn Affect Behav Neurosci. 2012;12(2):241–68. https://doi.org/10.3758/s13415-011-0083-5.
57. Derrfuss J, Brass M, Neumann J, von Cramon DY. Involvement of the inferior frontal junction in cognitive control: meta-analyses of switching and Stroop studies. Hum Brain Mapp. 2005;25(1):22–34. https://doi.org/10.1002/hbm.20127.
58. Rae CL, Hughes LE, Weaver C, Anderson MC, Rowe JB. Selection and stopping in voluntary action: a meta-analysis and combined fMRI study. Neuroimage. 2014;86:381–91. https://doi.org/10.1016/j.neuroimage.2013.10.012.
59. Cavanna AE, Trimble MR. The precuneus: a review of its functional anatomy and behavioural correlates. Brain. 2006;129(Pt 3):564–83. https://doi.org/10.1093/brain/awl004.
60. Jiang T, Soussignan R, Carrier E, Royet JP. Dysfunction of the mesolimbic circuit to food odors in women with anorexia and bulimia nervosa: a fMRI study. Front Hum Neurosci. 2019;13:117. https://doi.org/10.3389/fnhum.2019.00117.
61. Brooks SJ, O'Daly OG, Uher R, Friederich HC, Giampietro V, Brammer M, et al. Differential neural responses to food images in women with bulimia versus anorexia nervosa. Plos One. 2011;6(7):e22259. https://doi.org/10.1371/journal.pone.0022259.
62. Nikendei C, Friederich HC, Weisbrod M, Walther S, Sharma A, Herzog W, et al. Event-related potentials during recognition of semantic and pictorial food stimuli in patients with anorexia nervosa and healthy controls with varying internal states of hunger. Psychosom Med. 2012;74(2):136–45. https://doi.org/10.1097/PSY.0b013e318242496a.
63. Dockes J, Poldrack RA, Primet R, Gozukan H, Yarkoni T, Suchanek F, et al. NeuroQuery, comprehensive meta-analysis of human brain mapping. Elife. 2020;9. https://doi.org/10.7554/eLife.53385.
64. Alfano V, Mele G, Cotugno A, Longarzo M. Multimodal neuroimaging in anorexia nervosa. J Neurosci Res. 2020;98(11):2178–207. https://doi.org/10.1002/jnr.24674.
65. Steinglass J, Glasofer D, Dalack M, Attia E. Between wellness, relapse and remission: Stages of illness in anorexia nervosa. Int J Eat Disord. 2020; 53(7): 1088–96. https://doi.org/10.1002/eat.23237.
66. Nickel K, Joos A, Tebartz van Elst L, Matthis J, Holovics L, Endres D, et al. Recovery of cortical volume and thickness after remission from acute anorexia nervosa. Int J Eat Disord. 2018;51(9):1056–69. https://doi.org/10.1002/eat.22918.
67. von Schwanenflug N, Muller DK, King JA, Ritschel F, Bernardoni F, Mohammadi S, et al. Dynamic changes in white matter microstructure in anorexia nervosa: findings from a longitudinal study. Psychol Med. 2019; 49(9):1555–64. https://doi.org/10.1017/S003329171800212X.
68. Bernardoni F, King JA, Geisler D, Stein E, Jaite C, Natsch D, et al. Weight restoration therapy rapidly reverses cortical thinning in anorexia nervosa: a longitudinal study. Neuroimage. 2016;130:214–22. https://doi.org/10.1016/j.neuroimage.2016.02.003.
69. Martin Monzon B, Hay P, Foroughi N, Touyz S. White matter alterations in anorexia nervosa: a systematic review of diffusion tensor imaging studies. World J Psychiatry. 2016;6(1):177–86. https://doi.org/10.5498/wjp.v6.i1.177.
70. Cha J, Ide JS, Bowman FD, Simpson HB, Posner J, Steinglass JE. Abnormal reward circuitry in anorexia nervosa: a longitudinal, multimodal MRI study. Hum Brain Mapp. 2016;37(11):3835–46. https://doi.org/10.1002/hbm.23279.
71. DeGuzman M, Shott ME, Yang TT, Riederer J, Frank GKW. Association of elevated reward prediction error response with weight gain in adolescent anorexia nervosa. Am J Psychiatry. 2017;174(6):557–65. https://doi.org/10.1176/appi.ajp.2016.16060671.
72. Decker JH, Figner B, Steinglass JE. On weight and waiting: delay discounting in anorexia nervosa pretreatment and posttreatment. Biol Psychiatry. 2015; 78(9):606–14. https://doi.org/10.1016/j.biopsych.2014.12.016.
73. Doose A, King JA, Bernardoni F, Geisler D, Hellerhoff I, Weinert T, et al. Strengthened Default Mode Network Activation During Delay Discounting in Adolescents with Anorexia Nervosa After Partial Weight Restoration: A Longitudinal fMRI Study. J Clin Med. 2020;9(4). https://doi.org/10.3390/jcm9040900. Epub date 2020/03/29.

17

Predictors of illness course and health maintenance following inpatient treatment among patients with anorexia nervosa

Deborah R. Glasofer[1*†], Alexandra F. Muratore[1†], Evelyn Attia[1,2], Peng Wu[3], Yuanjia Wang[3], Hillary Minkoff[1], Teresa Rufin[4], B. Timothy Walsh[1] and Joanna E. Steinglass[1]

Abstract

Background: Anorexia nervosa (AN) is a life-threatening psychiatric disorder associated with significant medical and psychosocial impairment. Hospital-based behavioral treatment is an effective intervention in the short-term. However, relapse rates following discharge are high and thus, there is a need to identify predictors of longitudinal outcome. The current study provides information regarding illness course and health maintenance among patients with AN over 5 years following discharge from an eating disorder inpatient unit.

Methods: Participants were individuals with AN who were discharged from a specialized, inpatient behaviorally-based unit. Prior to discharge, height and weight were measured and participants completed self-report measures of eating disorder severity and general psychopathology (depression, anxiety, harm avoidance). Participants were contacted annually for self-report measures of weight, eating disorder severity and clinical impairment. Outcome was defined by illness course (body mass index (BMI) and clinical impairment during the 5 years) and health maintenance (categories of weight and eating disorder symptom severity) across follow-up, using all available data. Linear mixed models were used to examine whether demographic and clinical parameters at discharge predicted BMI and clinical impairment over time. Additional analyses examined whether these variables significantly influenced an individual's likelihood of maintaining inpatient treatment gains.

Results: One-hundred and sixty-eight individuals contributed data. Higher trait anxiety at discharge was associated with a lower BMI during follow-up ($p = 0.012$). There was a significant interaction between duration of illness and time, whereby duration of illness was associated with a faster rate of weight loss ($p = 0.003$) during follow-up. As duration of illness increased, there was a greater increase in self-reported clinical impairment ($p = 0.011$). Increased eating disorder severity at discharge was also associated with greater clinical impairment at follow-up ($p = 0.004$). Higher BMI at discharge was significantly associated with maintaining healthy weight across a priori BMI-based definitions of health maintenance.

(Continued on next page)

* Correspondence: deborah.glasofer@nyspi.columbia.edu
†Deborah R. Glasofer and Alexandra F. Muratore contributed equally to this work.
[1]Department of Psychiatry, Columbia University Irving Medical Center, New York State Psychiatric Institute, 1051 Riverside Drive, Unit 98, New York City, NY 10032, USA
Full list of author information is available at the end of the article

(Continued from previous page)
Conclusions: Weight status (higher BMI) and duration of illness are key factors in the prognosis of AN. Higher weight targets in intensive treatments may be of value in improving outcomes.

Keywords: Anorexia nervosa, Longitudinal study, Inpatients, Outcome, Body mass index, Duration of illness, Time course, Prognosis

Plain English summary

Anorexia nervosa (AN) is a life-threatening psychiatric disorder. Hospital-based behavioral treatment is an effective intervention in the short-term, but relapse rates following discharge are high. Here, we provide information on clinical features at the time of leaving the hospital that are related to illness course and health maintenance over the following five years. Prior to discharge, height and weight were measured and patients completed questionnaires about their eating disorder and associated symptoms. Participants were then contacted annually to answer questions about their eating disorder and health. One-hundred and sixty-eight individuals participated in at least one annual assessment. Longer duration of illness predicted faster weight loss after discharge, and was related to greater self-reported day-to-day impairment over time. Higher weight at discharge was associated with maintaining healthy weight over the follow-up period. High anxiety at discharge was associated with lower BMI over the 5-years of follow-up, while increased eating disorder severity was associated with greater day-to-day impairment. Results of this longitudinal study highlight that weight status at discharge and duration of illness are key factors in the course of AN. While duration of illness is not modifiable at the time of presentation for care, discharge weight is. Higher weight targets in intensive treatments may be of value in improving long-term outcomes.

Background

Anorexia nervosa (AN) is a serious psychiatric disorder associated with medical complications [1], impairments in psychosocial functioning [2, 3], and significant morbidity and mortality [4–7]. Behavioral treatment in intensive settings is effective in restoring weight and improving eating behavior and psychological functioning in the short-term [8, 9]. Recovery rates in AN differ depending on how recovery is defined, and range widely [10]. The rates of relapse following inpatient care are consistently high, with estimates ranging between 35 and 57% [10–13]. As AN is a not a common illness and long-term studies are few, more data are needed to fully understand the clinical factors that determine course of illness and promote health maintenance over time.

Several longitudinal studies have examined the course of illness in AN using different methodology and clinical parameters. Most [13–19], but not all [20], have identified longer duration of illness as a predictor of worse long-term outcome. Body mass index (BMI) is also related to outcome: most studies show associations between lower admission and discharge BMI and worse outcomes in adults [11, 14, 16, 17, 21–25], though research in adolescents suggests discharge BMI is less predictive of outcome when inpatient treatment is followed by structured outpatient treatment [26, 27]. AN subtype has also been associated with outcome, though this has not been a consistent finding [18, 28]. Compared to those with restricting subtype, some research suggests that patients with the binge-purge subtype appear more likely to drop out of treatment prematurely and may be at higher risk for relapse [12, 19, 29–32].

The impact of psychological factors such as depression, anxiety, harm avoidance, eating disorder psychopathology, and motivation for recovery have been mixed [12, 13, 33–38]. Though multiple longitudinal studies have examined the course of AN, the majority of studies focus on predictors and correlates of outcomes such as diagnostic status, mortality, and rates of relapse [5, 7, 10–12, 15, 16, 31, 33–36, 39–41]. Prior studies on inpatient samples specifically have tended toward examining predictors of outcome unrelated to treatment (e.g., age of onset, comorbidities, family support) and report overall prognosis categorically [42–47]. Fewer have studied continuous outcomes, such as weight, symptoms, and overall clinical impairment over time [13, 23, 38, 48, 49], and these have generally been limited to short-term follow up [13, 19, 49] or to a single assessment point [23, 25, 34]. Together, these studies suggest that higher BMI at discharge and shorter duration of illness are important factors in the course of AN. Evaluation of trajectory of change and other clinical measures across multiple time points is needed to better understand variables that predict both the course of illness and prognosis following behaviorally-based inpatient treatment.

The present study examined the association between clinical features at the time of hospital discharge and longer-term outcome among adolescents and adults with AN, the majority of whom had achieved weight restoration to a BMI within the normal range (18.5–24.9 kg/m^2). A longitudinal design, which allows for the examination of within-subject weight changes over multiple follow-up periods, was used to examine illness course over 5 years, and maintenance of health. We hypothesized that duration of illness and lower BMI at the time of hospital discharge would predict poorer longer-term outcome, and explored whether other clinical and psychological features impact outcome.

Methods

All patients with AN discharged from inpatient treatment at the New York State Psychiatric Institute (NYSP I) Eating Disorders Research Unit (EDRU) are offered enrollment in this ongoing 10-year longitudinal study. Participants are contacted annually following hospital discharge. The current study is an examination of data collected over the first 5 years following discharge, using all available data from patients enrolled beginning in 2009. This study was reviewed and approved by the NYSPI Institutional Review Board. All participants provided written informed consent (individuals under age 18 provided assent and a parent or guardian provided consent).

Participants

Participants were patients with AN who had been discharged from the EDRU between September 2009 and June 2018 and provided follow-up information on at least one occasion over the subsequent 5 years. Of the 196 patients discharged during this timeframe, 194 (99%) consented to participate. Diagnosis was established at hospital admission using the *Eating Disorder Assessment for DSM-5* (EDA-5) [50] or *Structured Clinical Interview for DSM-IV Axis I Disorders* (SCID-IV) [51], which also assessed co-occurring psychiatric illness.

Procedures

Treatment at the EDRU is behaviorally-based and aims for full weight restoration [52], corresponding to a BMI of ~ 20.0 kg/m^2 [9]. Prior to discharge, height and weight were measured and participants completed self-report measures of eating disorder severity (Eating Disorder Examination-Questionnaire – EDE-Q) [53], clinical impairment related to eating disorder symptoms (Clinical Impairment Assessment – CIA) [54], mood (Beck Depression Inventory – BDI) [55] and anxiety symptoms (Beck Anxiety Inventory – BAI) [56] and anxious traits (Spielberger State Trait Anxiety Inventory-Trait version – STAI-T) [57] and temperament (Temperament and Character Inventory – Harm Avoidance subscale – TCI-HA)) [58].

Procedures included annual phone interviews with participants and administration of self-report questionnaires. Weight was obtained by self-report during each annual assessment, in the context of an interview on psychosocial functioning, weight history (since last contact), current eating behavior, and medical status. In addition, patients were asked to provide permission for contact with a clinician to verify the reported weight. Clinician-reported weights were used when available; otherwise, self-reported weights were used. Self-report measures of eating disorder severity (EDE-Q) and eating disorder related psychosocial impairment (CIA) were sent for participant completion. Participants were paid $10 after completion of study questionnaires.

Data analysis

Data from a follow-up assessment were excluded if the individual had been receiving more than one week of structured treatment for AN (e.g., inpatient treatment, residential treatment; $n = 10$), or met criteria for bulimia nervosa or binge-eating disorder ($n = 8$) at the time of the assessment (as by BMI alone these individuals might otherwise have been considered healthy). Independent samples t-tests and Pearson chi-square tests were used to compare participants and non-contributors on demographic and clinical characteristics. Self-reported weights and clinician weights were compared using Pearson correlations. Independent samples t-tests compared demographic and clinical characteristics between individuals for whom both self-reported and clinician-reported weights were available and individuals for whom there was only one weight.

Illness course

Primary analyses examined BMI and CIA score (outcomes) at each year of follow-up with a linear mixed effects model fitting all available data. Age, time (year of follow-up), subtype, sex, duration of illness, BAI, BDI, STAI-T, EDE-Q (Global score), and TCI-HA were included as covariates in both models. Interaction between duration of illness and time was included to assess whether duration of illness predicted rate of change in BMI or CIA over 5 years. The number of annual assessments completed by each individual was included in both models to adjust for different number of observations available for each individual. Additionally, CIA at discharge was included as a predictor of BMI, and BMI at discharge was included as a predictor of CIA. Discharge BMI and discharge CIA were included as baseline (Year 0) outcomes and were therefore not included as predictors of BMI or CIA in their respective models. Of the total sample, 101 and 104 individuals had complete predictor data at discharge for inclusion in BMI and CIA analyses, respectively.

Health maintenance

To specifically assess factors associated with maintaining health after hospitalization, we tested the ability of the same variables to predict health maintenance ("good outcome") using a logistic regression model (TCI-HA was not included in this analysis due to small sample sizes in each category and missing data.). Health maintenance was defined in 3 ways: (1) maintenance of a BMI ≥ 18.5 kg/m^2 at all available time points, (2) maintenance of a BMI ≥ 19.5 kg/m^2 at all available time points, (3) maintenance of a BMI ≥ 18.5 kg/m^2 and an EDE-Q score of ≤ 2 at all available time points (maintenance of a BMI ≥ 19.5 kg/m^2 and an EDE-Q score of ≤ 2 at all available time points was not included due to insufficient data). BMI cutoffs were selected based on suggested diagnostic thresholds [59] and suggested recovery thresholds per previous reports [60, 61]. EDE-Q score cutoffs were selected to be within 1 SD of Global EDE-Q norms for young adult women [62], and consistent with existing conceptualizations of eating disorder health maintenance [60, 61]. Logistic regression models were fitted to the data to test whether there was a relationship between a patient's score on each variable and the likelihood of meeting criteria for each of the three health maintenance groups at follow up. Of the patients meeting criteria for health maintenance, three had been discharged from the hospital before reaching a BMI of 18.5 kg/m^2; as such, these individuals had *gained* weight, not *maintained* weight. Sensitivity analyses were conducted without these three participants.

SAS software, version 9.4, and SPSS, version 26.0, were used for all statistical analyses and modeling. Alpha level was set to 0.05.

Table 1 Demographic and Clinical Characteristics

	Participants $N = 168$	
Demographic Variables	**Mean**	**Range**
Age (years)	26.02 ± 8.20	14–64
Sex, female, *n* (%)	164 (98%)	n/a
Race, Caucasian, *n* (%)	148 (88%)	n/a
AN subtype, binge-purge, *n* (%)	82 (49%)	n/a
Duration of hospitalization (days)	78.82 ± 43.22	0–462
Duration of illness (years)	9.36 ± 7.70	0.25–50
Admission BMI (kg/m^2)	16.00 ± 1.86	10.7–20.8
Discharge BMI (kg/m^2)	20.02 ± 1.46	14.6–23.4
Psychological Measures – Discharge	**Mean ± SD**	**Range**
BAI (*n* = 135)	18.45 ± 11.45	0.00–61.00
BDI (*n* = 132)	17.89 ± 11.84	0.00–51.00
STAI-T (*n* = 131)	56.89 ± 12.18	25.00–80.00
CIA (*n* = 118)	23.53 ± 11.51	3.00–48.00
EDE-Q Global (*n* = 122)	2.67 ± 1.26	0.19–5.05
TCI-HA (*n* = 117)	21.60 ± 7.07	4.00–34.00

BMI body mass index. *BAI* Beck Anxiety Inventory, *BDI* Beck Depression Inventory, *STAI-T* Spielberger State Trait Anxiety Inventory-Trait version, *EDE-Q* Eating Disorder Examination – Questionnaire. *TCI-HA* Temperament and Character Inventory, Harm Avoidance Subscale

Results

Demographics, clinical characteristics and response rate

One-hundred ninety-four patients with AN (176 adults, 18 adolescents) were enrolled in the study, of whom 24 (12.4%) did not participate in any post-hospitalization assessments. Of the remaining 168, 42 individuals reported information at one time point, 31 individuals reported information at two time points, 35 individuals reported information at three time points, 26 individuals provided information at four time points, and 34 individuals provided information at five time points. Data from these 168 individuals were used in analyses (Table 1). Of these individuals, twenty participants (11.9%) were discharged at a BMI < 18.5 kg/m^2. Co-occurring diagnoses included current or past anxiety disorders ($n = 62$, 37%), major depressive disorder ($n = 80$, 48%), obsessive-compulsive disorder ($n = 17$, 10%), post-traumatic stress disorder (n = 17, 10%), and substance use disorders ($n = 22$, 13%) (Complete comorbidity data were missing for 11 participants).

The group that did not provide any follow up data (i.e., non-contributors) did not differ significantly in age, sex, race, admission BMI, or duration of illness (see Supplemental Table 1). Compared with participants, the non-contributors had a significantly lower BMI at discharge and a greater proportion of individuals with AN binge-purge subtype. Among the 168 participants, 56.5–67.3% provided BMI data each year (see Table 2). Of 457 total weights provided, 147 included both self-reported and clinician-verified weights. When weights from both sources were available, self-reported weights were highly correlated with clinician-provided weights ($r - .970$, $p - .000$). Participants who had weights from both sources and those who had weights from one source did not differ in age, weight, duration of illness, duration of hospitalization, admission BMI or discharge BMI (*ts* ≤± 1.82, *ps* = ≥ .069).

Primary analyses: longitudinal illness course

Of the 168 participants, 101 and 104 individuals had complete predictor data for BMI and CIA analyses, respectively. Table 3 reports results of linear mixed effects model analyses with BMI and CIA as outcomes. There was a significant interaction between time and duration of illness, such that as Duration of Illness increased, there was a greater decrease in BMI over time – meaning, a steeper slope of weight loss following discharge ($F(1,284) = 13.34$, $p = .0003$). Higher STAI-T score at discharge was associated with lower BMI during the follow-up timeframe ($F(1,284) = 6.36$, $p = .012$). Higher TCI-HA score at discharge was associated with higher BMI across time-points, $F(1,284) = 3.97$, $p = .047$. No other variables were associated with BMI. In the model predicting CIA, there was a significant interaction between time and duration of illness, such that as Duration of Illness

Table 2 Number of Individuals Providing Data at each Annual Assessment

	Year 1	Year 2	Year 3	Year 4	Year 5
Total Number Participants Eligible to Provide Information at Time Point	168	160	147	129	112
Number Participants Who Provided BMI (*n*, %)	113 (67%)	101 (63%)	98 (67%)	73 (57%)	71 (63%)
Number Participants Who Provided CIA (*n*, %)	88 (52%)	75 (47%)	74 (50%)	62 (48%)	55 (49%)
Number Participants Who Provided EDE-Q Global (*n*, %)	89 (53%)	81 (51%)	78 (53%)	73 (57%)	58 (52%)

Table listing the proportion of individuals who provided data at each of the five follow-up time points (Year 1-Year 5). Row 2 lists the total number of individuals who had reached the time point for data collection, and were therefore eligible. Rows 2–4 show the proportion of participants at each time-point who provided information with regard to body mass index (BMI), Clinical Impairment Assessment (CIA), and Eating Disorder Examination – Questionnaire (EDE-Q), respectively. Proportion of individuals who provided information are listed as numbers (n) and percent of total who were eligible (%)

increased, there was a greater increase in CIA scores (i.e., greater self-reported impairment) over time, $F(1, 232) = 6.65$, $p = .011$. Time was associated with CIA, such that across follow-up there was an overall decrease in CIA scores, $F(1,232) = 17.13$, $p < .0001$. The EDE-Q Global score was associated with CIA across time-points, with higher EDE-Q scores at discharge predicting increased CIA scores during follow-up ($F(1,232) = 8.38$, $p = .004$).

Health maintenance

Of the 168 participants, 77 individuals (45.8%) maintained a BMI ≥ 18.5 kg/m^2 at all available time points post-hospitalization, 54 maintained (32.1%) a BMI ≥ 19.5 kg/m^2, and 29 (17.3%) maintained a BMI ≥ 18.5 kg/m^2 and EDE-Q scores ≤ 2. After restricting participants to those with complete data at discharge (for model analyses), the sample included 53 (46.1%) with BMI ≥ 18.5 kg/m^2, 37 (34.8%) with BMI ≥ 19.5 kg/m^2, and 20 (13.2%) with BMI ≥ 18.5 kg/m^2 and EDE-Q scores ≤ 2. Table 4 provides Odds Ratio (OR) and 95% Confidence Intervals for the relationship between predictor variables and likelihood of meeting criteria for each of the three categorical outcomes.

Higher BMI at discharge significantly increased the likelihood of meeting criteria for two of the "good outcome" categories (Table 4). Specifically, a one unit increase in BMI at discharge led to a 2.21-fold increase in the odds of maintaining a BMI ≥ 18.5 kg/m^2 and a 3.18-fold increase in the odds of maintaining of a BMI ≥ 19.5 kg/m^2. Higher admission BMI also increased the likelihood of weight maintenance at follow-up, though the effect was less pronounced.

The number of annual follow-up assessments patients completed led to a 0.43-fold decrease in the odds of a participant maintaining a BMI of ≥ 19.5 kg/m^2, but did not contribute significantly to meeting criteria for the other categories. A sensitivity analysis was conducted including only participants who completed ≤ 4 annual assessments, and the pattern of results did not change (0.49-fold decrease in the odds of maintaining a BMI of ≥ 19.5 kg/m^2).

Table 3 Fixed Effects from Linear Mixed Model of Longitudinal Outcome

Variables	BMI ($n = 101$)				CIA ($n = 104$)			
	F	*ß*	*SE ß*	*p*	*F*	*ß*	*SE ß*	*p*
Intercept	–	21.959	1.326	<.0001	–	15.749	18.216	0.389
Time	3.55	0.178	0.094	0.060	17.13	−2.179	0.527	**< 0.0001**
AN subtype, binge-purge	2.31	0.565	0.372	0.129	0.01	0.209	1.756	0.905
Sex, female	0.02	0.132	0.922	0.887	0.01	0.328	4.424	0.941
Duration of Illness (years)	1.48	−0.038	0.032	0.225	0.78	0.136	0.154	0.378
CIA at Discharge	0.28	0.015	0.029	0.598	–	–	–	–
Discharge BMI (kg/m^2)	–	–	–	–	1.15	−0.851	0.793	0.284
BAI	2.59	0.034	0.021	0.109	1.56	0.124	0.099	0.213
BDI	0.33	−0.013	0.024	0.566	0.23	0.049	0.103	0.635
EDE-Q Global	0.15	−0.099	0.258	0.701	8.38	2.934	1.013	**0.004**
TCI-HA	3.97	0.061	0.030	**0.047**	0.01	−0.013	0.141	0.929
STAI-T	6.36	−0.071	0.028	**0.012**	2.68	0.213	0.129	0.103
Time x Duration of Illness	13.34	−0.033	0.009	**0.0003**	6.65	0.131	0.051	**0.011**

BAI Beck Anxiety Inventory, *BDI* Beck Depression Inventory, *BMI* body mass index, *CIA* Clinical Impairment Assessment, *EDE-Q* Eating Disorder Examination - Questionnaire, *STAI-T* Spielberger State Trait Anxiety Inventory-Trait version, *TCI-HA* Temperament and Character Inventory, Harm Avoidance Subscale. Bold values = $p < 0.05$

Table 4 Odds Ratios and Confidence Intervals for the Relationship between Predictors and Clinical Outcomes

	Outcome Category 1 BMI ≥ 18.5 (*n* = 53)			Outcome Category 2 BMI ≥ 19.5 (*n* = 37)			Outcome Category 3 BMI ≥ 18.5 and EDE-Q ≤ 2 (*n* = 20)		
	Odds Ratio	95% CI	*p*	Odds Ratio	95% CI	*p*	Odds Ratio	95% CI	*p*
Duration of Illness (years)	0.973	0.903–1.048	0.471	0.916	0.837–1.002	0.055	0.877	0.772–.996	**0.043**
BAI	1.026	0.973–1.082	0.345	1.041	0.976–1.111	0.225	1.005	0.922–1.095	0.914
BDI	0.956	0.900–1.015	0.139	0.927	0.854–1.005	0.066	0.953	0.854–1.063	0.385
STAI-T	1.009	0.950–1.072	0.769	1.019	0.953–1.090	0.586	1.043	0.950–1.144	0.377
EDE-Q Global	0.870	0.508–1.488	0.611	0.563	0.296–1.070	0.079	0.289	0.106–.788	**0.015**
AN subtype, binge-purge	1.148	0.425–3.100	0.785	0.857	0.268–2.736	0.794	0.319	0.074–1.380	0.126
Admission BMI (kg/m^2)	1.680	1.215–2.323	**0.002**	1.294	0.911–1.838	0.149	1.256	0.812–1.943	0.307
Discharge BMI	2.211	1.189–4.112	**0.012**	3.180	1.589–6.365	**0.001**	1.923	.925–3.996	0.079
Number of Annual Assessments Completed	0.740	0.514–1.065	0.105	0.426	0.255–.711	**0.001**	0.715	0.411–1.246	0.237

BAI Beck Anxiety Inventory, *BDI* Beck Depression Inventory, *BMI* body mass index, *EDE-Q* Eating Disorder Examination – Questionnaire, *STAI-T* Spielberger State Trait Anxiety Inventory-Trait version. Bold values = $p < 0.05$. Reported ns refer to number of individuals who met criteria for each outcome category

Longer duration of illness significantly decreased the likelihood of maintaining BMI of ≥ 18.5 kg/m^2 and an EDE-Q Global Score of ≤ 2 across all time points. Specifically, for every year increase in duration of illness, there was a 0.88-fold decrease in the odds of a participant maintaining weight within a normal range and reduced eating disorder symptoms. Higher EDE-Q score at discharge significantly decreased the likelihood of meeting criteria for this category, such that a one-point increase in EDE-Q Global score led to a 0.29-fold decrease in the odds of a participant maintaining a BMI ≥ 18.5 kg/m^2 and an EDE-Q score ≤ 2.

There were no differences in results of health maintenance analyses conducted with and without the three patients who did not achieve a BMI of 18.5 kg/m^2 prior to discharge.

Discussion

In this study, data collected post-hospitalization for 5 years from 168 patients with AN were examined to identify clinical factors that impact the course of illness. Two main factors emerged, one modifiable and one non-modifiable: BMI at discharge and duration of illness, respectively. More specifically, longer duration of illness was associated with more rapid weight loss after discharge and greater increase in reported clinical impairment, and higher BMI at discharge was associated with maintaining healthy weight. In addition, trait anxiety at discharge was associated with lower BMI across the 5 years of follow-up and surprisingly, harm avoidance at discharge was associated with higher BMI across the follow-up period. EDE-Q at discharge was associated with greater clinical impairment across the 5 years of follow-up.

The literature is reasonably consistent in finding that the BMI reached in treatment affects prognosis [13, 14, 21, 25, 63]. Although research with adolescents suggests lower discharge weight does not negatively influence outcomes [26, 27], individuals in these studies were discharged directly to a structured outpatient treatment, which likely influenced outcomes. This finding may also be specific to adolescents rather than adults, who comprise the majority of the current sample. As BMI is one of few potentially modifiable factors, the finding in the current study is important for treatment settings to consider. The majority of patients in this study (89.7%) were discharged from the hospital after full weight restoration. Excluding the twenty patients who left prior to achieving a BMI of ≥18.5 kg/m^2, the range of BMI at discharge was 19.0 to 23.4 kg/m^2, and in the health maintenance analyses, even including only patients in this normal range, a higher BMI at discharge predicted maintenance of a good outcome by two of the three definitions used. This is consistent with a prior study of weight-restored patients with AN (BMI = 19.2–22.0 kg/m^2, mean = 20.3 kg/m^2), which found that a higher BMI at the time of entry into relapse prevention treatment was associated with successful weight maintenance [13]. In an analysis of archival data of adults with AN participating in several outpatient treatment trials, weight restoration to above 85.8% of ideal body weight by the end of treatment was the best predictor of recovery (defined as a BMI > 19 kg/m^2, eating disorder severity scores within 1 standard deviation of community norms, and the absence of binge-purge behaviors) at one year follow-up [64]. Prior results and current findings highlight the value of adequate weight restoration in promoting health among patients with AN.

In this study, adequate weight restoration was possible within the scope of our behaviorally-based inpatient program for research participants [52], where length of stay was not determined by insurance coverage or financial status. The significance of length of stay and its relationship with other predictors included in the current analyses may be substantially different when subject to the constraints of financial coverage. Given that the majority of treatment settings are subject to these constraints, and that length of stay has been shown to be impacted by service setting [65], our findings may be limited in generalizability. However, the potent impact of discharge BMI on outcome in our sample emphasizes the importance of identifying factors that predict which individuals will remain in care to complete weight restoration. The interventions most helpful in facilitating this treatment engagement will be as to improving long-term outcome.

This study replicates and extends existing literature suggesting that longer duration of illness is associated with worse outcome in AN [13–19]. Our findings highlight the relationship between a longer duration of illness and an increase in impairment related to the eating disorder over time, as well as an association with rate of weight loss after hospital discharge. The significant impact of duration of illness on prognosis presents a clinical conundrum: intensive treatment seems indicated, yet it is burdensome to provide if relapse rates are high. As duration of illness is not modifiable at the time of presentation for care, this factor may be more relevant for consideration of treatment algorithms, including decision-making about sequencing levels of care or other interventions. Some studies have identified the period following hospitalization as an especially high-risk period [13], and it may be that for individuals with a longer illness it will be particularly valuable to focus resources on this phase. The efficacy of "step down" care in preventing relapse may merit further research. The more favorable prognosis associated with shorter duration of illness [14, 18, 20, 34, 35, 39, 41, 66] suggests that early intervention may be important, as well.

The role of psychological variables in the course of AN is less consistent across studies [12, 13, 33–38]. In the current study, greater trait anxiety as measured by STAI, but not anxiety at discharge as measured by BAI, predicted lower mean BMI during the following 5 years. The measure of clinical impairment used in this study, CIA, specifically addresses eating-disorder related psychosocial impairment, and therefore not surprisingly was related to EDE-Q scores at discharge (both measures assess the frequency and interference of eating habits, exercise, and overvaluation of shape and weight [53, 54]). Yet, EDE-Q scores were not related to health maintenance. Psychological symptom severity may be less reliable in determining long term prognosis. The anxiety finding in this study is of some interest because there are data to suggest that anxiety precedes illness onset [67, 68], is related to illness severity [34, 69], and may be a useful treatment target in its own right [70, 71]. On the other hand, harm avoidance is also a measure of anxiety, and this was associated with higher BMI during follow-up. This discrepancy underscores that psychological measures may be less reliable prognostic markers. Contrary to previous research [12, 19, 29–32], we found no effect of AN subtype on illness course or outcome. However, the non-contributors had a significantly greater proportion of patients with binge-purge subtype, suggesting individuals with this subtype were less likely to provide follow-up data. It is therefore impossible to assess whether this discrepancy may be indicative of a systematic difference (i.e., differential outcome or rates of relapse) between subtypes not captured in the participating sample.

One challenge for the current study was setting the a priori definition of "good outcome." A BMI of 18.5 kg/m^2 is the suggested lower threshold of normal BMI in the general population, and is commonly used as a guide for "underweight" status in meeting criteria for AN [59]. There is some consensus within the eating disorders field that achieving BMI ≥ 18.5 kg/m^2 is a required component of remission [72], and several studies support that this threshold is associated with sustained recovery [25, 73, 74]. In our sample, the rate of maintenance at or above a BMI of 18.5 kg/m^2 for the duration of follow-up, from one to five years, was 46.1%, similar to or slightly higher than rates reported in previous studies [12, 24, 41]. Notably, only 17.4% of individuals maintained a BMI ≥ 18.5 kg/m^2 and an EDE-Q score of ≤ 2. Clinically, patients with AN are commonly encouraged to consider a higher weight range in order to better mitigate other symptoms, and our data support this approach in that higher BMI reduced the risk of relapse. In the current study, the number of individuals who achieved a higher BMI in combination with lower EDE-Q scores was low, and so this study may not have been sufficiently powered to fully examine factors associated with this definition of health [60].

This study has several strengths. The vast majority of patients with AN admitted to the inpatient program agreed to participate and between one-half to two-thirds of those eligible responded to each annual follow-up. These annual assessments provide a rich longitudinal dataset of anthropometric and clinical measures during and in the years following inpatient weight restoration treatment for AN. The two statistical approaches are complementary in examining factors associated with illness course and with health maintenance.

The primary limitation of this study was the extent of missing data. Non-contributors in our sample were disproportionately individuals with binge-purge subtype who did not fully restore weight in the program, which could have introduced bias into the data. As the majority of individuals included in analyses had restricting subtype, it is possible our analyses do not fully capture the influence of binge-purge subtype on weight and clinical outcomes. Subtype was the sole characteristic that distinguished non-contributors from contributors. This is consistent with previous literature suggesting patients with binge-purge subtype may be more likely to drop out of treatment [29, 30] and may provide additional evidence suggesting a distinction between the two subtypes and their respective treatment outcomes. The assessments used in this study may have missed some potentially important variables with regard to long-term health, such as dietary intake patterns [75, 76], and it may be useful to obtain other measures of wellness, such as life satisfaction or health care utilization, to more broadly capture outcome. Though this study utilized clinician-reported weights where available, the majority of weights used in analyses were self-reported; this limitation is mitigated by the high correlation between clinician-reported and self-reported weights. Another notable limitation of this study is the finding that the number of annual assessments completed was associated with decreased likelihood of maintaining a weight of 19.5 kg/m^2, suggesting some of our a priori definitions of "good outcomes" may be confounded by number of assessments completed. Future studies may wish to define "outcome" differently or using a fixed number of assessments to control for this bias. Finally, the primary aim of the current study was to examine how clinical status at discharge predicts illness course over time. As such, the present analyses did not examine how *changes* to these predictors over time influence outcome. Future research utilizing longitudinal datasets may wish to examine how changes to these predictors impact illness course.

Conclusions

Longitudinal research conducted over an extended time period is critical to better understand illness course and prognosis in AN. Our findings reinforce the value of weight gain well within the normal range as a goal of treatment, and the importance of considering the role of duration of illness in overall prognosis and treatment planning.

Abbreviations

AN: Anorexia nervosa; BMI: Body mass index; NYSPI: New York State Psychiatric Institute; EDRU: Eating Disorders Research Unit; EDA-5: Eating Disorder Assessment for DSM-5; SCID-IV: Structured Clinical Interview for DSM-IV Axis I Disorders; EDE-Q: Eating Disorder Examination – Questionnaire; BDI: Beck Depression Inventory; BAI: Beck Anxiety Inventory; STAI-T: Spielberger State Trait Anxiety Inventory, Trait version; TCI-HA: Temperament and Character Inventory – Harm Avoidance Subscale; CIA: Clinical Impairment Assessment; OR: Odds Ratio

Acknowledgements

We would like to express gratitude for the repeated contributions of our longitudinal study participants, and acknowledge the ongoing efforts our research assistants for their help with data collection and entry.

Authors' contributions

DRG was involved in oversight of data collection, as well as drafting and revising the manuscript. AFM contributed to manuscript drafts and revisions, completed descriptive analyses, and assisted with interpretation of data. EA was involved in study design and serves as principal investigator for the 10-year longitudinal research study from which these data are compiled. PW completed data inspection and primary and secondary analyses (linear mixed effects and logistic regression models) and edited related sections of the manuscript. YW developed and oversaw the data analysis plan and edited related sections of the manuscript. HM and TR were involved in data collection, entry, and preparation for analysis. JES was involved in study design, oversight of data collection, interpretation of data, and drafting and revising the manuscript. BTW made substantial contributions to the data analysis plan, interpretation of data, and manuscript revisions. All authors read and approved the final manuscript.

Competing interests

DRG has received honoraria from Oxford University Press. EA and JES receive royalties from UpToDate. BTW has received royalties and honoraria from Guilford Press, McGraw-Hill, Oxford University Press, UpToDate, British Medical Journal, Johns Hopkins Press and Guidepoint Global.

Author details

[1]Department of Psychiatry, Columbia University Irving Medical Center, New York State Psychiatric Institute, 1051 Riverside Drive, Unit 98, New York City, NY 10032, USA. [2]Center for Eating Disorders, Weill Cornell Medical College, 21 Bloomingdale Road, White Plains, NY 10605, USA. [3]Department of Biostatistics, Mailman School of Public Health, 722 West 168th Street, New York, NY 10032, USA. [4]Harvard T.H. Chan School of Public Health, 677 Huntington Avenue, Boston, MA 02115, USA.

References

1. Mehler PS, Brown C. Anorexia nervosa - medical complications. J Eat Disord. 2015;3:11.
2. Mond JM, Owen C, Hay PJ, Rodgers B, Beumont PJV. Assessing quality of life in eating disorder patients. Qual Life Res. 2005;14(1):171–8.
3. Bohn K, Doll HA, Cooper Z, O'Connor M, Palmer RL, Fairburn CG. The measurement of impairment due to eating disorder psychopathology. Behav Res Ther. 2008;46(10):1105–10.
4. Arcelus J, Mitchell AJ, Wales J, Nielsen S. Mortality rates in patients with anorexia nervosa and other eating disorders. A meta-analysis of 36 studies. Arch Gen Psychiatry. 2011;68(7):724–31.
5. Fichter MM, Quadflieg N. Mortality in eating disorders - results of a large prospective clinical longitudinal study. Int J Eating Disord. 2016;49(4):391–401.
6. Smink FR, van Hoeken D, Hoek HW. Epidemiology, course, and outcome of eating disorders. Curr Opin Psychiatr. 2013;26(6):543–8.
7. Franko DL, Keshaviah A, Eddy KT, Krishna M, Davis MC, Keel PK, et al. A longitudinal investigation of mortality in anorexia nervosa and bulimia nervosa. Am J Psychiatry. 2013;170(8):917–25.
8. Olmsted M, McFarlane T, Carter J, Trottier K, Woodside D, Dimitropoulos G. The Treatment of Eating Disorders: A Clinical Handbook. 2010.
9. Attia E, Walsh BT. Behavioral Management for Anorexia Nervosa. N Engl J Med. 2009;360(5):500–6.
10. Khalsa SS, Portnoff LC, McCurdy-McKinnon D, Feusner JD. What happens after treatment? A systematic review of relapse, remission, and recovery in anorexia nervosa. J Eat Disord. 2017;5:20.
11. Carter JC, Mercer-Lynn KB, Norwood SJ, Bewell-Weiss CV, Crosby RD, Woodside DB, et al. A prospective study of predictors of relapse in anorexia nervosa: implications for relapse prevention. Psychiatry Res. 2012;200(2–3): 518–23.
12. Carter JC, Blackmore E, Sutandar-Pinnock K, Woodside DB. Relapse in anorexia nervosa: a survival analysis. Psychol Med. 2004;34(4):671–9.
13. Kaplan AS, Walsh BT, Olmsted M, Attia E, Carter JC, Devlin MJ, et al. The slippery slope: prediction of successful weight maintenance in anorexia nervosa. Psychol Med. 2009;39(6):1037–45.
14. Errichiello L, Iodice D, Bruzzese D, Gherghi M, Senatore I. Prognostic factors and outcome in anorexia nervosa: a follow-up study. Eating weight Disord. 2016;21(1):73–82.
15. Lo Sauro C, Castellini G, Lelli L, Faravelli C, Ricca V. Psychopathological and clinical features of remitted anorexia nervosa patients: a six-year follow-up study. Eur Eating Disord Rev. 2013;21(1):78–83.

16. Vall E, Wade TD. Predictors of treatment outcome in individuals with eating disorders: a systematic review and meta-analysis. Int J Eat Disord. 2015;48(7): 946–71.
17. Zipfel S, Löwe B, Reas DL, Deter H-C, Herzog W. Long-term prognosis in anorexia nervosa: lessons from a 21-year follow-up study. Lancet. 2000; 355(9205):721–2.
18. Wild B, Friederich H-C, Zipfel S, Resmark G, Giel K, Teufel M, et al. Predictors of outcomes in outpatients with anorexia nervosa – results from the ANTOP study. Psychiatry Res. 2016;244:45–50.
19. Le Grange D, Fitzsimmons-Craft EE, Crosby RD, Hay P, Lacey H, Bamford B, et al. Predictors and moderators of outcome for severe and enduring anorexia nervosa. Behav Res Ther. 2014;56:91–8.
20. Fichter MM, Quadflieg N, Crosby RD, Koch S. Long-term outcome of anorexia nervosa: results from a large clinical longitudinal study. Int J Eat Disord. 2017;50(9):1018–30.
21. Wales J, Brewin N, Cashmore R, Haycraft E, Baggott J, Cooper A, et al. Predictors of positive treatment outcome in people with anorexia nervosa treated in a specialized inpatient unit: the role of early response to treatment. Eur Eat Disord Rev. 2016;24(5):417–24.
22. Støving RK, Andries A, Brixen K, Bilenberg N, Hørder K. Gender differences in outcome of eating disorders: a retrospective cohort study. Psychiatry Res. 2011;186(2):362–6.
23. Strobel C, Quadflieg N, Naab S, Voderholzer U, Fichter MM. Long-term outcomes in treated males with anorexia nervosa and bulimia nervosa—a prospective, gender-matched study. Int J Eat Disord. 2019; 52(12):1353–64.
24. Casper RC, Jabine LN. An eight-year follow-up: outcome from adolescent compared to adult onset anorexia nervosa. J Youth Adolesc. 1996;25(4):499–517.
25. El Ghoch M, Calugi S, Chignola E, Bazzani PV, Dalle GR. Body mass index, body fat and risk factor of relapse in anorexia nervosa. Eur J Clin Nutr. 2016; 70(2):194–8.
26. Madden S, Miskovic-Wheatley J, Wallis A, Kohn M, Lock J, Le Grange D, et al. A randomized controlled trial of in-patient treatment for anorexia nervosa in medically unstable adolescents. Psychol Med. 2015;45(2):415–27.
27. Herpertz-Dahlmann B, Schwarte R, Krei M, Egberts K, Warnke A, Wewetzer C, et al. Day-patient treatment after short inpatient care versus continued inpatient treatment in adolescents with anorexia nervosa (ANDI): a multicentre, randomised, open-label, non-inferiority trial. Lancet (London, England). 2014;383(9924):1222–9.
28. Zeeck A, Hartmann A, Buchholz C, Herzog T. Drop outs from in-patient treatment of anorexia nervosa. Acta Psychiatr Scand 2005;111(1):29–37.
29. Gregertsen EC, Mandy W, Kanakam N, Armstrong S, Serpell L. Pre-treatment patient characteristics as predictors of drop-out and treatment outcome in individual and family therapy for adolescents and adults with anorexia nervosa: a systematic review and meta-analysis. Psychiatry Res. 2019;271:484–501.
30. Kahn C, Pike KM. In search of predictors of dropout from inpatient treatment for anorexia nervosa. Int J Eat Disord. 2001;30(3):237–44.
31. Zipfel S, Lowe B, Reas DL, Deter HC, Herzog W. Long-term prognosis in anorexia nervosa: lessons from a 21-year follow-up study. Lancet (London, England). 2000;355(9205):721–2.
32. Surgenor LJ, Maguire S, Beumont PJV. Drop-out from inpatient treatment for anorexia nervosa: can risk factors be identified at point of admission? Eur Eat Disord Rev. 2004;12(2):94–100.
33. Franko DL, Tabri N, Keshaviah A, Murray HB, Herzog DB, Thomas JJ, et al. Predictors of long-term recovery in anorexia nervosa and bulimia nervosa: data from a 22-year longitudinal study. J Psychiatr Res. 2018;96:183–8.
34. Zerwas S, Lund BC, Von Holle A, Thornton LM, Berrettini WH, Brandt H, et al. Factors associated with recovery from anorexia nervosa. J Psychiatr Res. 2013;47(7):972–9.
35. Eddy KT, Tabri N, Thomas JJ, Murray HB, Keshaviah A, Hastings E, et al. Recovery from anorexia nervosa and bulimia nervosa at 22-year follow-up. J Clin Psychiatr. 2017;78(2):184–9.
36. Keel PK, Dorer DJ, Franko DL, Jackson SC, Herzog DB. Postremission predictors of relapse in women with eating disorders. Am J Psychiatry. 2005; 162(12):2263–8.
37. Bulik CM, Sullivan PF, Fear JL, Pickering A. Outcome of anorexia nervosa: eating attitudes, personality, and parental bonding. Int J Eating Disord. 2000;28(2):139–47.
38. Segura-García C, Chiodo D, Sinopoli F, De Fazio P. Temperamental factors predict long-term modifications of eating disorders after treatment. BMC Psychiatr. 2013;13:288.
39. Andrés-Pepiñá S, Plana MT, Flamarique I, Romero S, Borras R, Julia L, et al. Long-term outcome and psychiatric comorbidity of adolescent-onset anorexia nervosa. Clin Child Psychol Psychiatr. 2020;25(1):33–44.
40. Dobrescu SR, Dinkler L, Gillberg C, Rastam M, Gillberg C, Wentz E. Anorexia nervosa: 30-year outcome. Br J Psychiatr. 2019:1–8.
41. Fichter MM, Quadflieg N, Hedlund S. Twelve-year course and outcome predictors of anorexia nervosa. Int J Eating Disord. 2006;39(2):87–100.
42. Seidensticker JF, Tzagournis M. Anorexia nervosa—clinical features and long term follow-up. J Chronic Dis. 1968;21(5):361–7.
43. Morgan HG, Russell GF. Value of family background and clinical features as predictors of long-term outcome in anorexia nervosa: four-year follow-up study of 41 patients. Psychol Med. 1975;5(4):355–71.
44. Nussbaum M, Shenker IR, Baird D, Saravay S. Follow-up investigation in patients with anorexia nervosa. J Pediatr. 1985;106(5):835–40.
45. Bryant-Waugh R, Knibbs J, Fosson A, Kaminski Z, Lask B. Long term follow up of patients with early onset anorexia nervosa. Arch Dis Child. 1988;63(1):5–9.
46. Steinhausen H-C, Seidel R. Outcome in adolescent eating disorders. Int J Eat Disord. 1993;14(4):487–96.
47. Halmi K, Brodland G, Loney J. Prognosis in anorexia nervosa. Ann Intern Med. 1973;78(6):907–9.
48. Boehm I, Finke B, Tam FI, Fittig E, Scholz M, Gantchev K, et al. Effects of perceptual body image distortion and early weight gain on long-term outcome of adolescent anorexia nervosa. Eur Child Adolesc Psychiatr. 2016; 25(12):1319–26.
49. Uniacke B, Attia E, Kaplan A, Walsh BT. Weight suppression and weight maintenance following treatment of anorexia nervosa. International journal of eating disorders. 2020.
50. Sysko R, Glasofer DR, Hildebrandt T, Klimek P, Mitchell JE, Berg KC, et al. The eating disorder assessment for DSM-5 (EDA-5): development and validation of a structured interview for feeding and eating disorders. Int J Eating Disord. 2015;48(5):452–63.
51. First MBS RL, Gibbon M, Williams JBW. Structured clinical interview for DSM-IV-TR axis I disorders, research version, patient edition. (SCID-I/P). New York: Biometrics Research, New York State Psychiatric Institute; 2002.
52. Company MLI. New weight standards for men and women. Stat Bull. 1959; 40:1–4.
53. Fairburn CG, Beglin S. Eating disorder examination questionnaire (EDE-Q 6. 0). In: Fairburn CG, editor. Cognitive behavior therapy and eating disorders. New York: Guilford Press; 2008.
54. Fairburn CG, Bohn K. Clinical impairment assessment questionnaire (CIA 3.0). In: Fairburn CG, editor. Cognitive behavior therapy and eating disorders. New York: Guilford Press; 2008.
55. Beck AT, Ward CH, Mendelson M, Mock J, Erbaugh J. An inventory for measuring depression. Arch Gen Psychiatry. 1961;4:561–71.
56. Beck AT, Steer RA. Beck anxiety inventory manual. San Antonio, TX: Psychological Corporation; 1993.
57. Spielberger CD, Gorsuch RL, Lushene R, Vagg PR, Jacobs GA. Manual for the state-trait anxiety inventory. Palo Alto, CA: Consulting Psychologists Press; 1983.
58. Cloninger CR. The temperament and character inventory (TCI): a guide to its development and use. St. Louis, MO: Center for Psychobiology of Personality, Washington University; 1994.
59. American Psychiatric Association. Diagnostic and Statistical Manual of Mental Disorders. 5th ed. Washington, DC. 2013.
60. Bardone-Cone AM, Hunt RA, Watson HJ. An overview of conceptualizations of eating disorder recovery, recent findings, and future directions. Curr Psychiatr Rep. 2018;20(9):79.
61. Bardone-Cone AM, Harney MB, Maldonado CR, Lawson MA, Robinson DP, Smith R, et al. Defining recovery from an eating disorder: conceptualization, validation, and examination of psychosocial functioning and psychiatric comorbidity. Behav Res Ther. 2010;48(3):194–202.
62. Mond JM, Hay PJ, Rodgers B, Owen C. Eating disorder examination questionnaire (EDE-Q): norms for young adult women. Behav Res Ther. 2006;44(1):53–62.
63. Steinhausen HC, Grigoroiu-Serbanescu M, Boyadjieva S, Neumärker KJ, Metzke CW. The relevance of body weight in the medium-term to long-term course of adolescent anorexia nervosa. Findings from a multisite study. Int J Eating Disord. 2009;42(1):19–25.
64. Lock J, Agras WS, Le Grange D, Couturier J, Safer D, Bryson SW. Do end of treatment assessments predict outcome at follow-up in eating disorders? Int J Eating Disord. 2013;46(8):771–8.

65. Kästner D, Löwe B, Weigel A, Osen B, Voderholzer U, Gumz A. Factors influencing the length of hospital stay of patients with anorexia nervosa - results of a prospective multi-center study. BMC Health Serv Res. 2018;18(1): 22.
66. Ratnasuriya RH, Eisler I, Szmukler GI, Russell GF. Anorexia nervosa: outcome and prognostic factors after 20 years. Br J Psychiatr. 1991;158:495–502.
67. Bulik CM, Sullivan PF, Fear JL, Joyce PR. Eating disorders and antecedent anxiety disorders: a controlled study. Acta Psychiatr Scand. 1997;96(2):101–7.
68. Kaye WH, Bulik CM, Thornton L, Barbarich N, Masters K. Comorbidity of anxiety disorders with anorexia and bulimia nervosa. Am J Psychiatry. 2004; 161(12):2215–21.
69. Marzola E, Porliod A, Panero M, De-Bacco C, Abbate-Daga G. Affective temperaments and eating psychopathology in anorexia nervosa: which role for anxious and depressive traits? J Affect Disord. 2020;266:374–80.
70. Steinglass JE, Sysko R, Glasofer D, Albano AM, Simpson HB, Walsh BT. Rationale for the application of exposure and response prevention to the treatment of anorexia nervosa. Int J Eat Disord. 2011;44(2):134–41.
71. Cardi V, Leppanen J, Mataix-Cols D, Campbell IC, Treasure J. A case series to investigate food-related fear learning and extinction using in vivo food exposure in anorexia nervosa: a clinical application of the inhibitory learning framework. Eur Eating Disord Rev. 2019;27(2):173–81.
72. Steinglass JE, Glasofer DR, Dalack M, Attia E. Between wellness, relapse, and remission: Stages of illness in anorexia nervosa. Int J Eat Disord. 2020;53(7): 1088–96.
73. Berends T, Boonstra N, van Elburg A. Relapse in anorexia nervosa: a systematic review and meta-analysis. Curr Opinion Psychiatr. 2018;31(6):445–55.
74. Rigaud D, Pennacchio H, Bizeul C, Reveillard V, Verges B. Outcome in AN adult patients: a 13-year follow-up in 484 patients. Diabetes Metab. 2011; 37(4):305–11.
75. Schebendach J, Mayer LE, Devlin MJ, Attia E, Walsh BT. Dietary energy density and diet variety as risk factors for relapse in anorexia nervosa: a replication. Int J Eating Disord. 2012;45(1):79–84.
76. Schebendach JE, Mayer LE, Devlin MJ, Attia E, Contento IR, Wolf RL, et al. Dietary energy density and diet variety as predictors of outcome in anorexia nervosa. Am J Clin Nutr. 2008;87(4):810–6.

18

Family members' reflections upon a family-based inpatient treatment program for adolescent anorexia nervosa: a thematic analysis

Jan-Vegard Nilsen[1,2*], Øyvind Rø[2,3], Inger Halvorsen[2], Hanne Weie Oddli[1] and Trine Wiig Hage[2]

Abstract

Background: Family-based outpatient treatment is usually recommended as the treatment of choice when a child develops anorexia nervosa. However, some young persons will inevitably require higher levels of care. Qualitative research on family perspectives may help inform strategies to adapt family-based practices into intensified treatment settings. Our overarching aim was to investigate family members' perspectives following a family-based inpatient treatment program for adolescent anorexia nervosa and to discuss clinical implications for treatment providers.

Methods: A subsample of eight families taking part in a naturalistic outcome study at a specialized eating disorder unit participated in the study (8 patients, 14 parents, and 10 siblings). The thematic analyses were inductive, predominantly descriptive, and guided by a multi-perspective framework.

Results: Five main themes were identified: 1: *Expectations and evaluation of needs. Entering treatment from different vantage points*, 2: *Interactions with peers during the admission as highly beneficial or problematic*, 3: *Perspectives on staff expertise and the eating disorder unit's structure*, 4: *Influencing within family relationships in different ways*, and 5: *Being admitted is at best only half the job: reflections on leaving the eating disorder unit.*

Conclusions: Our study offers insight into how former inpatients and their family members experienced an inpatient treatment program designed to align treatment with the central elements of an outpatient family-based treatment approach for adolescent anorexia nervosa. Overall, the findings support emerging research underlining the necessity of strengthening the family-based treatment approach within intensified treatment settings. Moreover, the results emphasized the need for more knowledge on how to optimize inpatient treatment as well as the importance of providing smooth transitions between care settings.

Keywords: Eating disorders, Anorexia nervosa, Family-based treatment, Inpatient treatment, Qualitative research, Higher levels of care, User perspectives

* Correspondence: uxnilj@ous-hf.no
[1]Department of Psychology, University of Oslo, Oslo, Norway
[2]Regional Department for Eating Disorders, Division of Mental Health and Addiction, Oslo University Hospital, Oslo, Norway
Full list of author information is available at the end of the article

Plain English summary

Inpatient treatment of anorexia nervosa has traditionally been individually based. At large, this has usually meant that the young person with anorexia nervosa has been separated from their family during a hospital admission, while parents and family-members have had the chance to visit for treatment meetings, support and therapy sessions. Inspired by the promising research on outpatient family-based treatment, a treatment model that put a lot of emphasis on supporting the parents and "the family as a whole" during treatment, some treatment centers around the globe has started to hospitalize parents and siblings together with the young person with anorexia nervosa. The present study offers insight into how family members have experienced taking part in such a family-based inpatient treatment program. The family members demonstrated considerable diversity in viewpoints. Without prescribing definitive answers, we believe the results have several important implications for treatment providers working within a family-based inpatient treatment approach.

Background

Outpatient family-based treatment, either the well-known "Maudsley approach" [1] or manualized family-based treatment (FBT-AN) [2], is usually recommended when a young person develops anorexia nervosa (AN) [3]. Still, inpatient treatment is often required for child- and adolescent AN, both because of the complexity and symptom severity, but also due to the lack of accessible recommended outpatient treatments in many regions [4, 5]. Inpatient treatment is also frequently used when a young person with severe AN does not achieve adequate progress at an outpatient treatment facility [6, 7]. For some, a more intensive level of care is required even when the young person and their family receives highly specialized, evidence-based outpatient treatment, as no treatment is a panacea [8].

Inpatient treatment demands a lot of resources, including human and financial [4, 9]. Availability is typically limited, as most specialized treatment centers have strict admission criteria and offers only a few beds for a large catchment area [7, 10]. Inpatient care is recognized as a highly multifaceted and complex endeavor, and to date, no internationally agreed upon treatment guidelines for AN exist to guide clinicians on how to efficiently and effectively provide and manage inpatient care [4, 11]. Importantly, inpatient care has shown to have uncertain long-term effects, as many of the patients fail to maintain improvements achieved during admission [4, 12]. The latter is mirrored in the relative high relapse rates for this population-at-large, and underscores the importance of improving inpatient care as well as collaboration with the referral system to facilitate transitions [13].

Developing better ways to optimize the inpatient treatment setting for young persons with AN has been called for by recent ED studies [4, 11]. Due to promising evidence from the last two decades of development and research on outpatient family-based treatments, some treatment centers around the globe have begun to incorporate key tenets of outpatient family-based treatment into higher levels of care [6, 7, 10, 14, 15]. Most developments have been pioneered by highly specialized treatment centers aiming to align the core features embedded in evidence-based FBT within intensified treatment programs. This work aims to both optimize the provision of care during hospitalizations and importantly, to enhance the maintenance of effects following discharge [7, 10, 11, 14].

Research investigating the potential benefits of adapting family-based interventions at higher levels of care is emerging, yet remains scarce [7, 16–19]. A recent study from an Australian context investigated the effects of a brief admission prior to outpatient FBT and showed that admitting the family for an intensified two-week program offered the families an opportunity for relational strengthening and re-unification, thereby providing a stronger foundation for outpatient FBT [18]. Another study found that although outpatient FBT cannot be replicated at higher levels of care, treatment principles can be effectively adapted to a day treatment program [6, 16]. Our own research on outcome following admission to a family-based inpatient treatment program also found that enhancing the family-based focus during hospitalization is a promising approach for those who fail to respond to outpatient treatment [7].

With the current study, we aimed to extend our prior research on a family-based inpatient treatment approach for adolescent AN, which has to date focused upon outcome [7], treatment satisfaction [20], siblings' experiences [21], and user experiences [19]. In the present study, we provided a multiperspectival approach to extend our knowledge beyond the single-position approach previously applied in our qualitative studies [19, 21, 22]. Specifically, the research question focused upon how to characterize the multiple user perspectives of parents, siblings and patients' belonging to a single family following admission to a family-based inpatient treatment program at a specialized eating disorder unit (EDU) for adolescents with AN.

Methods

Research design

The study was a qualitative descriptive study and formed part of a larger naturalistic outcome study investigating different aspects related to a family-based inpatient program.

Ethics

Ethics approval was obtained from the Regional Committee for Medical Research ethics, South East Norway [REK2014/2223]. All participants provided written consent to take part in this research. All names in the results section are pseudonyms.

Participants and sampling procedure

Post-treatment perspectives from eight former inpatients and their family members were included (8 former patients, 14 parents, and 10 siblings). All participants took part in a family-based inpatient treatment program at a specialized EDU between 2008 and 2014. This subsample was purposively derived from the complete data set of thirty-seven inpatients participating in the main outcome study [7]. The eight families were selected because we had post-treatment interview data from patients, as well as their siblings and parents. This sampling choice mirrored our aim to investigate user perspectives from multiple positions within a single family and enable within and between family comparisons.

Mean age at admission was 15 years (range: 12–18) and mean age at follow up was 19 years (range: 16–21). Mean length of stay was 21.4 weeks (range: 8–58), including planned leaves as part of the treatment program. All patients had an admission diagnosis of AN. No statistically significant differences existed between the 8 participants and the 29 non-participating patients for the following variables: age at admission, duration of ED before admission, length of stay, weight and BMI percentile at admission and discharge, time elapsed between discharge and follow up and EDE-Q global score at follow up.

All patients had received previous outpatient treatment at specialized mental health services, as well as prior inpatient treatment at a medical and / or psychiatric unit. During the follow-up interviews, 5 of the former patients did not meet the criteria for any DSM-5 ED diagnosis. In seven of the eight families, the parents were married. Six of the parent interviews were conducted with both parents together; two of the interviews were conducted only with the mother. Siblings' mean age at admission was 11 years (range: 6–16) and mean age at follow up was 15.4 years (range: 11.9–23). None of the siblings reported any previous treatment experiences beyond visitation during hospitalization of their sibling. Only one of the siblings had attended a family session at the local outpatient clinic.

Overall, our sampling strategy was guided by the acknowledgement that each and every participant inevitably represented themselves and their subjective opinions and perspectives, and further, that the themes generated through the qualitative analysis would be judged more or less as representative or relevant within different clinical contexts by the reader, an approach to generalization often recognized as a case-to-case transferability [23].

Treatment setting

In 2008, the EDU changed the treatment program in order to provide a family-based inpatient treatment program. This restructuring was guided by a) the promising evidence-base from research on outpatient family-based therapy for AN, b) the wish to prevent separating the ill child from caregivers during hospitalizations and c) the specific legal situation in Norway, where children have a legal right to be accommodated by a parent during hospitalization. Since then, up to 5 families have been treated at the same time [7].

As outpatient FBT was originally a manualized version of the family-based treatment approach developed at the Maudsley hospital, the EDUs inpatient treatment program has undoubtedly been influenced by both sources. Although these two outpatient treatment models are today recognized by some differences, they share the common core features that, taken together, have been influential for treatment adaptations at the EDU. These features include charging parents with more responsibility during the admission (i.e., continually aiming to facilitate parental empowerment throughout treatment), externalizing the ED, together with aligning treatment with the non-blaming/non-etiological/non-authoritarian therapeutic stances embedded in both outpatient treatment models. Although the EDU has not adhered to a strict manualized FBT approach, the EDU has continually aimed to align treatment with the core features and therapeutic stances associated with outpatient FBT [2, 11, 24]. Generally, the treatment program corresponds to the first phase of outpatient FBT, as the main aim during admissions has been to enable AN symptom improvement. Contrary to standard outpatient FBT, however, the treatment team has had the final say on the meal plans during admissions. This decision-making process has commonly been done in close collaboration with the parents and only when viewed appropriate involved the patient, during the weekly treatment meetings (i.e., dependent on progress). During later phases of hospitalization, the focus has gradually shifted towards encouraging the adolescent to assume more responsibility for eating, with continued parental supervision. All families had weekly treatment meetings with a multidisciplinary team. Parents were provided with parental counseling. Staff had daily scheduled meetings with both parents and the young person. Families were usually offered family therapy sessions twice a week and some of the patients were offered individual sessions. Supplementary sessions were typically arranged in collaboration with the patient and parents. As a rule these individual sessions were intended to align with the overarching family therapeutic approach and could be viewed as predominantly supportive or motivational sessions, aiming to support the young person's treatment engagement together with helping them appreciate the greater responsibilities obtained by the parents. During some phases between 2008 and 2014, parents have been offered a parenting course inspired by the skills-based parent program developed at the Maudsley hospital [25], and for the majority of the time period (i.e., between 2008 and 2014) the EDU has provided weekly parent groups facilitated by staff, where the parents themselves were in charge of the content.

At discharge, all patients and families were transferred back to their local mental health services. Although siblings were welcome to take part in the admission, most families arranged for siblings to remain at home during the majority of the hospital admission. Siblings, however, could participate in family therapy sessions and family meals during visits to the EDU. Occasionally, a sibling group has been offered at the EDU led by a senior nurse or clinical psychologist.

Interview guides and interviews

Interview guides were developed separately for patients, parents and siblings by a group of experienced clinicians led by a senior researcher [IH]. Interview guides were piloted and revised before the final completion. Despite subtle differences, all interview guides were semi-structured and organized into three broad sections to cover perspectives related to the pre- admission phase, admission, and post discharge. Patients and siblings were interviewed individually. Parents were given the opportunity to choose whether they wanted to be interviewed separately or together.

Interviews were administered in 2015. A team of 5 senior clinicians and one advanced psychology student conducted the interviews, with one of the co-authors [IH] administering the majority of interviews (i.e., 14 of 26). The rest of the interviews were administered by the psychology student (i.e., 6 of the sibling interviews), and four specialist nurses (i.e., three specialist nurses conducted one interview each, and one specialist nurse and family therapist administered three interviews). Interviews were transcribed verbatim. Questions included how the participants had experienced the admission, whether they would have preferred any changes based on their experiences, an invitation to give their advice to the treatment providers and peers, together with questions on how they experienced the pre-treatment phase and transitioning back home. The interview guides are available upon request.

Qualitative analyses

Starting out our analysis was inspired by a multiperspectival interpretative phenomenological analysis (IPA) framework [26]. During the initial process of conducting the analysis according to the steps outlined in multiperspectival IPA, we [JVN & TWH] encountered several dilemmas. In particular, we were concerned whether our data were sufficiently rich enough to utilize an interpretative or hermeneutic approach such as multiperspectival IPA. After thoroughly discussing these important dilemmas we concluded that the raw data, together with the original research question, were most likely better managed while applying a predominantly pragmatic descriptive thematic analysis (TA) approach [27].

Both TA and IPA share much in common. They offer the researcher a set of steps, or a road map, for conducting the analysis, they can both be multiperspectival (i.e., involve participants from different positions as including parents, siblings and patients) and they both aim to generate themes based on the original data. Still the most striking difference, we believe, and this became crucial for our conclusions, is that while IPA has strong historic roots in specifically hermeneutics and phenomenology [26], TA represents a more pragmatic, a-theoretic framework that enables the analytic team to position the analysis in more flexible ways [27]. Critical for the current study was hence the assessment that our data was judged as more suitable for a descriptive TA approach, compared with the more interpretative stance recognizing the IPA framework.

Although unavoidably influenced by our initial analysis, we started over by re-familiarizing ourselves with the raw material while retaining the original multiperspectival approach. The first author [JVN] read and re-read all transcripts together with preliminary coding, applying a more descriptive stance. At the same time, co-author TWH read the complete data set in order assist and collaborate in the evolving process, performing the role as a "critical friend" [28]. Again, we read and coded [chiefly performed by JVN] individual transcripts, one family at the time. We started out with the parents, followed by the index patient, and finally the siblings. Before finalizing the analysis, we scheduled weekly meetings to discuss the iterative process over a 2-month period. This work was done in accordance with the 6 steps outlined in TA [27]. After analyzing the individual interviews case- by- case, we used substantial time to explore whether we could find any thematic development that supported a shared family narrative, that is, we searched for themes potentially shared within the family as a whole, and also for similarities and discrepancies between families.

Results

A thematic structure of 5 main themes captured 14 subthemes, as outlined below (cf. Table 1 for a brief summary). During the analysis, we did not find evidence of a shared family narrative within the current sample. Rather than constructing "a shared family narrative" or mapping out themes on the "family level," it was interpreted that the participants' perspectives were predominantly influenced by both the position in the family (i.e., on an individual or between individuals level) and what we understood as the relationship to the ED. As outlined below, some of the subthemes were related to all family members, and these reflections are captured collectively under the same subtheme, whereas some subthemes represent views from one position alone (i.e., only the parents). All 8 families are represented with data excerpts.

Main theme 1: expectations and valuation of needs. Entering treatment from different vantage points

This main theme reflected the perspective that young persons with AN (hereafter abbreviated as YP-AN) and their family members entered treatment from very different vantage points. This variation was predominantly interpreted as contingent on roles and responsibilities at the time of the admission, together with what we determined as the relationship to the ED.

Subtheme 1: "We needed a time-out": parents appreciating the admission as a much needed restart for the family

> We couldn't handle the situation at home, we clearly needed help [...] it's obvious. You feel very powerless as a parent when your child stops eating [Anna, *a mother reflecting back on a sensation resonating with most parents prior to the admission. Although engaged in treatment prior to the family-based admission; expressing strong feelings of being disempowered as parents, combined with a growing sense of that "somebody" has to intervene as things were beyond parental control*]

Although some of the parents recalled initial skepticism and ideally wanted to manage the situation at home without intensified treatment efforts, parents entered treatment with an overall high degree of readiness, as most "longed for the admission to finally start." Generally, parents recalled the pre-admission phase by interpersonal tension and high levels of within-family conflicts. They voiced multiple examples of how the family and individual family members had accommodated to the ED over time. Simultaneously, most parents

Table 1 Results

Main themes	Subthemes
1: Expectations and evaluation of needs. Entering treatment from different vantage points	Subtheme 1: "We needed a time-out": parents appreciating the admission as a much needed restart for the family – *parents* (*N* = 14) Subtheme 2: From opposition to realizing that "something had to happen" – *patients* (*N* = 8) Subtheme 3: The admission arriving as a surprise – *siblings* (*N* = 8)
2: Interactions with peers during the admission as highly beneficial or problematic	Subtheme 1: Sharing, learning and recognition of oneself in the other – *parents* (*N* = 14) and *siblings* (*N* = 5) Subtheme 2: Peer interactions as problematic: heightened pressure and symptom contagion – *patients* (*N* = 6) and *parents* (*N* = 2)
3: Perspectives on staff expertise and the EDU structure	Subtheme 1: Improved understanding of ED and insight into the young patients challenges – *parents* (*N* = 14) and *siblings* (*N* = 7) Subtheme 2: Strengthening parental authority and re-establishing normalized meal routines – *parents* (*N* = 9) Subtheme 3: Enabling necessary weight gain – *parents* (*N* = 8), *patients* (*N* = 3) and *siblings* (*N* = 4) Subtheme 4: The unintended potential of treatment keeping parents in a bystander position – *parents* (*N* = 5)
4: Influencing within-family relationships in different ways	Subtheme 1: Strengthening within family relationships – *siblings* (*N* = 5), *parents* (*N* = 10) and *patients* (*N* = 6) Subtheme 2: The potential of maintaining or increasing fragmentation – *siblings* (*N* = 5) and *parents* (*N* = 4)
5: Being admitted is at best only half the job: reflections on leaving the EDU	Subtheme 1: Leaving the EDU while the ED is still on board – *parents* (*N* = 10) and *patients* (*N* = 4) Subtheme 2: Being transferred back to where it did not work out in the first place – *parents* (*N* = 8) and *patients* (*N* = 5) Subtheme 3: For siblings, leaving the EDU meant leaving treatment for good: calling for better sibling involvement – *siblings* (*N* = 8) and *parents* (*N* = 10)

Note: To indicate the robustness of findings, the number of participants sharing views within each subtheme is listed in parenthesis recollected feeling renewed hope when reflecting on the time prior to the admission; anticipating that this new treatment effort could be helpful, "finally we were going to get help." Looking back, all parents described "a sense of relief" when the referral to the EDU was accepted. Most parents also recalled they found it important that the EDU was deliberately providing space for the whole family, "as this was a family issue."

Subtheme 2: from opposition to realizing that "something had to happen"

Contrary to their parents, all but one of the YP-AN remembered opposing treatment at the time of the admission.

> I was kind of... forced... I was really fed up with treatment and did not want to be there [Brenda, 20 years, 14 during the admission, *an extract resonating with most YP-AN at the time of the admission, as they overall recalled low readiness for a new treatment effort*]

Reflecting back from a more distant position, all eight former patients acknowledged that something had to happen at the time of the admission, as they remembered things were not working out at home or even at the treatment facility where they had received therapy.

> I guess I thought, "I'm not going to go there". That it was totally unacceptable. I guess I didn't imagine that I needed another admission, after [recently] being discharged at the medical ward... [...] It was necessary, I see that *now*. That I got help somewhere, so, if it was at [name of unit] or a different place, I don't know, but it was nevertheless essential that they stopped me from losing further weight... [Molly, 18 years, 15 during the admission, *although her vantage point was characterized by initial opposition, the excerpt showed how her perspectives on being admitted had changed over time*]

One YP-AN reflected contrary views, as she voiced high levels of pre-admission readiness, recalling that she felt extremely exhausted, and "ready for somebody to take over control," as she recognized that everything pertaining to food and meals was far beyond control. She also remembered thinking that although she really wanted change, she was unable to make the necessary changes alone.

Subtheme 3: the admission arriving as a surprise

> I thought it was very peculiar. Very extraordinary, that my family had to be hospitalized. That my sister, that *she* had any problems? She was very conscientious and was feeling really, very well, I thought [...] that she needed help, that there was a problem, that I found very strange [Sister, Catherine, 14 years, 10 during the admission, *reflecting back on the admission arriving as a surprise*]

None of the siblings had previously been involved in family-based treatment for AN. In general, siblings described that the admission came as a big surprise. For the two siblings that did not express this viewpoint, one was apparently well-informed and also very eager to take part in the admission. Resonating with the YP-AN views captured in subtheme 2, some of the siblings recalled feeling oppositional when they learned the admission was family-based and they were expected to participate. For some, the sensation of surprise thus developed into sheer resistance.

> I was very negatively inclined. I did not like the fact that we were supposed to be admitted, that I had to stay there. I never stayed there. Me and my little brother were always at home together with either mom or dad [...] I remember they asked if I wanted to stay over, but I didn't want to, I didn't feel it was right... [Sister, Jenna, 15 years, 12 during the admission, *reflecting back on her immediate reactions when learning she was supposed to be admitted too*]

Main theme 2: interactions with peers during admission as highly beneficial or problematic

This main theme captured participants' views on being admitted to a treatment setting in which they had the opportunity to interact with peers. Common for all participants was that the family-based admission represented the first time they were admitted together with other families. The subthemes revealed that peer interactions were viewed as predominantly beneficial (subtheme 1) or problematic (subtheme 2).

Subtheme 1: sharing, learning and recognition of oneself in the other

> I think everybody felt that it was really useful to recognize that others had, in fact, experienced the same, or at least something in the same way. That it wasn't all about us. I believe that is important for parents too, to know that you're not alone on this [Father, Paul, *reflecting back on the peer group for parents. Although facilitated by staff, the group focused on issues the parents raised on that particular day*]

Parents and siblings both viewed being admitted together with other families as largely supportive and meaningful. Parents emphasized that having weekly meetings scheduled with other parents was a very supportive experience. They typically recognized that their own within-family struggles, as well as the numerous challenges with the health care system, resonated with others, i.e., "increased feeling of connection," "we were not the only ones," "others held similar experiences as ours," "it was not only us that reacted to such behaviors." Additionally, some parents remarked that it was often easier to discuss issues with other parents compared to professionals.

For siblings who interacted with other siblings during the admission, the prospect of meeting others was viewed favorably, especially among siblings of the same age with shared interests. Whereas few parents spontaneously interacted with other parents or family members during the admission, siblings reported more frequent encounters.

> I think it was pretty nice. Then I understood that it wasn't only me that had it like that. Somebody else had the same, like me. It felt, I think it was a good thing to be together with somebody else that had similar challenges [Brother, Kenneth, 15.5 years, 12 during the admission; *on the perceived benefit of meeting other siblings during the stay*]

Subtheme 2: peer interactions as problematic: heightened pressure and symptom contagion

> For me, the surroundings were very negative... and I guess I was very susceptible too, and that I think everybody was [YP-AN, Jane, 21 years, 16 during the admission, *on being admitted with peers with severe challenges in a vulnerable phase, a sensation resonating with the majority of the YP-AN when reflecting back on interactions with peers*]

None of the patients shared stories of supportive interactions with fellow patients or other families. Quite the contrary, the YP-AN seemed to strongly feel that being admitted with peers was problematic. They recalled peer interactions frequently led to comparisons and negative competition. Some also acknowledged they, too, likely exerted negative pressure on others. Several of the YP-AN concluded that being admitted with peers with AN is potentially very problematic and should be handled carefully. Overall, parents perceived peer interactions between YP-AN as less problematic, although some did recollect that their child probably learned new and negative symptom behaviors, most likely due to observing and imitating peers during the admission.

Main theme 3: perspectives on staff expertise and the EDU structure

Both parents and siblings voiced that interacting with, and getting support from, experienced staff together within a structured treatment setting was beneficial for understanding the ED, strengthening parental authority, and re-establishing normalized meal routines. Several also emphasized that the EDU structure and staff expertise were crucial factors enabling weight gain and ED symptom improvement. Finally, this main theme also captured that, although staff expertise and the structure of the EDU were viewed as beneficial overall (especially voiced by parents), some aspects could, in certain instances, be interpreted as non-intentionally maintaining the ED.

Subtheme 1: improved understanding of the ED and insight into the young patients challenges

> That we learned more about the ED. That we could be present... and maybe that mom and dad learned to be more firm when telling my sister that she needed to eat [Brother, Kenneth, *on what he believed was especially valuable for the family; both a better understanding and that the parents were able to manage the meals more efficiently*]

Most of the parents, and some of the siblings, recalled benefiting from the staff's expertise, which improved their general knowledge of EDs, as well as their specific understanding of the unique challenges facing the YP-AN. Several of the parents, and siblings, implied that greater knowledge and awareness enhanced empathy, i.e. "when we were able to see how difficult it was, we could understand better how it really was for her." Despite having undergone extensive prior treatment, including previous hospitalizations, quite a few parents and siblings emphasized this was the first time they truly had the opportunity to learn about the ED. The educational program for parents was viewed as particularly beneficial in improving knowledge about the ED, and how the ED challenged the parental role.

> Attending the parenting courses was very helpful. Then you got something concrete to relate things to, and that helped, I think [Mother, Caroline, *recalling how learning more about ED and being introduced to how the ED typically challenges parenting was useful for her*]

Subtheme 2: strengthening parental authority and re-establishing normalized meal routines

> To learn to be calmer during meals. I think we were able to manage the meals more peacefully while on

> the unit, compared with previously, then there was no such thing as a calm meal! And we got rid of weighing the food [Mother, Ruth, *reflecting on the potential benefit of breaking patterns while being socialized into a meal structure compatible with a more normalized family life, and the prospect of unlearning of non-supportive behaviors*]

Parents highlighted several aspects of the EDU structure as particularly beneficial for breaking patterns and in re-establishing normalized meal routines.

> That I felt *so* secure, that the [meal] structure was so firm [...] that was the first thing I was very satisfied with, that somebody, like, took the responsibility from us, so we could have some real help, since we didn't manage it [at home] [Mother, Sarah, *on the potential benefit of parents being able to lean on a structure administered by the professionals*]

Following Sarah's excerpt, the father continued to describe how the established routines and structure at the EDU aided in re-installing parental authority, which had more or less vanished under the pressures of the ED.

> It was a very welcome feeling of not standing alone with everything [...] We were, in a way, defeated as parents, and how should I put it? Ehm, we had no authority, no influence; we were no longer defined by our daughter as caregivers in relation to food. I think our daughter didn't perceive that we had anything reasonable to say concerning food, because she was so convinced she was right. So, to come here and get support for the parenting, that felt very meaningful [Father, Peter, *on the EDUs potential of reinstalling and supporting parental authority*]

Sarah (wife) later joined in and summed it up:

> We regained a belief in our ability to function as parents [...] we recovered self-confidence and a belief in that we can be parents and authority figures for our daughter [Mother, Sarah]

Subtheme 3: enabling necessary weight gain

Although some of the YP-AN retrospectively acknowledged the necessity of weight gain to recover, parents and some siblings strongly emphasized the benefits of the admission in facilitating improvement on physical parameters. Weight gain and medical outcomes were predominantly ascribed to staff expertise, and enabled by the structure of the EDU, more than fueled by increased parental self-efficacy. Yet weight gain and related improvements were not uniformly perceived as linked with improved psychological well-being, as reflected in Caroline's quote below:

> To gain weight, you talked a lot about that, that it was supposed to help, and then you were supposed to get a clearer mind. We've witnessed quite the contrary with her [Mother, Caroline, *referring to how she remembered that although emphasizing the inevitable necessity of weight gain; how difficult it was when her daughter Jane actually gained weight, and that psychological symptoms did not immediately recede as she felt she had been told over and over again*]

Subtheme 4: the unintended potential of treatment keeping parents in a bystander position

> We didn't perceive ourselves as so important [during the admission]. It was more that our son was prioritized. That was most important [Father, Steven]

Although most parents voiced an initial need to step back and "let the experts take care of an unmanageable situation," the majority retrospectively perceived that treatment strengthened their role and position as caregivers (i.e., as reflected by the majority in subtheme 2 above). Still, we interpreted some parental views as acknowledging the potential of the treatment to maintain them in a bystander or sidelined position. For some, it was as if treatment failed to co-construct a collaborative relationship that strengthened their parental authority and relational agency.

> Paul [Father]: I think, for my part, that it was reassuring that somebody could help my daughter, like, "Now we know she gets what she needs", "Now she's going to get better", that I felt was very reassuring [...] still I felt that it was difficult. I didn't feel that *I* took part. I don't know if this was because I opted out or not, but I don't think so, it was like, you were supposed to join in and take part, still you were on the sideline [...] It was like, the one who controlled everything and had the direction, it was that therapist, or the one being present at that moment [that were in charge] and I was in a way set aside, as I felt it...
>
> Inger [Interviewer]: The therapist took over?
>
> Paul [Father]: Yes, it was like that in a way, and further, I noticed on my daughter too [...] like, she really needed to hear it from somebody [else] what she should do too, and it became much easier for

> her to listen to somebody else, of course, that knows this.

As we read this excerpt, together with other parental excerpts that touched upon Paul's perspectives, we recognized the potential of the YP-AN becoming dependent upon staff instructions and / or authority. This development could ultimately become a hindrance in aiding parental efficacy, and reinforce the idea that staff members are the "true" experts, thereby maintaining parents in a bystander position.

Main theme 4: influencing within-family relationships

This main theme captured contrasting views on how the admission was perceived as supportive and strengthening within-family relationships, while others viewed the admission as maintaining or increasing fragmentation.

Subtheme 1: strengthening within-family relationships

Parents and siblings shared a range of views relating to reduced relational distance, i.e., "we came closer," improved collaboration," "we managed to collaborate better." Several voiced enhanced within-family understanding of each other and the ED, i.e. "by being together we learned together and understood better," and reduced within-family conflicts, i.e., "things became calmer."

> Sarah [Mother]: We felt we came closer to each other, that our collaboration improved, or...
>
> Peter [Father]: Mhm... we experienced that as a family, too. All these conversations we had, and the groups and, yes, both the individual family sessions and couple sessions we had, and these group meetings with the other parents. Everything helped us to sort things out between us... so our relationship and to our daughter... I think it became a closer relationship [*Both parents reflecting on noticing improved collaboration and strengthened relationships*]

Although few of the YP-AN emphasized that having been admitted was aiding them directly (i.e., as personally perceived as supportive at the time), some reflected as Jane below, that although the admission paralleled an extremely difficult time period, looking back she had come to appreciate that the admission was of benefit for her parents, the family, and in strengthening relationships:

> When I think back, I do believe it is the worst thing I've ever experienced [reflecting back on the time of the admission] [still] I did observe, there, that my parents seemed a bit happier, calmer. At home, I felt it was like, police and thief, and our relationship was suffering when we were at home [prior to the admission], and I felt it was strengthened when we were there. They became more my supporters [...] I would say it was of benefit for my family... [Jane, 21 years, 16 during the admission, *recalling that although the admission represented the worst of memories, it was beneficial for the family*]

Subtheme 2: the potential of maintaining or increasing fragmentation

Although we assume that "living with the ED" had contributed to an increased sense of separateness for the afflicted families, some of the participants voiced concerns that the organization of the admission might represent a further division for some families, i.e., "as we did not stay there together, we became even more divided".

> I feel in a way that we came closer to each other, but also that we in ways became divided. Mom was with my sister all the time [at the EDU], and then it was us three [at home]. We too came a bit closer, still it was a bit divided [Sister, Angie, 15 years, 12 during the admission, *reflecting on the feeling of both getting closer with some family-members, and at the same time; a sensation of being divided*]

This sense of disconnectedness was particularly echoed in some of the siblings' accounts. In particular, some of the youngest siblings found it challenging to spend less time with the parent who was frequently at the EDU; typically this was their mother. On the other hand, some siblings voiced the benefits of an improved relationship with their father as a consequence. This feeling of disconnectedness also resonated with some of the parents, who emphasized that if they could do "one thing over again," it would be to be admitted earlier to the specialized EDU, and to stay together as an entire family. These parents now believed that "they" as parents and "we" as the family would have benefited more from an earlier admission that included all family members.

Main theme 5: being admitted is at best only half the job: reflections on leaving the EDU

This main theme captured realizations that discharge did not represent the end of living with an ED, or even signify the end of treatment, as some of the family members may have anticipated or hoped for initially when admitted. Although many viewed several aspects of hospitalization as beneficial, both for themselves and their family, it was clear that discharge from the EDU represented at best only half the job.

Subtheme 1: leaving the EDU while the ED is still on board

> It was very final, at least for us, when we were discharged, it was like "goodbye" and that's it. We never made any calls and I guess there were no openings either? We never heard that we could, and we didn't do it anyhow. I guess we probably could have done it, and maybe have the chance to have a conversation with somebody, but we felt it was very final, that we were not supposed to make any calls [to the EDU] and I guess it often feels like this, that it is a bit abrupt after such a long admission [Mother, Linda, *reflecting back on discharge*]

The majority of the participants remembered the immediate phase following discharge as very difficult. The ED was still present and exerted a great influence on the YP-AN and daily life as a family. Despite practice managing the recommended meal structure at the EDU during planned leaves, several parents acknowledged a prolonged admission or additional follow-up at the EDU as potentially beneficial after discharge. Some parents suggested that a scheduled brief "booster" re-admission would be beneficial, without having to undergo a full relapse to gain re-admission at the EDU or inpatient treatment elsewhere. Although discharge was known in advance and planned to a certain extent, several of the parents still perceived discharge as occurring suddenly and implied that it was not properly planned.

Even some of the YP-AN who initially resisted hospitalization felt the admission ended abruptly with insufficient planning and predictability. Some even reflected that a longer admission would have been beneficial, as they realized they had remaining ground to cover.

> When I was admitted, at the time I didn't eat by myself [nasogastric tube] ... Nor did I start with serving myself, and [thus] did never practice that, so, that I think was something we could have worked on... [Diana, 20 years, 17 during the admission, *on the potential benefit of having progressed further before being discharged*]

Subtheme 2: being transferred back to where it did not work out in the first place

> I didn't feel they had sufficient expertise; they didn't follow up appropriately [Father, Anthony, *on the decision of not going back to the local outpatient clinic after discharge*]

Most parents voiced concerns related to a treatment impasse at the local outpatient clinic prior to the admission, and found it difficult to accept a referral back to a treatment setting "where it did not work out in the first place." The majority had lost confidence in the local outpatient clinic and doubted the treatment team could provide assistance following admission to the family-based inpatient program. Skepticism was probably fueled by previous encounters and likely reinforced by receiving highly specialized treatment at the EDU. Similarly, several of the YP-AN also reflected on the paradox of being referred back to the same treatment setting where treatment had previously failed.

> I was sent back to the outpatient clinic where I had been prior to the admission and that did not work out at all. And the fact that I was sent back to that place, that was kind of... yes, it did not work out to say it bluntly. So, I'm having a hard time figuring out that one, why it was like that [...] And I met a person at the outpatient clinic that didn't know much, and that was very frustrating and contributed to the ED growing and gained more space again [Molly, 18 years, 15 during the admission, *on finding it difficult to accept that she had to go back to where it did not work, while implying how crucial expertise can be to prevent things getting worse*]

One solution for some families involved seeking treatment at a private practice instead of returning to the local outpatient clinic. Although initiated by parents, the decision resonated with the YP-AN's skepticism in returning to treatment at the local outpatient clinic.

> We didn't go back to the outpatient clinic, because we couldn't see that there was any therapist there that understood anything of this, and I have to say that we were very lucky to get in touch with a private practitioner, so we started there [Mother, Caroline, *on the difficulties with trusting the local outpatient clinic for further follow up post discharge, and recalling how all in all satisfied she was with finding an experienced private practitioner for her daughter and their family*]

Subtheme 3: for siblings, leaving the EDU meant leaving treatment for good: calling for better sibling involvement

Siblings also recalled continued hardships for the families following discharge. None of the siblings received additional involvement in treatment post-discharge. Upon reflection, parents and siblings called for a greater focus on siblings during the admission, as "siblings are an equally important part of the family," including siblings beyond chance meetings and an occasional session with a therapist.

Discussion

The current study contributes novel knowledge regarding user experiences which can supplement emerging research on adapting core aspects of evidence-based outpatient FBT into higher levels of care [6, 7, 16, 17]. Findings revealed five main themes capturing 14 subthemes (cf. Table 1 for brief summary). No evidence was found of any shared post-treatment family narrative. Participants demonstrated considerable diversity in viewpoints, which was interpreted as being contingent upon their role in the family, responsibilities and relationship to the ED. Without prescribing definitive answers, we believe the results have several implications for treatment providers working within a family-based inpatient treatment approach.

Main theme 1: *Expectations and evaluation of needs. Entering treatment from different vantage points.* This main theme is a useful reminder of the importance of recognizing and valuing the individual needs of families, and refraining from making immediate generalizations of YP-AN and their family members. Families are inevitably constituted by individuals that think, feel and behave differently, even while navigating the apparent "same" social phenomena such as hospitalization. During the pre-admission phase, we believe it is critical to allow sufficient time to explore central issues together with the YP-AN, their family, and the referral system. The findings suggest that different levels of readiness for change, knowledge of the ED as well as preparedness for the admission, in addition to varied expectations and needs are important to explore in-depth prior to an admission. Therefore, we strongly recommend that pre-admission sessions move beyond simply sharing information about the treatment program. The treatment team should enable sufficient time to transparently explore the mutual expectations of family members and treatment providers, investigate previous treatment experiences in-depth, and begin negotiating roles and responsibilities aligning with the overarching family-based treatment approach. Theme 1 also suggests the potential of providing YP-AN and their family members more structured or planned interventions prior to the admission. Without prescribing specific types of interventions, we would recommend the consideration of motivational enhancement sessions for the YP-AN [29, 30] in addition to a brief education program for parents aligning with the skills and content espoused by a family-based approach [25, 31]. It is feasible that an investment in greater resources prior to the admission may optimize the starting point and help the admission become more efficient. Lastly, the first theme emphasizes the importance of enhancing the focus on sibling involvement prior to the admission. Parents should not be left alone in determining how siblings should be informed and / or involved, as sibling involvement should naturally constitute a part of pre-treatment planning for a family-based admission for adolescent AN.

Main theme 2: *Interactions with peers during the admission as highly beneficial or problematic.* The finding that parents valued the mutual support and sharing of experiences with other families is consistent with prior studies of parental peer support and treatment satisfaction in multi-family group therapy [1]. Similarly, the difficulties in navigating peer relationships experienced by YP-AN during admission have also been reported in previous studies [19, 32, 33]. Siblings' perspectives indicated the benefit of engaging with other siblings, highlighting the importance of enhanced sibling interactions during admissions. Overall, the second main theme suggests the importance of strengthening multi-family work during admissions [34]. Inspired by these findings, we recommend that treatment providers carefully review how peer interactions are enabled and managed during admissions, and to evaluate how the inpatient context can be further optimized to utilize the rich knowledge base embedded in the family members' lived experiences [1, 35]. Specifically, results remind treatment providers to carefully identify and counter negative peer dynamics between the YP-AN during admissions, and to create opportunities to facilitate peer support. The latter is a potential direction of further investigation in collaboration with YP-AN who have prior inpatient treatment experience.

Main theme 3: *Perspectives on staff expertise and the EDU structure.* The majority of parents viewed the EDU structure and staff expertise as aiding their perceived parental self-efficacy, which is one of the proposed mechanisms of change in family-based treatments [6]. It is encouraging that most parents reported observable behavior change or symptom improvement, not simply treatment satisfaction. Such improvements tended to generally be ascribed to the opportunity to interact with knowledgeable staff and being supported by the EDU structures. Although encouraging, we believe the EDU needs to continue focusing on enabling parental empowerment during admissions [6, 11]. Importantly, the current findings suggest that perceived enhanced parental self-efficacy was not universally experienced. Similar to outpatient FBT [8], inpatient admission is not a panacea, and there is no "one way" to empower all parents. As parents and families enter treatment with unique vulnerabilities, experiences and needs, the therapeutic task of empowering parents must be continually negotiated and tailored to the individual parent's needs and vantage point.

Main theme 4: *Influencing within-family relationships in different ways.* Findings indicated that treatment was generally perceived to strengthen within-family relationships. This is a reassuring finding, as preventing fissures in relationships and strengthening collaboration within families comprise the core tenants of family-based treatment. Findings are also in accordance with an Australian study of an intensive 2-week family admission program [18]. Although findings generally aligned with the rationale for offering a family-based inpatient program, findings also question the family-based foundation of the program design, as none of the participating families stayed for the entire length of the admission. Thus, it is reasonable to question how family-based the program "really" is, when important members of the family system were rarely represented at the EDU, and thus not actively engaged in treatment. Involving the "whole" family is usually advocated in the literature, as this constitutes a pillar when providing treatment. Still, the prominent stance of "including the family" is often far removed from the day-to-day realities. This seems to resonate with research showing that clinicians regularly fail to sufficiently involve family members even when providing standard FBT, a treatment model that explicitly aims to include the family [36, 37]. Admitting a family for a prolonged time period is obviously demanding on resources and represents a highly complex treatment situation for which clear evidence to guide treatment providers is scarce. Research is sorely needed to understand how to best optimize the inpatient setting and to investigate whether engaging the whole family to a greater extent during hospitalizations can improve outcome and facilitate successful transitions after discharge.

Main theme 5: *Being admitted is at best only half the job: reflections on leaving the EDU.* In accordance with previous literature [12, 38], transitioning between services represented a vulnerable phase for our families. In general, findings suggested that clinicians carefully plan discharge with the family, and maintain a collaborative relationship with the referral system during the admission. As suggested by our findings, we believe that planning for discharge, and the vulnerable phase after the admission, needs to be properly addressed early during the admission. This includes exploring the expectations of family members, as well as the treatment providers responsible for referral and aftercare, regarding the goals of admission. This effort ensures expectations and goals are transparent, and can help orient everyone involved about the "reality" of the admission being a temporary part of the journey toward recovery [4]. All YP-AN, by definition, will need further specialized care after participation in the family-based admission, and therefore, a plan for the follow-up phase should ideally be decided upon prior to the admission and negotiated based on treatment progression. Collaboration with the referral system should be given more attention prior to the admission, and during treatment, in order to minimize the likelihood of families perceiving discharge as abrupt and poorly planned.

Strengths and limitations

Investigating user perspectives from three different positions (patient, parents, and siblings) is viewed as a strength. Throughout the analysis, we maintained a focus on the family. In our view, the experience of families is perhaps paradoxically lacking in many qualitative studies of family-based interventions, which often focus on the single views of the patient, parents, or siblings. An obvious limitation is the retrospective nature of the study. Unquestionably, the time elapsed between discharge and follow-up interviews may influence participants' recollections. Still, time has also enabled participants to reflect from a potentially more mature, self-reflexive, and thus, less emotionally-laden position, compared to being interviewed shortly after discharge. Another limitation is the sampling strategy. As few intact families were available in the dataset ($N = 8$), results cannot be generalized broadly, and different families may have provided difference responses. Thus, the analysis does not claim to provide a narrative on how family members generally experience family-based inpatient treatment. In addition, the specialized EDU treatment setting which offered treatment comprises a specific context not necessarily generalizable to other regions and countries. Still, we believe the findings, in addition to clinical implications derived, offer valuable insight and are relevant for treatment providers aiming to optimize family-based treatment at higher levels of care. Another limitation is that several interviewers with varying levels of interview skills took part in conducting the interviews. This may have affected the richness of the data. We also question whether the retrospective interview data, as in the current study, provides the best data source to inform further treatment development, which is the overarching aim for our qualitative research projects. Future research should aim to generate more detailed descriptions to guide the development of family-based treatment for adolescent AN at higher levels of care. We suggest improving the system for administering interviews (e.g., to administer interviews both during treatment and soon after discharge), together with ethnographic fieldwork in order to study practice as it unfolds in real time. Lastly, a potential limitation worth mentioning is that the patient and sibling transcripts have been utilized in our previous research, although with a different research purpose. This can have influenced both analysis and findings in the current study.

Conclusions

Our study offers insight into how former inpatients and their family members experienced an inpatient treatment program designed to align treatment with the central elements of an outpatient family-based treatment approach for adolescent anorexia nervosa. Overall, the findings support emerging research underlining the necessity of strengthening the family-based treatment approach within intensified treatment settings. Moreover, the results emphasized the need for more knowledge on how to optimize inpatient treatment as well as the importance of providing smooth transitions between care settings.

Abbreviations

AN: Anorexia nervosa; FBT: Family-based treatment; EDU: Eating disorder unit; YP-AN: Young person with anorexia nervosa; TA: Thematic analysis; IPA: Interpretative phenomenological analysis

Acknowledgements

The authors would like to thank all the participants for their greatly appreciated contributions to this research. We also would like to thank Anne-Lise Kvakland, Cathrine Olsen Voldnes, Tore William Larsen and Annika Rø for their contributions in conducting interviews. Special thanks to PhD Deborah Lynn Reas for the English proofreading.

Authors' contributions

Together with JVN, IH made a substantial contribution to developing the interview guides. IH was leading and supervising the data collection. JVN transcribed the interviews, read and re-read the whole data set several times. TWH read all transcripts. The process of developing the theme structure and analyzing and interpreting the data material was a collaborative effort between JVN and TWH, and done in dialogue with HWO, with JVN taking the lead throughout the process. JVN wrote the first draft of the manuscript. HWO supervised the whole process together with ØR and TWH, and all authors made substantial contributions to the final paper. All listed authors are accountable for all aspects of the work, including issues related to accuracy and integrity. All authors read and approved the final version of the manuscript.

Competing interests

The authors declare that they have no competing interests.

Author details

[1]Department of Psychology, University of Oslo, Oslo, Norway. [2]Regional Department for Eating Disorders, Division of Mental Health and Addiction, Oslo University Hospital, Oslo, Norway. [3]Institute of Clinical Medicine, University of Oslo, Oslo, Norway.

References

1. Eisler I, Simic M, Hodsoll J, Asen E, Berelowitz M, Connan F, et al. A pragmatic randomised multi-Centre trial of multifamily and single family therapy for adolescent anorexia nervosa. BMC Psychiatry. 2016;16:422.
2. Lock J, Le Grange D. In: Le Grange D, Russell G, editors. Treatment manual for anorexia nervosa : a family-based approach. 2nd ed. New York: Guilford Press; 2013.
3. Hilbert A, Hoek H, Schmidt R. Evidence-based clinical guidelines for eating disorders: international comparison. Curr Opin Psychiatr. 2017:423–37.
4. Isserlin L, Spettigue W, Norris M, Couturier J. Outcomes of inpatient psychological treatments for children and adolescents with eating disorders at time of discharge: a systematic review. J Eat Disord. 2020;8(1):32.
5. Lock J, Le Grange D. Family-based treatment: where are we and where should we be going to improve recovery in child and adolescent eating disorders. Int J Eat Disord. 2019;52(4):481–7.
6. Hoste RR. Incorporating family-based therapy principles into a partial hospitalization programme for adolescents with anorexia nervosa: challenges and considerations. J Fam Ther. 2015;37(1):41–60.
7. Halvorsen I, Reas DL, Nilsen JV, Ro O. Naturalistic outcome of family-based inpatient treatment for adolescents with anorexia nervosa. Eur Eat Disord Rev. 2017.
8. Le Grange D, Lock J. Family-based treatment is overvalued: reply to Strober. Adv Eat Disord. 2014;2(3):297–9.
9. Toulany A, Wong M, Katzman DK, Akseer N, Steinegger C, Hancock-Howard RL, et al. Cost analysis of inpatient treatment of anorexia nervosa in adolescents: hospital and caregiver perspectives. CMAJ Open. 2015;3(2): E192–E7.
10. Wallis A, Alford C, Hanson A, Titterton J, Madden S, Kohn M. Innovations in Maudsley family-based treatment for anorexia nervosa at the Children's Hospital at Westmead: a family admission programme. J Fam Ther. 2013;35: 68–81.
11. Murray SB, Anderson LK, Rockwell R, Griffiths S, Le Grange D, Kaye WH. Adapting family-based treatment for adolescent anorexia nervosa across higher levels of patient care. Eat Disord. 2015;23(4):302–14.
12. Treasure J, Schmidt U, Hugo P. Mind the gap: service transition and interface problems for patients with eating disorders. Br J Psychiatry. 2005; 187:398–400.
13. Khalsa SS, Portnoff LC, McCurdy-McKinnon D, Feusner JD. What happens after treatment? A systematic review of relapse, remission, and recovery in anorexia nervosa. J Eat Disord. 2017;5:20.
14. Rockwell RE, Boutelle K, Trunko ME, Jacobs MJ, Kaye WH. An innovative short-term, intensive, family-based treatment for adolescent anorexia nervosa: case series. Eur Eat Disord Rev. 2011;19(4):362.
15. Fjelkegård M, Hausswolff-Juhlin Y, Olsen EM. Hur påverkar involvering av familjen heldygnsbehandling av barn och tonåringar med restriktiv ätstörning? Fokus på familien. 2020;48(1):22–31.
16. Rienecke RD, Richmond RL. Three-month follow-up in a family-based partial hospitalization program. Eat Disord. 2018;26(3):278–89.
17. Spettigue W, Norris ML, Douziech I, Henderson K, Buchholz A, Valois DD, et al. Feasibility of implementing a family-based inpatient program for adolescents with anorexia nervosa: a retrospective cohort study. Front Psychiatry. 2019;10:887.
18. Fink K, Rhodes P, Miskovic-Wheatley J, Wallis A, Touyz S, Baudinet J, et al. Exploring the effects of a family admissions program for adolescents with anorexia nervosa. J Eat Disord. 2017;5:51.
19. Nilsen J-V, Hage TW, Rø Ø, Halvorsen I, Oddli HW. Family-based inpatient treatment for adolescent anorexia nervosa: a thematic analysis of former patients' post-treatment reflections. Eat Disord. 2019:1–18.
20. Halvorsen I, Ro O. User satisfaction with family-based inpatient treatment for adolescent anorexia nervosa: retrospective views of patients and parents. J Eat Disord. 2019;7:12.
21. Fjermestad KW, Rø AE, Espeland KE, Halvorsen MS, Halvorsen IM. "Do I exist in this world, really, or is it just her?" Youths' perspectives of living with a sibling with anorexia nervosa. Eat Disord. 2020;28(1):80-95.
22. Nilsen J-V, Hage TW, Rø Ø, Halvorsen I, Oddli HW. Minding the adolescent in family-based inpatient treatment for anorexia nervosa: a qualitative study of former inpatients' views on treatment collaboration and staff behaviors. BMC Psychol. 2019;7(1):72.
23. Maxwell J, Chmiel M. Generalization in and from qualitative analysis. 2014 2018/10/12. In: The SAGE handbook of qualitative data analysis [internet]. London: SAGE Publications Ltd. Available from: http://methods.sagepub.com/book/the-sage-handbook-of-qualitative-data-analysis. Accessed 10 Nov 2020.
24. Rienecke RD. Family-based treatment of eating disorders in adolescents: current insights. Adolesc Health Med Ther. 2017;8:69–79.
25. Toubøl A, Koch-Christensen H, Bruun P, Nielsen DS. Parenting skills after participation in skills-based training inspired by the New Maudsley Method: a qualitative study in an outpatient eating disorder setting. Scand J Caring Sci. 2019;33(4):959-68.
26. Larkin M, Shaw R, Flowers P. Multiperspectival designs and processes in interpretative phenomenological analysis research. Qual Res Psychol. 2019; 16(2):182–98.
27. Braun V, Clarke V. Using thematic analysis in psychology. Qual Res Psychol. 2006;3(2):77–101.
28. Smith B, Sparkes AC. Narrative inquiry in psychology: exploring the tensions within. Qual Res Psychol. 2006;3(3):169–92.
29. Vitousek K, Watson S, Wilson GT. Enhancing motivation for change in treatment-resistant eating disorders. Clin Psychol Rev. 1998;18(4):391–420.
30. Geller J. What a motivational approach is and what a motivational approach isn't: reflections and responses. Eur Eat Disord Rev. 2002;10:155–60.
31. Goodier GH, McCormack J, Egan SJ, Watson HJ, Hoiles KJ, Todd G, et al. Parent skills training treatment for parents of children and adolescents with eating disorders: a qualitative study. Int J Eat Disord. 2014;47(4):368-75.

32. Vandereycken W. Can eating disorders become 'contagious' in group therapy and specialized inpatient care? Eur Eat Disord Rev. 2011;19(4): 289–95.
33. Espíndola C, Blay S. Anorexia Nervosa's meaning to patients: a qualitative synthesis. Psychopathology. 2009;42(2):69–80.
34. Depestele L, Claes L, Dierckx E, Colman R, Schoevaerts K, Lemmens GMD. An adjunctive multi-family group intervention with or without patient participation during an inpatient treatment for adolescents with an eating disorder: a pilot study. Eur Eat Disord Rev. 2017;25(6):570–8.
35. Engman-Bredvik S, Carballeira Suarez N, Levi R, Nilsson K. Multi-family therapy in anorexia nervosa--a qualitative study of parental experiences. Eat Disord. 2016;24(2):186–97.
36. Hughes EK, Burton C, Le Grange D, Sawyer SM. How well are we engaging the family in family-based treatment for adolescent anorexia nervosa? J Eat Disord. 2015;3(Suppl 1):O49.
37. Hughes EK, Burton C, Le Grange D, Sawyer SM. The Participation of Mothers, Fathers, and Siblings in Family-Based Treatment for Adolescent Anorexia Nervosa. J Clin Child Adolescent Psychol. 2018;47(sup1):S456-S66.
38. Dimitropoulos G, Toulany A, Herschman J, Kovacs A, Steinegger C, Bardsley J, et al. A qualitative study on the experiences of young adults with eating disorders transferring from pediatric to adult care. Eat Disord. 2015;23(2):144–62.

19

Sharing and connecting with others – patient experiences of radically open dialectical behavior therapy for anorexia nervosa and overcontrol

Martina Isaksson[1*], Ata Ghaderi[2,3], Martina Wolf-Arehult[1,4], Caisa Öster[1] and Mia Ramklint[1]

Abstract

Background: Recovery rates after psychological treatments for anorexia nervosa are low to moderate, and in adults, no treatment outperforms any other. The aim of this study was to evaluate patient experiences of Radically open dialectical behavior therapy (RO DBT), a treatment developed for disorders related to maladaptive overcontrol.

Methods: Eleven female patients with anorexia nervosa were interviewed after either treatment completion (eight patients) or drop-out (three patients) from RO DBT. Interviews were transcribed and analyzed with inductive thematic analysis.

Results: The analysis yielded five main themes: 1) a comprehensive treatment, 2) the benefits of sharing and connecting with others, 3) growing trust, 4) moving toward valued goals – but some remain, and 5) doing well in treatment.

Conclusion: Patients appreciated what they described as a comprehensive treatment and holistic view of their problems, which helped them reduce both maladaptive overcontrol and eating disorder symptoms. Gradually sharing personal experiences both in- and outside therapy was described as essential and led to enhanced social connectedness.

Keywords: Eating disorder, Anorexia, Qualitative analysis, Thematic analysis, Radically open dialectical behavior therapy, RO DBT

* Correspondence: martina.isaksson@neuro.uu.se
[1]Department of Neuroscience, Psychiatry, Uppsala University, Entrance 10, Floor 3B, SE-751 85 Uppsala, Sweden
Full list of author information is available at the end of the article

Plain English summary

Anorexia nervosa is a severe psychiatric disorder and recovery rates after psychological treatments are low to moderate. Both patients and clinicians have raised criticism of the treatments that are most frequently offered, suggesting that there is too much focus on food and weight, with little emphasis on psychological and social needs and what may have caused the disorder. Excessive overcontrol, characterized by e.g., rigidity, inhibition of showing feelings, and social distancing, has been suggested as an important mechanism for developing the disorder. In the present study, we evaluated how patients that had participated in Radically open dialectical behavior therapy (RO DBT), a psychological treatment developed for disorders related to excessive overcontrol, experienced the treatment. Eleven patients with anorexia were interviewed after they either had completed (eight patients) or dropped out (three patients) from the treatment. Their experiences were recorded and the recordings transcribed to written text. After, the text was analyzed and the content was categorized in overarching themes. Patients appreciated what they described as a comprehensive treatment. They described that the treatment had a holistic view of their problems, beyond mere focus on food and weight, which helped them reduce both maladaptive overcontrol and eating disorder symptoms. Patients also described that they wanted to do well in treatment, and that their trust in the treatment and their therapists improved as therapy progressed. Finally, gradually sharing personal experiences both in- and outside therapy was described as important for recovery.

Introduction

There is no superior psychological treatment for adults with anorexia nervosa (AN) [1]. Recovery rates are generally low to moderate, varying between around 10 and 40%, and attrition and relapse rates are high [2]. Clinical guidelines recommend a combination of psychotherapeutic treatment and re-nourishment, and that the majority of patients with AN should be treated in outpatient care [1, 3]. However, severe AN or lack of improvement indicate a need for meal support in a day program or inpatient care. Among other things, it has been recommended that new interventions be developed to improve treatment outcome [1, 4].

When evaluating new treatment approaches, experimental designs are essential [5]. However, information on the patients' own experiences may supplement quantitative data, which is of particular importance in early phases of complex intervention evaluation [6]. Qualitative research may promote a better understanding of treatment effect and fidelity and aid identification of potential mechanisms of change [6]. However, little is known about patient experiences of outpatient treatments for AN. Patients often experience that AN treatments in general (both in- and outpatient) are too rigid, with an excessive focus on food and weight [7] and too little emphasis on psychological and social needs and what may have caused the disorder [8, 9]. Some researchers have raised similar criticisms, suggesting that the treatments most frequently offered focus too much on symptom reduction, while failing to address the core psychopathology of AN [10–12].

Overcontrol has been suggested as a potentially important mechanism for development and maintenance of AN [13, 14]. While self-control, or overcontrol, is defined as the ability to inhibit emotional urges, impulses, and behaviors to pursue long-term goals [15, 16], *excessive* overcontrol is when self-control, emotion inhibition, and rigidity reach a degree that severely affects the individual's well-being [16]. Radically open dialectical behavior therapy (RO DBT) is a treatment developed for patients with psychiatric disorders linked to excessive overcontrol difficulties. In RO DBT, emotional loneliness is regarded as the core problem, resulting from low openness (e.g., rigidity and dismissing feedback) and deficits in social signaling (e.g., smiling when distressed or inhibited sharing of personal experiences). Thus, both openness and social signaling are considered to be potentially important mechanisms of change to enhance social connectedness and increase well-being [14, 16]. The capacity to openly adapt to situational demands and to express emotions is practiced and reinforced during treatment. Also, an open, self-disclosing, genuine, and relaxed therapeutic stance is used to model adaptive social signaling and increase patient engagement (Lynch [17], page 406).

There have been studies evaluating treatment effect of RO DBT for AN [18–20]. However, no evaluation assessing both treatment effect and patient experiences has been performed. Studies evaluating patient experiences of outpatient AN treatments are few, in particular for treatment approaches with a broader focus than mainly ED symptoms. The aim of the present study was to evaluate patient experiences of RO DBT for AN and overcontrol in a clinical outpatient setting. Details on quantitative results are reported in an experimental, multiple baseline single-case experimental design study that can be found elsewhere [21], preregistered in the ISRCTN registry (no: ISRCTN47156042, URL: https://www.isrctn.com/ISRCTN47156042).

Methods

Research design

Patient experiences were evaluated using an inductive qualitative thematic analysis as described by Braun and Clarke [22]. Analyses were performed using the following steps: familiarizing with the text, coding, generating themes, reviewing themes, defining and naming themes, and writing and exemplifying themes. The method was chosen because it is suitable for evaluating patient experiences, and because it is flexible and appropriate for managing rich data material.

Participants, setting, and procedure

All thirteen patients who had participated in the experimental evaluation of RO DBT for AN at the eating disorder (ED) clinic at Uppsala University Hospital were eligible for participation. Because the study sought to evaluate the effects of outpatient treatment, only patients with a BMI $\geq 16\,kg/m^2$ were included, as patients with severe AN are generally treated with inpatient care or with extensive meal support in a day program. In addition, because RO DBT is only relevant for patients with overcontrol tendencies, each patient's personality style was identified based on the prototype rating by Lynch ([17], p. 81–82). Excluded were patients 1) in need of intense care for ED or treatment for another disorder, 2) participating in psychological treatment within three months before study start, or 3) with cognitive difficulties or difficulties with the Swedish language, based on if a patient could not independently fill out questionnaires or answer questions during interviews.

A research assistant not involved in the treatment contacted the patients via phone to provide information about the qualitative interview. Each patient who was willing to participate was booked for a face-to-face interview within a month from treatment termination. Eleven patients accepted – all eight completers and three out of five non-completers from the single-case study of treatment effect. Written informed consent was obtained from all 11 participants.

Participants were diagnosed with mild to moderate AN (ten patients) or atypical AN (one patient). Full criteria for AN and atypical AN diagnoses were met at the start of treatment. Mean age was 25 years, standard deviation (*SD*) = 6.02, range 18–41. Mean ED onset was at 15 years of age (*SD* = 2.64), range 10–20. The mean duration of the ED was 9 years (*SD* = 6.42), range 1–27. The number of comorbid diagnoses was between one and three. All eight completers were in remission after treatment, with BMI within a healthy range and ED psychopathology within one SD of the community mean. The non-completers were either in partial remission or not improved. Ethical approval was obtained by the Regional Ethics Committee in Uppsala (Ref. no. 2014/252).

The treatment

RO DBT is a transdiagnostic treatment developed for people with excessive overcontrol, identified in a spectrum of disorders such as AN, chronic depression, and cluster A and C personality disorders [14, 17]. Long-term goals in RO DBT are to form warm and intimate relationships and to reduce emotional loneliness. RO DBT differs from other treatments for AN. For example, rather than mainly focusing on weight restoration and ED symptoms – openness, flexibility, and social signaling are emphasized as key mechanisms of the treatment. A comprehensive description of the RO DBT treatment is provided in the textbook [17] and skills training manual [23] by professor Lynch. Material essential for providing RO DBT was translated to Swedish and used in the present study [24, 25].

The RO DBT intervention at the ED clinic in Uppsala was performed in outpatient care. It consisted of two phases: 1) an initial engagement phase of 6 weeks, orientating the patient to the RO DBT treatment and taking the first steps toward healthy eating and weight, and 2) 34 weeks of both individual therapy and skills class, focusing on enhancing openness, flexibility and social connectedness.

The interviews

A semi-structured interview guide was developed to explore the patients' overall experiences of the treatment, and began with an open question asking participants to describe their experiences. Subsequent questions covered the experiences of the treatment's contents and structure, the therapeutic relationship, potential differences from previous treatments, potential areas for improvement of the treatment, and the participant's changes or lack of changes during treatment. Probing questions were used throughout each interview to get the participant to develop their answers or give examples. Interview time ranged between 25 and 85 min. A research assistant who had training and experience in interview technique performed the interviews. The interviewer had no involvement in the preceding treatment, and had no knowledge of the outcome for any of the patients. Prior to the interviews, subjects were informed that interviews would be anonymized, with identifiers removed before analyses. Interviews were audio-recorded and transcribed verbatim by another research assistant not otherwise involved in this project. Identifiers such as patient and therapist names were removed.

Data analysis

To ensure methodological quality, transcripts were reviewed separately by two independent reviewers, the first author (one of the RO DBT therapists) and the fourth author (with extensive experience in qualitative analyses and no involvement in the ED clinic). First, interviews were read and reread to give the reviewers familiarity with the contents. Second, text relevant for the research question and aim was coded with appropriate labels. Third, themes and subthemes were generated by identifying patterns among the labels. To make sure the themes represented the data, interviews were reread several times. Fourth, the first and fourth author compared their findings, discussed and resolved any differences, and came up with preliminary names for the themes. Fifth, the process of reviewing the themes, going back to the interviews, recoding under the new themes, and discussing was performed a second time. Lastly, themes with codes were presented to the other authors and disagreements were discussed until agreement was achieved.

Because we only had a limited number of potential participants (i.e., 13), analysis of data saturations was not used in the recruitment procedure. However, no new categories emerged when going through the last interviews.

Results

Five main themes were identified: 1) a comprehensive treatment, 2) the benefits of sharing and connecting with others, 3) growing trust, 4) moving toward valued goals – but some remain, and 5) doing well in treatment. Between two and four subthemes were identified within each main theme. Themes and subthemes are described below and presented in a summary in the Additional file 1.

A comprehensive treatment

A flexible and complex approach

Patients expressed appreciation for the fact that the treatment was intense and comprehensive with a holistic view on their problems, both in response to the initial open question and when they contrasted it to previous treatments. The treatment was also experienced as flexible, with interventions adapted to individual needs.

> *I felt that this treatment is more thorough than previous treatments ... you see the whole person and nothing fell through the cracks ... you're not only focusing too narrowly on the eating disorder. (Participant 9)*

Patients also said they liked that RO DBT included both individual therapy and skills training. Some highlighted that it was helpful with text message contact between sessions, others appreciated that contact through text messaging was available, even if they did not use it. Individual therapy was described as essential for adapting the therapy to fit individual needs. Descriptions mentioned that the treatment dealt with the ED from multiple perspectives, that it was adequately long, and that the balance between working with overcontrol in general, such as social signaling, relationships and emotions, and working with ED symptoms, was helpful.

> *There has been a lot of focus on feelings and relationships, which is very different from previous treatments. I've been to day programs several times, focusing only on eating, but that has not been therapy ... and once I went to regular therapy with no focus on the food - which made me sink like a stone. This therapy has been a good balance. I was allowed to talk about food if I felt "I have to talk about this and get a structure!" ... It's been a very good combination. (Participant 4)*

Even though most participants highlighted the flexibility of the treatment as a strength, one description included a wish for even more flexibility. It was also mentioned that severe ED symptoms, such as starvation, were sometimes an obstacle to working with overcontrol and participating in the skills class, as they made it hard to grasp the essence and the sometimes demanding material and training. Both the lack of flexibility in receiving more help if needed, and the preoccupation with food and weight, was experienced as a hinder for completing the treatment. Some experienced the contents and the materials in skills class as extensive or complicated, while others felt they were overly simplified.

> *It was hard to focus on other things because I was so caught up in the eating disorder and everything else became less interesting, I was kind of hijacked by the eating disorder ... I think it would be easier if you are more stable. (Participant 1)*

Following, or not following, the treatment wholeheartedly

Following the treatment wholeheartedly was necessary for it to be helpful. It was also essential to make the decision to challenge your fears and actually practice applying the skills. Some participants described that they did not put enough time and effort into the treatment, and experienced that fear and not being receptive to change prevented them from getting better.

> *It is important to try to be actively involved and let the treatment come first, to do it at a hundred percent. (Participant 10)*

Skills for moving toward valued goals

Values were highlighted as being important for recovery, and skills as helpful for moving toward valued goals. Recurrent and continuous emphasis on values and valued goals helped patients remember and reflect on why they were doing certain things, such as gaining weight or challenging their fears.

> *It's like, what do I want to be like? Do I want to sit there when I'm 65, by myself, because no one wants to hang out with you any more, that's not how you want your life to be. You want to be able to see that you've done fun stuff. (Participant 7)*

Various skills were pinpointed as helpful. Examples included working with chain analyses to learn how to see patterns, activating their parasympathetic nervous system in order to feel safe in social situations, participating without planning ahead, and using self-enquiry to learn more about oneself. Another example was enhancing intimacy in relationships through sharing personal experiences, e.g., by using a skill called "Match + 1" that helped the patient increase interpersonal warmth and closeness.

> *I think it is called match, when you start small and go deeper and deeper in the relationship when you talk to someone ... I did this when I met a friend, for like half a year, and in the end I was able talk about almost anything. (Participant 4)*

Patients described that not gaining adequate skills, for example for reducing anxiety, not following up on homework assignments, or not generalizing enough to the home environment might have hindered progress. Some felt that the material in skills class did not always fit their needs.

The benefits of sharing and connecting with others

A trusting and genuine therapeutic relationship

A trusting, honest and open therapeutic relationship was important in the therapy. In particular, the open and genuine atmosphere was highlighted by the participants as being essential for sharing personal experiences and connecting with the therapist.

> *It was nice that we had a genuine tone, If I did something my therapist thought was strange, she told me. And if I thought she did anything that was strange, I told her ... that was helpful. (Participant 3)*

Patients also stated that they liked their therapist and felt that the therapist cared for and understood them. Several patients described the therapists as relaxed. It was seen as important that the therapist believed it was possible to get better; hope could fade if the therapist no longer communicated that change was possible. One description mentioned feelings of being reserved in therapy because of being scared of not being good enough or not being liked by the therapist.

> *I don't think it had anything to do with the therapist, I have trust issues and am afraid of not being liked ... When I finally let my guard down and dared to show what I felt, then it was easier to feel trust. (Participant 1)*

Not being open to the therapist and not feeling like the therapist believed in change, could contribute to treatment drop-out.

Sharing and connecting with others in the group

The skills group provided an opportunity to practice sharing personal information and opinions with others. In particular, patients described sharing as important, saying it helped them recognize themselves in others and gain new perspectives and social connectedness. The experience of opening up and showing weakness – and still being accepted in the group – was seen as helpful.

> *It was hard at first because you talked about sensitive stuff, but it was really rewarding hearing the others and recognizing myself in them ... It was nice, you could help each other out, many of the things they said to me when I told them about things, I still remember and carry with me. (Participant 2)*

Patients welcomed that the instructors encouraged openness, and felt that the more they got to know the group, the better things got. If a new member joined, the group became more closed again for a while. Though most patients appreciated that the group was focused on life outside the ED, others wished for more opportunities to talk about the ED. One description mentioned not feeling safe in the group, contributing to treatment drop-out.

Growing trust

Initial skepticism

There was an initial skepticism regarding various aspects of the therapy, e.g., sharing experiences and thoughts with the therapists and peers in the skills training. However, trust grew as the therapy progressed thanks to the perceived open and non-judgmental approach. Some questioned the contents of the treatment in the beginning, but this changed as the therapy progressed.

> *In the beginning I felt like "these questions are really uncomfortable, I don't want to do this", that's why I was skeptical in the beginning ... I wanted solutions right away, like "This is what you should do" and "if I do that everything will be fine". I know it doesn't really work like that, but that's what I wanted ... But looking back it was really helpful. (Participant 5)*

Initial skepticism was partly based on the participants' feelings of agony that came with exposure to something stressful. However, aversive feelings and physiological reactions also helped patients realize that something needed to be challenged. Openness in the group and the therapeutic relationship, as well as skills, helped them overcome such skepticism.

> *In the beginning I was really suspicious and did not feel that I trusted my therapist ... But the better I got, the more proof I got that what she did was good. And also ... the more you open up to someone, a bond grows, whether you want it to or not. (Participant 3)*

Change takes time

Patients who completed treatment mentioned that change was not immediate, but growing as therapy progressed. It was important to highlight that things might get harder first and that the benefits could come later. Initially, confronting anxiety and gaining weight was difficult and it was important to highlight that a change in well-being would not come just because the weight began stabilizing.

> *I did a lot of comparing: how fat I was, and if I had breakfast and felt full, that was the only thing I could think of. But then it gradually changed, and like in November I noticed "It's been several days and I have been sitting on my bus and didn't think about it, I've been thinking about other stuff" — but this was after several months of struggles. (Participant 2)*

Moving toward valued goals – but some remain

Getting to know myself in a kind, but sometimes painful, way

Getting to know oneself in a kind way, even though it was sometimes painful, was perceived as a helpful process. The treatment gave the participants new perspectives, self-knowledge and self-awareness through self-enquiry. Reflecting on oneself was perceived as difficult: seeing who you really were, not just what you presented to others. Patients also described the experience of learning to embrace the pain and reflect, rather than escape. Many descriptions mentioned that participants liked themselves more and were kinder toward themselves after the treatment.

> *Self-enquiry was one of the most positive things for me, to try and find the core, like "why does this make me sad or upset?" "What is this about?" Previously I kind of moved on and just dealt with things ... but to take the time and find the essence is kind of a starting point to actually change, because you find out what really needs to change. (Participant 11)*

Receiving feedback on their social signaling was described as helpful to improve self-awareness and change overcontrolled behaviors.

> *It's like with the body language, like "yeah I have a quite closed body language ... oh, so of course people don't find it enjoyable to talk to me" ... now I know that about myself and how to handle it. (Participant 3)*

A journey from rigidity to more flexibility, openness, and connectedness

Patients reported that they had gained improved flexibility and freedom, acting more from personal values than from a desire to be perfect and avoid distress. Some felt that the perfectionistic tendencies remained, but they became more able to make mistakes and did not act based on their fears to the same extent. Examples of participating without planning ahead and letting others do things in their own way were described. Changing from avoiding things to showing vulnerability, being more open and being able to show their real feelings, helped improve and deepen relationships.

> *Even if it is hard to show it or talk about it, I really try to do it anyway ... with some friends. Before, I tried to control other people's picture of me a lot, I do that less now, I really try to show more of who I am ... because I noticed that it has brought me stronger and better relationships. (Participant 4)*

Changes in the eating disorder

Patients described a normalization of their weight and less ED symptoms, improved flexibility and new perspectives on their body. For example, they described that their body was healthy, that they learned to listen to their body, and that their body was better suited for life in accordance with their personal values. Patients also described that they saw the connection between the ED and their overcontrol and relational difficulties, and that the eating had changed due to changes in the overcontrol behaviors.

> *I've been able to let go of these thoughts about having a certain body and a certain weight, there are other things in life that are more important. There are days where I want to go with the eating disorder, but then I remind myself ... "there are friends and school and things that I enjoy doing" ... yeah, it's really nice to have a life. (Participant 6)*

> *There is nothing I can't eat anymore, that is a huge difference ... and when you don't have as many*

"don'ts" you can be more social ... and eat lunch with a friend, and it's not so strict where and when. (Participant 8)

... but some remain

Descriptions related to an absence of improvement mentioned that the ED changed character but had not improved, that it was too difficult to make changes, or an unwillingness to continue weight restoration, resulting in treatment drop-out. One description mentioned an intention of coming back to treatment after additional care. Patients sometimes described that they were healthier than before, but that some problems, such as weighing and measuring food at times or having issues with their body, remained. It was also noted that it was challenging to try new things, to start sharing experiences in social situations, and that it was scary and difficult to get closer to others.

... there are some left, and I think it will take some time before that goes away too. I can get a lot of feelings of being fat at times ... I guess that is what's still left, and the fact that I need an approximate plan for my meal routines. (Participant 5)

Doing well in treatment

Not wanting to be a bother

The idea of potentially bothering the therapist was described as an obstacle to seeking contact and asking for help, especially in between sessions and through text messaging. Participants experienced that their difficulties with wanting to perform well or that they felt they were not doing well enough or were not liked by the therapist might have hindered them from seeking as much contact as they would have wanted.

It felt difficult to contact her in between sessions, I felt like I was bothering her ... I called a few times when I panicked and really wanted to deal with something. But this way of working between sessions was totally new to me ... it could have been clearer, like "It's not that I'm being nice to you, this is a part of my job, I want you to call". (Participant 4)

Being the best of patients

Wanting to be a good patient and do well in treatment was common, especially in comparison with others in the skills class. These ideas could be either helpful (e.g., pushing yourself in doing the homework or sharing in skills class) or unhelpful (e.g., not feeling like you were doing enough, or wanting to do too much, making the treatment stressful which might have contributed to treatment drop-out).

It was good that there were other people in the group ... it felt a bit like you're not only disappointing yourself if you're not working on a homework assignment, but the others in the group as well. (Participant 3)

It was also considered helpful that it was seen as acceptable not to do everything perfectly in treatment. Social comparison in that area could be beneficial at times, since it was focused on adaptive skills, not on food or the ED.

If someone hadn't done something as well as the others in skills class, it was okay. I think that was a relief, since there wasn't so much pressure on doing things perfectly. It's like, what is a perfect treatment, should you be the perfect RO patient, or what?". (Participant 5)

Discussion

The aim of this study was to evaluate patient experiences of RO DBT in outpatient treatment for AN.

In general, RO DBT was described as a flexible and complex treatment with a holistic view of the patients' difficulties. More specifically, the combination of different treatment components, as well as the broader focus beyond ED symptoms, were highlighted as helpful. Indeed, treatments of AN have often been described by patients as having an excessive focus on food and weight, lacking a broad focus beyond the ED [7–9]. At the same time, it is known that re-nourishment and weight gain are essential to recover from AN [1, 3]. The findings in this study, with patients expressing appreciation for the fact that both their ED symptoms and their rigid, emotional, and relational difficulties were addressed, might indicate that RO DBT is a treatment that both is in line with the clinical guidelines and appeal to the patients.

Nevertheless, like in other outpatient treatments for AN [26–28], a significant number of patients ($n = 5$, 38%) dropped out from RO DBT. Three of those who dropped out participated in the interviews. There were no descriptions of the treatment per se as a bad fit. However, the interviews suggest that social comparison and not feeling safe in skills class might increase the risk for drop-out. Drop-out was also described as a consequence of difficulties in understanding the demanding material and in keeping a focus on overcontrol while being preoccupied with food and weight. These findings may correspond to research suggesting that a brain in starvation is less plastic and receptive to psychological treatments [29, 30]. However, day treatment programs [20] and inpatient treatment [19] with RO DBT for more severe AN have shown positive results. Further, it has been suggested that weight restoration and medical issues should be supported with appropriate interventions (e.g., medical management) while providing the RO DBT treatment [31, 32]. Based on the results in this study and in the single-case study of treatment effect, as well as previous research, it is reasonable to assume that RO DBT as outpatient treatment only (e.g., without additional meal support) might be sufficient for mild to moderate levels of AN and overcontrol. Patients with severe or enduring AN might be highly affected by starvation or other ED symptoms, making it difficult to fully engage in the RO DBT if delivered as the sole intervention. These patients are likely in need of additional support, e.g., by providing initial inpatient treatment or day program before or along the RO DBT treatment. A more flexible approach could have the potential to both reduce drop-out and improve clinical utility. Whether these adaptations affect drop-out and outcome has, however, not been evaluated. Moreover, the field is in need of additional evaluation. In particular, larger studies evaluating the efficacy of RO DBT for AN, in addition to contrasting it to other treatments, are warranted.

Another important aspect that emerged across several themes was the open and sharing atmosphere in both skills class and individual therapy. Most patients described the therapeutic relationship as good and helpful, highlighting that the therapists were genuine, open, relaxed, and able to understand them and that this helped them open up to their therapist and engage in treatment. This is in line with previous research, underlining the importance of an authentic and strong therapeutic relationship [7, 33] and its association with positive treatment outcome [34]. In RO DBT, enhanced openness and social signaling are also hypothesized to be important mechanisms for change toward a healthier life [16]. The patients' perceptions of the value of sharing personal experiences in this study supported these ideas.

While some patients reported no improvement or merely a shift in how their ED difficulties appeared, several areas of improvement – such as a healthier weight, less ED symptoms, and stronger relationships – were described in most interviews. This also corresponds to the result from the single-case study of treatment effects [35], in which all eight completers, all of whom participated in this qualitative evaluation, displayed both healthy weight and ED symptoms within one SD of the community mean (i.e., no or minor residual ED symptoms) after treatment. Patients described increased self-awareness, more openness in their personal relationships, and increased flexibility. Interestingly, the effect on outcomes related to overcontrol was small in the single-case study of treatment effect. By reviewing qualitative data in addition to quantitative results, a more comprehensive picture of patient experiences of changes or lack of changes might be gained. For example, it is possible that the small effects in overcontrol in the quantitative evaluation were a result of unsatisfactory quantitative self-rating measurements. Moreover, it is likely easier to measure distinct ED symptoms such as restrictive or rigid eating, where validated instruments exist, than factors related to psychological well-being in general, and overcontrol in particular – such as flexibility and usage of social signaling. Findings in the present study underline the importance of developing quantitative instruments that can assess behavioral changes in relation to social signaling and an overcontrolled personality style.

Strengths and limitations

Demographic and clinical data do not allow for any conclusions regarding severely underweight or male participants. Limitations also include the relatively low number of participants, especially patients dropping out from treatment. Thus, even though saturation was reached overall, it is likely that data on reasons for treatment drop-out were incomplete. Also, one of the therapists participated in the qualitative analyses, which might have affected how data were interpreted and analyzed. To address this issue, an experienced researcher without any involvement in the study was invited to perform the analyses. The diverse research group is also a strength, providing different backgrounds and perspectives.

Conclusion and future research

This study is the first to provide a qualitative evaluation of outpatient RO DBT for AN, and one of few to evaluate the experiences of treatment for outpatient AN in general. The results indicated that patients appreciated the comprehensive treatment and the holistic view of their difficulties. In particular, patients described sharing as important for progress in all aspects of therapy: individual therapy, skills class, and in relationships outside therapy. Thus, patient experience suggest that a treatment with a main focus on overcontrol in AN is promising for treating the disorder. Future research should continue evaluating reasons for treatment drop-out, and identify valid quantitative measurements that can be used to assess behavioral changes in overcontrol. Research should also include evaluation of potential mechanisms of change – e.g., change in social signaling behaviors.

Abbreviations

AN: Anorexia nervosa; BMI: Body mass index; DSM: Diagnostic and statistical manual of mental disorders; ED: Eating disorder; RO DBT: Radically open dialectical behavior therapy; SD: Standard deviation

Acknowledgments

We would like to thank all the participants for their involvement in the study, Region Uppsala for providing a salary to the first author, and Märta and Nicke Nasvell foundation for financial support. Additionally, we thank Ann-Charlotte Fält and Ylva Walldén and for their contributions.

Consent to participate
Informed consent was obtained from all individual participants included in the study.

Authors' contributions
All authors contributed substantially to each part of the manuscript. The first draft of the manuscript was written by Martina Isaksson and all authors commented on previous versions of the manuscript. All authors read and approved the final manuscript.

Competing interests
The authors declare that they have no conflict of interest.

Author details
[1]Department of Neuroscience, Psychiatry, Uppsala University, Entrance 10, Floor 3B, SE-751 85 Uppsala, Sweden. [2]Division of Psychology, Department of Clinical Neuroscience, Karolinska Institutet, SE-171 77 Stockholm, Sweden. [3]Stockholm Centre for Eating Disorders, Stockholm Health Care Services, Stockholm County Council, SE-171 77 Stockholm, Sweden. [4]Psychiatry Northwest, Region Stockholm, Clinical Management, PO Box 98, SE-191 22 Sollentuna, Sweden.

References

1. Zipfel S, Giel KE, Bulik CM, Hay P, Schmidt U. Anorexia nervosa: Aetiology, assessment, and treatment. Lancet Psychiatry. 2015;2:1099–111. https://doi.org/10.1016/S2215-0366(15)00356-9.
2. Brockmeyer T, Friederich HC, Schmidt U. Advances in the treatment of anorexia nervosa: a review of established and emerging interventions. Psychol Med. 2018;48:1228–56. https://doi.org/10.1017/S0033291717002604.
3. National Institute for Health and Care Excellence. Eating disorders: recognition and treatment. (NICE guideline No. 69) [Internet]. 2017.
4. Holmes EA, Ghaderi A, Harmer CJ, Ramchandani PG, Cuijpers P, Morrison AP, et al. The lancet psychiatry commission on psychological treatments research in tomorrow's science. Lancet Psychiatry Elsevier Ltd. 2018;5:237–86. https://doi.org/10.1016/S2215-0366(17)30513-8.
5. Craig P, Dieppe P, Macintyre S, Michie S, Nazareth I, Petticrew M. Developing and evaluating complex interventions: the new Medical Research Council guidance. Int J Nurs Stud Elsevier Ltd. 2013;50:587–92. https://doi.org/10.1016/j.ijnurstu.2012.09.010.
6. Crawford MJ, Weaver T, Rutter D, Sensky T, Tyrer P. Evaluating new treatments in psychiatry: the potential value of combining qualitative and quantitative research methods. Int Rev Psychiatry. 2002;14:6–11. https://doi.org/10.1080/09540260120114005.
7. Rance N, Moller NP, Clarke V. "Eating disorders are not about food, they're about life": client perspectives on anorexia nervosa treatment. J Health Psychol. 2017;22:582–94. https://doi.org/10.1177/1359105315609088.
8. Eivors A, Button E, Warner S, Turner K. Understanding the experience of drop-out from treatment for anorexia nervosa. Eur Eat Disord Rev. 2003;11: 90–107. https://doi.org/10.1002/erv.492.
9. Westwood LM, Kendal SE. Adolescent client views towards the treatment of anorexia nervosa: a review of the literature. J Psychiatr Ment Health Nurs. 2012;19:500–8. https://doi.org/10.1111/j.1365-2850.2011.01819.x.
10. Watson HJ, Bulik CM. Update on the treatment of anorexia nervosa: review of clinical trials, practice guidelines and emerging interventions. Psychol Med. 2013;43:2477–500. https://doi.org/10.1017/S0033291712002620.
11. Martinez MA, Craighead LW. Toward person(ality)-centered treatment: how consideration of personality and individual differences in anorexia nervosa may improve treatment outcome. Clin Psychol Sci Pract. 2015;22:296–314. https://doi.org/10.1111/cpsp.12111.
12. Lynch TR, Hempel RJ, Whalley B, Byford S, Chamba R, Clarke P, et al. Refractory depression - mechanisms and efficacy of radically open dialectical behaviour therapy (RefraMED): findings of a randomised trial on benefits and harms. Br J Psychiatry. 2020;216:204–12. https://doi.org/10.11 92/bjp.2019.53.
13. Westen D, Harnden-Fisher J. Personality profiles in eating disorders: rethinking the distinction between Axis I and Axis II. Am J Psychiatry American Psychiatric Association. 2001;158:547–62. https://doi.org/10.1176/a ppi.ajp.158.4.547.
14. Hempel R, Vanderbleek E, Lynch TR. Radically open DBT: targeting emotional loneliness in anorexia nervosa. Eat Disord Routledge. 2018;26:92–104. https://doi.org/10.1080/10640266.2018.1418268.
15. Letzring TD, Block J, Funder DC. Ego-control and ego-resiliency: Generalization of self-report scales based on personality descriptions from acquaintances, clinicians, and the self. J Res Pers. 2005;39:395–422. [cited 2013 Dec 30]. https://doi.org/10.1016/j.jrp.2004.06.003.
16. Lynch TR, Hempel RJ, Dunkley C. Radically open-dialectical behavior therapy for disorders of over-control: signaling matters. Am J Psychother. 2015;69: 141–62. https://doi.org/10.1176/appi.psychotherapy.2015.69.2.141.
17. Lynch TR. Radically open dialectical behavior therapy: theory and practice for treating disorders of Overcontrol. Oakland, CA: New Harbinger Publications; 2018.
18. Chen EY, Segal K, Weissman J, Zeffiro TA, Gallop R, Linehan MM, et al. Adapting dialectical behavior therapy for outpatient adult anorexia nervosa-a pilot study. Int J Eat Disord. 2015;48:123–32. https://doi.org/1 0.1002/eat.22360.
19. Lynch TR, Gray KLH, Hempel RJ, Titley M, Chen EY, O'Mahen H a. Radically open-dialectical behavior therapy for adult anorexia nervosa: feasibility and outcomes from an inpatient program. BMC Psychiatry. BMC Psychiatry; 2013 [cited 2014 Jan 31];13:293–209. doi:https://doi. org/10.1186/1471-244X-13-293
20. Baudinet J, Simic M, Griffiths H, Donnelly C, Stewart C, Goddard E. Targeting maladaptive overcontrol with radically open dialectical behaviour therapy in a day programme for adolescents with restrictive eating disorders: an uncontrolled case series. J Eat Disord. J Eat Disord; 2020;8:1–13. doi:https:// doi.org/10.1186/s40337-020-00338-9.
21. Isaksson M, Ghaderi A, Ramklint M, Wolf-Arehult M. Radically open dialectical behavior therapy for anorexia nervosa: A multiple baseline single-case experimental design study across 13 cases. J Behav Ther Exp Psychiatry. 2021;71. https://doi.org/10.1016/j.jbtep.2021.101637.
22. Braun V, Clarke V. Using thematic analysis in psychology. Qual Res Psychol. 2006;3:77–101. https://doi.org/10.1191/1478088706qp063oa.
23. Lynch TR. The Skills Training Manual for Radically Open Dialectical Behavior Therapy. New Harbinger Publications; 2018.
24. Lynch TR. RO-DBT Terapeutinstruktioner: Radikalt öppen dialektisk beteendeterapi (L. Roosdorp, Trans.). Stockholm: Natur & Kultur; 2020.
25. Lynch T. RO-DBT Arbetsmaterial: Radikalt öppen dialektisk beteendeterapi (L. Roosdorp, Trans.). Stockholm: Natur & Kultur; 2020.
26. Fassino S, Pierò A, Tomba E, Abbate-Daga G. Factors associated with dropout from treatment for eating disorders: a comprehensive literature review. BMC Psychiatry. 2009;9:67. [cited 2014 Jan 10]. https://doi.org/10.11 86/1471-244X-9-67.
27. Byrne S, Wade T, Hay P, Touyz S, Fairburn CG, Treasure J, et al. A randomised controlled trial of three psychological treatments for anorexia nervosa 2017;2823–2833. doi:https://doi.org/10.1017/S0033291717001349.
28. Fairburn CG, Cooper Z, Doll HA, Connor MEO, Palmer RL, Dalle R. Enhanced cognitive behaviour therapy for adults with anorexia nervosa : a UK–Italy study. Behav Res Ther Elsevier Ltd. 2013;51:R2–8. https://doi.org/10.1016/j. brat.2012.09.010.
29. Treasure J, Schmidt U. The cognitive-interpersonal maintenance model of anorexia nervosa revisited: a summary of the evidence for cognitive, socio-emotional and interpersonal predisposing and perpetuating factors. J Eat Disord. 2013;1. https://doi.org/10.1186/2050-2974-1-13.
30. Hay PJ, Sachdev P. Brain dysfunction in anorexia nervosa: cause or consequence of under-nutrition? Curr Opin Psychiatry. 2011;24:251–6. https://doi.org/10.1097/YCO.0b013e3283453775.
31. Gilbert K, Hall K, Codd RT. Radically open dialectical behavior therapy: social signaling, transdiagnostic utility and current evidence. Psychol Res Behav Manag. 2020;13:19–28. https://doi.org/10.2147/PRBM.S201848.
32. Ben-Porath D, Duthu F, Luo T, Gonidakis F, Compte EJ, Wisniewski L. Dialectical behavioral therapy: an update and review of the existing treatment models adapted for adults with eating disorders. Eat Disord. Routledge. 2020;28:101–21. https://doi.org/10.1080/10640266.2020.1723371.
33. Wright KM, Hacking S. An angel on my shoulder: a study of relationships between women with anorexia and healthcare professionals. J Psychiatr Ment Health Nurs. 2012;19:107–15. https://doi. org/10.1111/j.1365-2850.2011.01760.x.
34. Flückiger C, Del AC, Wampold BE, Horvath AO. The Alliance in adult psychotherapy: a meta-analytic synthesis. Psychotherapy. 2018;55:316–40. https://doi.org/10.1037/pst0000172.
35. Isaksson M, Ghaderi A, Ramklint M, Wolf-Arehult M. Radically open dialectical behavior therapy for anorexia nervosa: a multiple baseline single-case experimental design study across 13 cases. J Behav Ther Exp Psychiatry. 2021;71. https://doi.org/10.1016/j.jbtep.2021.101637.

20

A preliminary exploration of the effect of concurrent antidepressant medication on responses to high-frequency repetitive transcranial magnetic stimulation (rTMS) in severe, enduring anorexia nervosa

Bethan Dalton[1], Jessica McClelland[1], Savani Bartholdy[1], Maria Kekic[1], Iain C. Campbell[1] and Ulrike Schmidt[1,2*]

Abstract

Background: Repetitive transcranial magnetic stimulation (rTMS) is a promising treatment option for people with severe, enduring anorexia nervosa (SE-AN). As depression is often comorbid with AN, antidepressant medication is commonly prescribed to this patient group. Concurrent antidepressant medications may affect the rTMS treatment response. Therefore, in a secondary analysis of data from a feasibility trial, we explored the effect of antidepressant medication on responses to rTMS in people with SE-AN.

Methods: Twenty-six participants with SE-AN received 20 sessions (over 4 weeks) of neuronavigated high-frequency real rTMS to the left dorsolateral prefrontal cortex. Eating disorder (ED) and general psychopathology symptoms were assessed at baseline, post-treatment and at a 4-month follow-up.

Results: Participants taking antidepressants (n = 16) for the duration of the rTMS treatment had a greater reduction in ED symptoms at the 4-month follow-up, compared to those not taking antidepressants (n = 10). Antidepressant status was not however associated with significant changes in mood outcomes.

Conclusions: In people with SE-AN receiving rTMS treatment, preliminary findings suggest a potential synergistic effect of antidepressant medication in reducing ED symptomatology. There was however no associated reduction in affective symptoms i.e., the effect does not seem to be related to changes in mood. The sample in this exploratory study was small and heterogenous. However, the preliminary results provide a basis for hypothesis generation for future studies.

Keywords: Repetitive transcranial magnetic stimulation, Anorexia nervosa, eating disorders

* Correspondence: ulrike.schmidt@kcl.ac.uk
[1]Section of Eating Disorders, Department of Psychological Medicine, Institute of Psychiatry, Psychology & Neuroscience, King's College London, London SE5 8AF, UK
[2]South London and Maudsley NHS Foundation Trust, Maudsley Hospital, Denmark Hill, London SE5 8AZ, UK

Plain English summary

Approximately 20–30% of patients with anorexia nervosa have a severe and enduring form of the illness. Therefore, new treatment approaches are needed. Repetitive transcranial magnetic stimulation (rTMS) is a promising treatment option for people with severe, enduring anorexia nervosa. Research in people with depression suggests that taking antidepressants may affect a person's response to rTMS treatment. People with anorexia nervosa often experience depression and antidepressants are commonly prescribed to this patient group. This study explored the effect of antidepressants on responses to rTMS in people with severe, enduring anorexia nervosa. Participants received 20 sessions (over 4 weeks) of rTMS. We found that those taking antidepressants during rTMS treatment showed a greater reduction in eating disorder symptoms at follow-up, compared to those not taking antidepressants. Participants not taking antidepressants and those taking antidepressants showed similar improvements in depression and anxiety symptoms. This suggests that the improvement in eating disorder symptoms associated with the combination of rTMS and antidepressants was not related to changes in mood. The study sample was small, and we were unable to explore the effect of other medications on response to rTMS treatment. Further research is needed to investigate the effect of antidepressant medication on response to rTMS treatment in this patient group.

Background

Repetitive transcranial magnetic stimulation (rTMS) is a promising treatment option for severe, enduring anorexia nervosa (SE-AN; [1]). In a recent feasibility clinical trial (the TIARA study; [2]), we found small effects of rTMS on body mass index (BMI) and eating disorder (ED) symptoms, together with moderate to large positive effects on mood outcomes at follow-up (Cohen's $d = 0.61$ to 1.0; 4-months post-randomisation), favouring real rTMS over sham, in people with SE-AN [3]. It has been proposed that concurrent antidepressant medication use may influence rTMS treatment outcomes in major depressive disorder (MDD; [4]). A higher proportion of participants (61.7%) in the original TIARA trial were taking antidepressant medication, compared to those in other treatment trials in AN (e.g., [5, 6]). Therefore, using data from the TIARA trial (and the subsequent open trial), we explored whether rTMS treatment response was affected by concurrent antidepressant medication.

Methods

Full methods of the TIARA trial are described elsewhere ([2, 3]; trial registration number: ISRCTN14329415, pre-results). The study was a double-blind, randomised sham-controlled feasibility trial in adult women with SE-AN. Participants were randomly allocated to 20 sessions of real or sham neuro-navigated high-frequency rTMS delivered to the left dorsolateral prefrontal cortex (DLPFC). Participants in the real group received rTMS at the following parameters: 110% resting motor threshold; 10 Hz frequency consisting of twenty 5-s trains with 55-s inter-train intervals (1000 pulses/session) with a total duration of 20 min (see Supplementary S1 for further details). Sham stimulation was administered at the same parameters as real rTMS; however, a sham coil was used. Ethical approval was given by the London – City Road & Hampstead Research Ethics Committee (Reference: 15/LO/0196).

Clinical outcomes were assessed in all participants at baseline (pre-randomisation), within 1 week of completing rTMS treatment (post-treatment; 1-month post-randomisation) and at a follow-up (4-months post-randomisation). Outcomes used in the present analyses were related to ED symptoms, assessed by BMI and the Eating Disorder Examination – Questionnaire (EDE-Q; [7]), and mood, as measured by the Depression Anxiety Stress Scales – Version 21 (DASS-21; [8]). Medication status was recorded at screening and confirmed at start of rTMS treatment.

Participants were unblinded following completion of data collection at the follow-up assessment. If they remained eligible, those who completed sham treatment were given the opportunity to receive real rTMS treatment (using the identical protocol and rTMS parameters to that used in the main trial, described above). Participants who took this opportunity were re-screened and completed baseline, post-treatment, and follow-up assessments at the same schedule as described above as part of an open study. For the present study, only participants who received real rTMS, either in the initial trial (originally allocated to real rTMS) or the associated open study (originally allocated to sham rTMS but completed real rTMS), were included.

Data analyses were performed in Stata 15 [9]. Depending on the distribution of the data, between-subjects t-tests or Mann-Whitney U tests were used to assess group differences in baseline demographic and clinical characteristics. A chi-squared test was used to examine group differences in AN-type. The post-treatment and follow-up group means and SDs for the clinical outcomes were adjusted for baseline (post-treatment/follow-up scores minus baseline scores) and have been presented with between-group effect sizes (Cohen's *d*) alongside 95% confidence intervals.

Results

Twenty-six participants received real rTMS and were included in this study ($n = 16$ initially randomised to real rTMS treatment, $n = 10$ completed real rTMS treatment as part of the open study after initially being randomised to sham rTMS). Sixteen participants were taking a stable dose of antidepressant medication for the duration of rTMS treatment (data from one participant is missing at follow-up) and ten were not taking antidepressants. In the antidepressant group, ten were taking only a selective serotonin reuptake inhibitor (n = 1 Fluvoxamine, n = 2 Fluoxetine, n = 7 Sertraline), two were taking both a norepinephrine–dopamine reuptake inhibitor and a selective serotonin reuptake inhibitor (n = 1 Bupropion and Sertraline, n = 1 Bupropion and Fluoxetine), two were taking a selective serotonin and norepinephrine reuptake inhibitor (Duloxetine), one was taking a monoamine oxidase inhibitor (Phenelzine), and one was taking a tetracyclic antidepressant (Mirtazapine).

Full medication details and other concurrent treatments are detailed in Supplementary S2. Baseline demographics for both groups are shown in Table 1. Groups did not significantly differ in demographic or clinical characteristics at baseline ($p > 0.05$), although the antidepressant group reported more severe ED, depression and anxiety symptoms. Clinical characteristics at post-treatment and follow-up are presented in Supplementary S3.

The means, standard deviations and between-group treatment effect sizes (with confidence intervals) for change scores (baseline to post-treatment and baseline to follow-up) of the clinical outcomes are shown in Table 2. Post-treatment group differences in clinical outcomes were of small effect: ED symptom outcomes favoured rTMS with concurrent antidepressant medication whereas BMI and mood outcomes favoured rTMS alone (i.e., no concurrent antidepressant medication). At follow-up however, there were large between-group effect sizes in measures of ED symptoms and small to medium effect sizes for BMI and mood outcomes. These all favoured rTMS treatment with concurrent antidepressant medication.

We further explored the association between antidepressant use and changes in ED symptoms by calculating ED symptom recovery rates (EDE-Q Global Score < 2.77, i.e., < 1 SD above community mean; [10]) for each group. In the antidepressant group at baseline, no participants were classed as recovered in terms of ED symptoms. ED symptom recovery was reported in 3/16 (18.75%) participants at post-treatment and 6/15 (40%) participants (including the n = 3 recovered at post-treatment) at follow-up. In the no antidepressant group, of those who did not report ED symptom recovery prior to rTMS treatment (n = 7, 70%), one additional participant reported ED symptom recovery at post-treatment only (1/7, 14.29%) and one further participant at follow-up only (1/7, 14.29%).

Discussion

This small exploratory study examined the potential effects of antidepressant medication on responsiveness to rTMS treatment in people with SE-AN. These preliminary findings show that concurrent antidepressant medication is not associated with ED outcomes immediately post-rTMS treatment nor with mood-related outcomes at post-treatment or follow-up. In fact, at follow-up, in the antidepressant group, depression scores remained in the severe range (according to clinical cut-off scores on the DASS-21; [8]). However, in relation to ED symptoms, there were large between-group effect sizes on change scores from pre-treatment to follow-up: these favoured the group with real rTMS and concurrent antidepressant medication. Furthermore, following rTMS treatment, a greater number of participants in the antidepressant group reported ED symptom recovery compared to those who were not on concurrent antidepressant medication. This is of particular relevance

Table 1 Baseline demographics and clinical characteristics for the antidepressant and no antidepressants groups

	Antidepressants (n = 16)	No antidepressants (n = 10)	Group comparison
Age (years) (mean ± SD)	29.56 ± 9.15	33.20 ± 13.29	U = 64.5, z = 0.82, p = 0.413
Illness duration (years) (mean ± SD)	14.16 ± 9.38	19.40 ± 14.13	U = 61.5, z = 0.98, p = 0.328
AN-R / AN-BP (n)	10 / 6	6 / 4	$\chi^2(1)$ = 0.02, p = 0.899
BMI (kg/m^2) (mean ± SD)	16.36 ± 1.50	15.95 ± 1.85	t(24) = −0.62, p = 0.540
EDE-Q Global (mean ± SD)	4.31 ± 0.82	3.64 ± 1.58	t(24) = − 1.45, p = 0.164
EDE-Q Restraint (mean ± SD)	4.20 ± 1.34	3.42 ± 1.86	t(24) = − 1.25, p = 0.225
EDE-Q Eating Concern (mean ± SD)	3.69 ± 0.80	3.28 ± 1.88	t(24) = − 0.77, p = 0.449
EDE-Q Shape Concern (mean ± SD)	4.83 ± 1.02	4.08 ± 1.68	U = 59, z = − 1.11, p = 0.266
EDE-Q Weight Concern (mean ± SD)	4.53 ± 0.98	3.78 ± 1.64	t(24) = − 1.46, p = 0.157
DASS-21 Total (mean ± SD)	74.00 ± 24.61	62.60 ± 29.33	t(24) = − 1.07, p = 0.296
DASS-21 Depression (mean ± SD)	29.13 ± 9.72	22.00 ± 10.71	t(24) = − 1.75, p = 0.093
DASS-21 Anxiety (mean ± SD)	17.38 ± 10.22	12.60 ± 10.96	t(24) = − 1.13, p = 0.865

Abbreviations: *SD* Standard deviation, *AN-R* Anorexia nervosa restricting type, *AN-BP* Anorexia nervosa binge-eating/purging type, *n* Number, *BMI* Body mass index, *EDE-Q* Eating Disorder Examination – Questionnaire, *DASS-21* Depression, Anxiety and Stress Scales – Version 21

Table 2 The mean change scores (post-treatment and follow-up scores adjusted for baseline[a]) for the clinical outcome measures, including the number of participants (N), means, and standard deviations (SD) for the antidepressant and no antidepressant groups, and the estimated between-groups effect size (Cohen's *d* with 95% confidence intervals)

Measure	Antidepressants			No antidepressants			Between- subject *d* (95% CI)
	N	Mean	SD	*N*	Mean	SD	
Post-treatment (adjusted for baseline[a])							
BMI	16	0.03	0.72	10	0.16	0.36	0.22 (− 0.58 to 1.01)
EDE-Q Global	16	− 0.34	0.68	10	− 0.09	0.56	0.40 (−0.41 to 1.19)
EDE-Q Restraint	16	−0.18	0.73	10	0.14	0.67	0.45 (−0.36 to 1.24)
EDE-Q Eating Concern	16	−0.43	0.83	10	−0.12	0.84	0.37 (−0.43 to 1.16)
EDE-Q Shape Concern	16	−0.45	0.74	10	−0.10	1.11	0.38 (−0.42 to 1.18)
EDE-Q Weight Concern	16	−0.33	0.83	10	−0.30	0.94	0.03 (−0.76 to 0.82)
DASS-21 Total	16	−9.00	22.14	10	−16.2	19.31	−0.34 (−1.13 to 0.46)
DASS-21 Depression	16	−1.25	8.61	10	−4.80	8.34	−0.42 (−1.21 to 0.39)
DASS-21 Anxiety	16	−3.63	8.86	10	−4.20	4.76	−0.08 (− 0.87 to 0.72)
Follow-up (adjusted for baseline[a])							
BMI	15	0.27	1.17	10	0.06	0.89	−0.20 (−1.00 to 0.91)
EDE-Q Global	15	−0.88	0.85	10	−0.03	0.62	**1.10 (0.23 to 1.96)**
EDE-Q Restraint	15	−0.75	1.29	10	0.18	0.68	**0.85 (0.001 to 1.67)**
EDE-Q Eating Concern	15	−0.67	1.06	10	0.06	0.95	0.71 (−0.12 to 1.53)
EDE-Q Shape Concern	15	−1.06	0.83	10	−0.09	0.83	**1.17 (0.29 to 2.03)**
EDE-Q Weight Concern	15	−1.04	1.01	10	−0.28	0.67	**0.85 (0.006 to 1.68)**
DASS-21 Total	15	−17.33	23.80	10	−14.4	18.40	0.13 (−0.69 to 0.93)
DASS-21 Depression	15	−8.13	10.43	10	−4.20	8.24	0.41 (−0.41 to 1.21)
DASS-21 Anxiety	15	−4.40	7.57	10	−3.00	7.13	0.19 (−0.62 to 0.99)

Abbreviations: *N* Number, *SD* Standard deviation, *CI* Confidence intervals, *BMI* Body mass index, *EDE-Q* Eating Disorder Examination - Questionnaire, *DASS-21* Depression Anxiety and Stress Scales - Version 21

[a]Post-treatment/follow-up scores minus baseline scores. Bold font signifies that the CI do not include 0

given the somewhat limited treatment success usually seen in SE-AN.

Antidepressants are commonly prescribed to adults with AN [11]. There is some evidence that they improve symptoms of comorbid depression in AN [12], but limited data for them being effective in improving ED symptoms [13]. In the TIARA trial, ~ 60% of our participants were taking antidepressants and in fact, the total group had somewhat higher depression scores compared to other treatment studies of AN (e.g., [5]). In the present analyses, those taking antidepressants reported more severe ED, depression and anxiety symptoms at baseline i.e., they appeared to be more psychologically unwell (though none of the differences were statistically significant). In this context, it is of note that none of the participants in the antidepressant group, but 3/10 (30%) of the participants in the no antidepressant group, reported ED symptom recovery prior to rTMS treatment.

In MDD, rTMS is typically administered as an augmentation therapy to antidepressant medication (e.g., [14]). However, little is known about the potential impact of antidepressants on the clinical efficacy of rTMS (and vice versa). Data on the effects of concurrent antidepressant medication during rTMS treatment for MDD is mixed, reporting either an enhancement of the rTMS response [4, 15] or no effect [16]. In terms of potential synergistic mechanisms, it is of note that both rTMS and antidepressant medication (including those with rapid onset effects) have been reported to alter neuronal plasticity and cortical excitability [17–20]. To an extent, this is suggested by our data. It is unclear however, why antidepressant status was associated with improvements in ED outcomes, but not with significant changes in mood following the rTMS treatment, especially as symptoms of depression are the typical target of antidepressants and these medications are reported to have little efficacy in treating ED symptoms [13].

Our study has some limitations: our sample size was small and it is an exploratory analysis of pre-existing data, i.e., concurrent antidepressant medication and dose were not standardised across participants and a proportion in both groups were also taking other psychotropic medications. It was not possible to explore whether other concurrent medications (e.g., benzodiazepines) were associated with rTMS response in SE-AN due to the small number of participants taking these. Recent research suggests that in response to rTMS treatment in MDD, benzodiazepine use is associated with less improvement and psychostimulants with greater improvement [16, 21]. For these exploratory analyses, we combined participants who received real rTMS from the original randomised controlled trial (i.e., participants were blinded) with those who received real rTMS as part of the open label follow-up (i.e., participants were unblinded). However, there was approximately equal distribution of these across the no antidepressant and antidepressant groups (e.g., 60–62.5% in both groups received real rTMS in the original randomised controlled trial). In addition, we identified a possible floor effect in the no antidepressant group in terms of ED symptom recovery, where a limited potential for further symptom reductions in these participants may have contributed to the findings. Furthermore, we did not systematically assess comorbid psychiatric diagnoses (e.g., depression). Given the relatively short follow-up period, longer term follow-ups are needed to examine whether the observed effects persist and/or extend to other clinical features. There is likely also value in exploring the combination of rTMS with other treatment approaches, aside from medication in SE-AN, such as psychotherapy or cognitive training [22].

Conclusions

In people with SE-AN, who received 20 sessions of high-frequency rTMS to the left DLPFC, we have obtained preliminary findings that at follow-up, antidepressant medication appears to enhance the response to rTMS with respect to ED symptoms but not to affective symptoms. The impact of concurrent medication on rTMS efficacy needs to be more rigorously tested in larger samples of people with SE-AN and these preliminary results provide the basis for hypothesis generation for these future studies.

Abbreviations

AN: Anorexia nervosa; BMI: Body mass index; DASS-21: Depression Anxiety and Stress Scales – Version 21; ED: Eating disorder; EDE-Q: Eating Disorder Examination Questionnaire; MDD: Major depressive disorder; rTMS: Repetitive transcranial magnetic stimulation; SE-AN: Severe enduring anorexia nervosa

Acknowledgements

We would like to thank the individuals who participated in this study for their time and commitment.

Authors' contributions

US conceived the study. Data collection was performed by BD, JM, SB, and MK. BD analysed and interpreted the data and drafted and prepared the manuscript. ICC assisted with drafting the manuscript and data interpretation. All authors critically reviewed and approved the final manuscript.

Competing interests

The authors declare that they have no competing interests.

References

1. Dalton B, Bartholdy S, Campbell IC, Schmidt U. Neurostimulation in clinical and sub-clinical eating disorders: a systematic update of the literature. Curr Neuropharmacol. 2018;16(8):1174–92. https://doi.org/10.2174/1570159X16666180108111532.
2. Bartholdy S, McClelland J, Kekic M, O'Daly OG, Campbell IC, Werthmann J, et al. Clinical outcomes and neural correlates of 20 sessions of repetitive transcranial magnetic stimulation in severe and enduring anorexia nervosa (the TIARA study): study protocol for a randomised controlled feasibility trial. Trials. 2015;16:548. https://doi.org/10.1186/s13063-015-1069-3.
3. Dalton B, Bartholdy S, McClelland J, Kekic M, Rennalls SJ, Werthmann J, et al. Randomised controlled feasibility trial of real versus sham repetitive transcranial magnetic stimulation treatment in adults with severe and enduring anorexia nervosa: the TIARA study. BMJ Open. 2018;8(7):e021531. https://doi.org/10.1136/bmjopen-2018-021531.
4. Berlim MT, Van den Eynde F, Daskalakis ZJ. High-frequency repetitive transcranial magnetic stimulation accelerates and enhances the clinical response to antidepressants in major depression: a meta-analysis of randomized, double-blind, and sham-controlled trials. J Clin Psychiatry. 2013;74(2):e122–9. https://doi.org/10.4088/JCP.12r07996.
5. Byrne S, Wade T, Hay P, Touyz S, Fairburn CG, Treasure J, et al. A randomised controlled trial of three psychological treatments for anorexia nervosa. Psychol Med. 2017;47(16):2823–33. https://doi.org/10.1017/S0033291717001349.
6. Schmidt U, Magill N, Renwick B, Keyes A, Kenyon M, Dejong H, et al. The Maudsley Outpatient Study of Treatments for Anorexia Nervosa and Related Conditions (MOSAIC): comparison of the Maudsley Model of Anorexia Nervosa Treatment for Adults (MANTRA) with specialist supportive clinical management (SSCM) in outpatients with broadly defined anorexia nervosa: a randomized controlled trial. J Consult Clin Psychol. 2015;83(4):796–807. https://doi.org/10.1037/ccp0000019.
7. Fairburn CG, Beglin SJ. Appendix: eating disorder examination questionnaire (EDE-Q version 6.0). In: Fairburn CG, editor. Cognitive behaviour therapy and eating disorders. New York: Guilford Press; 2008.
8. Lovibond SH, Lovibond PF. Manual for the depression anxiety stress scales. 2nd ed. Sydney: Psychology Foundation; 1995.
9. StataCorp. Stata statistical software: release 15. College Station: StataCorp LLC; 2017.
10. Mond JM, Hay PJ, Rodgers B, Owen C. Eating disorder examination questionnaire (EDE-Q): norms for young adult women. Behav Res Ther. 2006;44(1):53–62. https://doi.org/10.1016/j.brat.2004.12.003.
11. Garner DM, Anderson ML, Keiper CD, Whynott R, Parker L. Psychotropic medications in adult and adolescent eating disorders: clinical practice versus evidence-based recommendations. Eat Weight Disord. 2016;21(3):395–402. https://doi.org/10.1007/s40519-016-0253-0.
12. Marvanova M, Gramith K. Role of antidepressants in the treatment of adults with anorexia nervosa. Ment Health Clin. 2018;8(3):127–37. https://doi.org/10.9740/mhc.2018.05.127.
13. Crow SJ. Pharmacologic treatment of eating disorders. Psychiatr Clin North Am. 2019;42(2):253–62. https://doi.org/10.1016/j.psc.2019.01.007.
14. Mutz J, Vipulananthan V, Carter B, Hurlemann R, Fu CHY, Young AH. Comparative efficacy and acceptability of non-surgical brain stimulation for the acute treatment of major depressive episodes in adults: systematic review and network meta-analysis. BMJ. 2019;364:l1079. https://doi.org/10.1136/bmj.l1079.
15. Sehatzadeh S, Daskalakis ZJ, Yap B, Tu H, Palimaka S, Bowen JM, et al. Unilateral and bilateral repetitive transcranial magnetic stimulation for treatment-resistant depression: a meta-analysis of randomized controlled trials over 2 decades. J Psychiatry Neurosci. 2019;44(3):151–63. https://doi.org/10.1503/jpn.180056.
16. Hunter AM, Minzenberg MJ, Cook IA, Krantz DE, Levitt JG, Rotstein NM, et al. Concomitant medication use and clinical outcome of repetitive transcranial magnetic stimulation (rTMS) treatment of major depressive disorder. Brain Behav. 2019;9(5):e01275. https://doi.org/10.1002/brb3.1275.
17. Duman RS, Aghajanian GK, Sanacora G, Krystal JH. Synaptic plasticity and depression: new insights from stress and rapid-acting antidepressants. Nat Med. 2016;22(3):238–49. https://doi.org/10.1038/nm.4050.

18. Duman RS, Shinohara R, Fogaca MV, Hare B. Neurobiology of rapid-acting antidepressants: convergent effects on GluA1-synaptic function. Mol Psychiatry. 2019;24(12):1816–32. https://doi.org/10.1038/s41380-019-0400-x.
19. Zanos P, Thompson SM, Duman RS, Zarate CA Jr, Gould TD. Convergent mechanisms underlying rapid antidepressant action. CNS Drugs. 2018;32(3): 197–227. https://doi.org/10.1007/s40263-018-0492-x.
20. Minzenberg MJ, Leuchter AF. The effect of psychotropic drugs on cortical excitability and plasticity measured with transcranial magnetic stimulation: implications for psychiatric treatment. J Affect Disord. 2019;253:126–40. https://doi.org/10.1016/j.jad.2019.04.067.
21. Deppe M, Abdelnaim M, Hebel T, Kreuzer P, Poeppl T, Langguth B, et al. Concomitant lorazepam use and antidepressive efficacy of repetitive transcranial magnetic stimulation in a naturalistic setting. Eur Arch Psychiatry Clin Neurosci. 2020. https://doi.org/10.1007/s00406-020-01160-9.
22. Sathappan AV, Luber BM, Lisanby SH. The dynamic duo: combining noninvasive brain stimulation with cognitive interventions. Prog Neuro-Psychopharmacol Biol Psychiatry. 2019;89:347–60. https://doi.org/10.1016/j.pnpbp.2018.10.006.

21

Are poor set-shifting and central coherence associated with everyday function in anorexia nervosa?

Kelly M. Dann[1*], Phillipa Hay[2] and Stephen Touyz[3]

Abstract

Background: There is increasing interest in associations between cognitive impairments and clinical symptoms in Anorexia Nervosa (AN), however, the relationship with everyday function is unclear. The current review synthesizes existing data regarding associations between scores on tests of set-shifting and central coherence and functional outcome measures for individuals with AN.

Method: A systematic electronic database search yielded 13 studies which included participants with current or lifetime AN where scores on a neuropsychological test of set-shifting or central coherence were directly or indirectly compared to a functional outcome measure.

Results: Associations between set-shifting and central coherence performance measures and functional outcomes were limited in number and noted only in adult or mixed-age cohorts. Associations were noted at subscale level, suggesting they are specific in nature. In younger cohorts, assessments of executive functioning in everyday life appear sensitive to cognitive-behavioral flexibility issues.

Conclusions: Associations between cognitive performance and functional outcome have not been as systematically assessed in AN as in other psychiatric disorders. Key factors to address in future research include: (a) the use of function measures which are sensitive to both the level of impairment, and specific rather than general impairments (b) the ecological validity of measures, (c) the task impurity problem, especially in regard to cognitive flexibility assessment, and (d) the need to measure both cognitive deficits and strengths, because tests of specific cognitive processes may underestimate the ability to function in daily life due to compensatory strategies.

Keywords: Anorexia Nervosa, cognition, set-shifting, cognitive flexibility, central coherence, executive function, functional outcome, neuropsychology, quality of life, eating disorders

Plain English summary

The current review gathers existing evidence regarding whether poor performance on tests of cognitive flexibility and detail-oriented processing are associated with difficulties in everyday function for people with Anorexia Nervosa. A literature search identified 13 articles which included data which address this question. The associations between poor performance on cognitive tests and day-to-day function were not strong, and were noted only in adult and mixed-aged groups. In younger samples, self-report measures of everyday cognitive skills appear to be more sensitive to function issues. Overall this review suggests that more research is needed to better understand how group differences on cognitive flexibility and detail-oriented processing tests relate to daily functioning for individuals with Anorexia Nervosa. It is

* Correspondence: kelly.dann@sydney.edu.au
[1]School of Psychology, University of Sydney, Sydney, Australia
Full list of author information is available at the end of the article

recommended that future research should also measure cognitive strengths which may be used to compensate for cognitive weaknesses in everyday life.

Background

Anorexia Nervosa (AN) is an eating disorder (ED) characterized by extreme dietary restriction and other weight-loss behaviors, and a persistent fear of weight-gain despite significantly low weight [1]. The complex and serious physical and psychological health issues associated with AN result in significant health-related disability. Individuals with AN experience severe impairment in their social and occupational function [83], and longitudinal research highlights poor psychosocial functioning as a significant predictor of mortality [30].

In the past 10 years there has been increasing interest in neurocognitive functioning in ED research, with a recent 'review of reviews' finding 28 systematic and meta-analytic publications since 2010 [73]. A consistent finding in the literature is that adults with AN perform more poorly on neuropsychological tests of set-shifting and central coherence than healthy control groups [45, 100]. Set-shifting is the ability to shift focus between mental sets in response to changing demands, and is a measure of cognitive flexibility [21]. Central coherence refers to the normal tendency to process information in a global or holistic manner, rather than with excessive attention to detail. In contrast, a focus on detail at the expense of overall conceptual and contextual understanding, is an attentional bias known as weak central coherence [37]. Poor performance in these two areas forms a cognitive profile of inflexible, detail-focused processing which is consistent with clinical observations of cognitive-behavioral rigidity in individuals with AN. The Cognitive-Interpersonal Maintenance Model for AN [72] proposes poor set-shifting and weak central coherence underlie obsessive-compulsive traits, and together with socio-emotional avoidance, are key risk factors in both the aetiology and maintenance of the disorder. This inflexible cognitive style is further suggested to contribute to poor treatment engagement and response [84].

Taking a broader perspective, deficits in set-shifting and/or central coherence are present in other psychiatric disorders, prompting suggestions that the impairments may be a trans-diagnostic marker, or general risk-factor for a range of disorders. Within this wider psychiatric literature, cognitive deficits across the domains of attention, memory and executive function have been shown to predict both clinical and functional outcomes. Meta-analytic results suggest a substantial effect of general cognitive deficits on overall functional outcome in Schizophrenia [34], Bipolar Disorder [20], and a more limited general effect in Major Depressive Disorder [26]. In AN there has been no synthesis of the existing evidence of the effect of cognitive impairments on functional outcomes. However, a substantial body of research has focused on the measurement of cognitive impairments and possible associations with clinical characteristics of the disorder.

Set-shifting and central coherence impairments in AN

Set-shifting

A comprehensive meta-analysis which included 1394 participants with AN [100], found set-shifting deficits across a range of tasks of small to medium effect (Hedges' $g = -0.44$). The effect was not consistent across included studies; 29 of 49 studies did not find significant differences between AN participants and healthy control cohorts. Effect sizes also varied greatly by measure; performance was most impaired in the Haptic Illusion task [87] ($g = -1.02$), but not significantly different to controls in the Intra-Extra Dimensional Set Shift test [71] ($g = -0.17$). There are suggestions that shifting is not impaired in all domains; participants with AN have demonstrated superior category switching compared to controls on tests of verbal fluency [77, 78].

Set-shifting is most commonly assessed using the Wisconsin Card Sort Task (WCST; [32]) on which individuals with AN often perform poorly. A meta-analysis of 22 studies which assessed set-shifting using the WCST found significant effect for adults (Cohen's $d = .48$) but not children ($d = .25$) [95]. This is consistent with meta-analysis across a range of executive function tasks which found effects were not significant for children with AN [40], however other meta-analytic results have not yielded significant differences between adolescent and adult participants [100] suggesting further clarification is needed.

Differences in shifting ability between AN Restricting subtype (AN-R) and Binge-Purge subtype (AN-BP) are inconsistent [73], however studies are often limited in their power to detect effects by sub-type. Splitting by sub-type, meta-analytic results of 11 studies including participants with AN-R suggest set-shifting deficits of medium effect ($g = -0.51$) but across 6 studies the effect size for AN-BP was not significant ($g = -0.18$) [100]. Overall, the literature suggests the presence of set-shifting impairments, but effects are not consistent, and vary greatly by measure.

Weak central coherence

Meta-analytic results of 7 studies using the Rey Osterreith Complex Figure Test (ROCFT; [61]) in AN indicate difficulties with global processing of medium to large effect ($d = 0.63$) [45, 47]. A synthesis of 5 studies using the Group Embedded Figures Test (GEFT; [98, 99]) shows a bias towards local processing, also of medium to large effect ($d = 0.63$) [45, 47]. Taken together, these results indicate weak central coherence in participants with AN. Significant differences in central coherence by AN subtype have been suggested, with AN-R participants noted to perform more poorly than AN-BP on the Wechsler Block Design and Object Assembly tasks [88], however the validity of the Block Design task as a central coherence measure has been questioned [45, 47, 50]. A meta-synthesis of studies using the ROCFT found participants with AN, and a group of unaffected relatives of AN patients both scored significantly lower on the central coherence index than healthy controls, but participants recovered from AN performed similarly to controls [46]. These findings are difficult to interpret, since poor performance by unaffected relatives suggest deficits may be trait-based, while similar performance to controls by the recovered group suggests issues may be state-dependent.

Associations between cognitive impairments and clinical characteristics of AN

Associations between cognitive impairments and clinical characteristics of the disorder provide support for the Cognitive-Interpersonal Maintenance Model for AN [72]. Poor set-shifting has been associated with a longer duration of illness, more severe ED rituals [69] and illness severity [84]. Weak central coherence has been associated with severity of illness, BMI and ED-related compulsions [70]. However, evidence regarding the relationship between cognitive impairments and clinical characteristics is quite inconsistent, which has prompted suggestions that deficits may be "clinically silent" [67]. The direction of causality is also difficult to interpret since cognitive flexibility is impacted by even short-term starvation in healthy participants [8, 63].

Cognitive Remediation Therapy (CRT) for AN is a treatment augmentation which aims to improve set-shifting and central coherence [81]. Since difficulties in these areas are thought to be both a risk factor in the maintenance of the disorder and also a barrier to engagement with treatment, remediation may improve clinical outcomes. Early reviews showed encouraging results and good patient acceptance in both adult and adolescent cohorts [82, 85]. However, a recent meta-analysis of randomized controlled trials of CRT versus control treatments showed no improvement in central coherence, ED symptoms or BMI, and mixed results for set-shifting which were unable to be synthesized due to the wide variety of measures used [35]. These results require cautious interpretation; since CRT is a relatively new intervention they include participants across a wide age group and both AN subtypes. Part of the CRT program involves applying new thinking styles to everyday life, and two studies which have included quality of life (QoL) outcomes [22, 90] have shown CRT is associated with improvement in ED-related QoL [35].

Functional outcome in AN

Functional impairment, or limitation in ability in areas of everyday living such as social, academic and occupational function, does not form part of the diagnostic criteria of AN. However, improvement in function is widely acknowledged as a key marker of recovery, and a self-report measure of function or QoL is often included as a secondary outcome in empirical research.

The Clinical Impairment Assessment (CIA; [10]), is a widely-used ED-specific self-report measure designed to assess functional impairments secondary to eating disorder symptoms. Weight and shape concerns and binge eating frequency have been shown to significantly predict CIA scores [66], and impairment on the CIA has also been demonstrated to increase as a function of illness severity according to BMI [18]. A recent network analysis of data from participants with AN found moderate correlations between ED symptoms at baseline and post-treatment CIA scores [24].

Results from assessments of QoL in AN are somewhat mixed, and may be complicated by the ego-syntonic nature of the disorder, wherein aspects of the disorder are perceived as congruent with the ideal self. Participants with AN-R have been noted to score similarly to healthy controls on a subjective QoL scale, possibly because items may be interpreted differently by AN patients whose concerns are not associated with low weight, and where weight increases towards a healthy range may be associated with a reduction in QoL ratings [58]. Mixed results appear to be more associated with shorter term follow-up measures, and shorter duration of illness [55], but in participants with severe and enduring AN, a close association between QoL, BMI and ED symptom severity has been demonstrated [5].

Functional impairment in AN is most commonly assessed as a secondary outcome, however longitudinal research has demonstrated that health-related QoL has a bi-directional relationship with ED symptoms - lower QoL scores predicted increases in ED symptoms over periods up to 4 years - suggesting QoL is a valid treatment target [55]. QoL, mood and social adjustment were the primary outcome measures in a randomized controlled trial of two alternative treatments for severe and enduring AN which demonstrated an unusually high retention rate, suggesting the approach may also increase patient engagement [86]. As mentioned earlier, CRT has been associated with preliminary, yet encouraging improvements in self-reported QoL in two studies [35]. These results suggest QoL could be more broadly explored as a treatment target in future CRT interventions.

The current review

Understanding the possible impact of cognitive factors on everyday function is important because functional improvements are milestones of recovery. Cognitive Remediation Therapy (CRT) is being implemented in AN, and it has been suggested that further evaluation of CRT should include whether it supports improvement in everyday functioning [11, 49]. To support the inclusion of broader functional outcomes in the evaluation of current therapies, a clearer understanding of the impact of cognitive inefficiencies on day-to-day function in AN is needed. To address this need, we conducted a systematic review of the literature to answer the question: Are poor set-shifting and central coherence associated with everyday function in Anorexia Nervosa?

Method

Inclusion and exclusion criteria

Inclusion criteria for studies were:

(a) Participants met the criteria for current or lifetime Anorexia Nervosa.
(b) Comparison between scores on a neuropsychological test of set-shifting or central coherence and scores on a measure of everyday function, or concurrent measurement of these variables compared to a healthy control group was reported.

A broad definition of everyday function which included social function, quality of life scales and measures of cognitive flexibility or detail-oriented processing in everyday life was used to maximize the breadth of studies included. We did not apply any age limit on participants because studies in AN often include a wide age range to maximize power.

Literature search

A search was conducted in November 2019 and updated in February 2021. Embase, Medline, PsychInfo and Scopus databases were searched using the following general and Medical Subject Headings (MeSH) search terms:

"anorexia nervosa" AND.

"daily function" OR "quality of life" OR "activities of daily living" OR "functional outcome" OR "employment" OR "independent living" OR "work and social adjustment scale" OR "Clinical impairment assessment" OR "eating disorders quality of life" OR "inventory of interpersonal problems" OR "Health related quality of life in eating disorders" OR "SF-36" OR "social function" OR "psychosocial function" OR "socio-emotional function" OR "social cognition" OR "ecological validity" OR "ecologically valid" OR "Behavioural assessment of dysexecutive syndrome" OR "Behaviour rating inventory of executive function" OR "detail and flexibility questionnaire" OR "D-Flex" AND.

Neurocogniti* OR neuropsych* OR "cognitive assessment" OR "neuropsychological assessment" OR "cognitive style" OR "cognitive deficit" OR "cognitive flexibility" OR "executive function" OR " set shifting" OR "task switching" OR "central coherence" OR "Rey-Osterreith" OR "Wisconsin card sort" OR "Group embedded figures" OR "trail making" OR "Fragmented pictures" OR "Hayling" OR "Brixton" OR "Ravello Profile" OR "Delis Kaplan" OR "NEPSY*".

Initial results were limited to English language, human subjects and peer-reviewed articles where possible. The database search was supplemented by a ProQuest Dissertations and Theses search using the above terms to search the full bibliographic record excluding the full text (NOFT), and a manual reference list search to identify any further articles relevant to the review. The review was performed according to the Preferred Reporting Items for Systematic reviews and Meta-Analyses (PRISMA) standards. Two reviewers (K.D. & S.T.) independently reviewed a subset of the articles at both abstract and full-text stage to determine eligibility.

Results

Thirteen articles met the inclusion criteria. The systematic search process is illustrated in Fig. 1. Included studies used a variety of measures of set-shifting, central coherence and functional outcome, and different methods of analysis, therefore a descriptive review was conducted. The included studies are summarized in Table 1. The table is organized according to the type of functional outcome measure used. The first section includes studies which used general function, social function and quality of life measures. The second section includes studies which employed measures of executive functioning in daily life.

Quality assessment

Methodological quality of the included studies was assessed using a modified version of the Downs & Black Quality Index [23]. Items excluded from the original index were items relating to randomized controlled trials, as revised by Ferro and Speechley [28], and one item relating to description of response rate which were not useful assessment criteria for the current review. The amended 14-item index is presented in Table 2. Items were scored 1 for Yes (✓), and 0 for No (x) or Unable to determine (?). Maximum score was 14. The overall methodological quality of the studies included in the review was high. Two items were not well fulfilled; only two studies included a power calculation and less than half included information regarding the proportion of participants vs. those who were invited to participate.

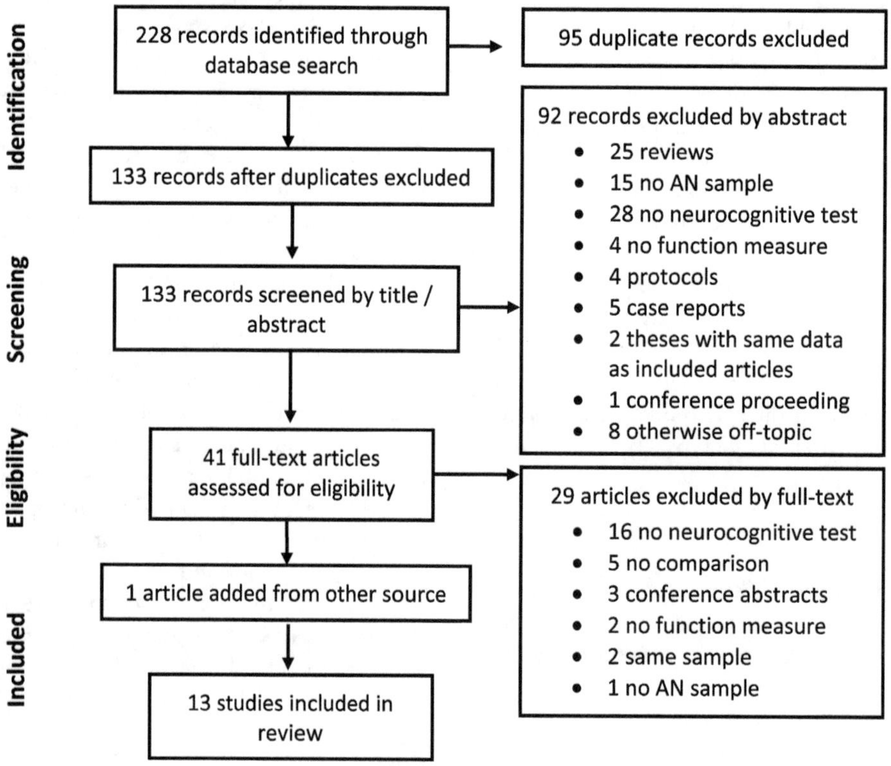

Fig. 1 PRISMA flow diagram for study selection

Sample characteristics and measures

Participants in the studies included in the review were demographically heterogeneous. Most studies included only female participants, one study included two males [79] and two did not specify [39, 60]. Five studies included only adult participants and six studies describe their cohorts as children, adolescents or young people. One study included participants 16–42 years [75], and one included participants 12–47 years [94]. Eight studies included a healthy control comparison group.

Participants were also clinically heterogeneous. Most studies included only participants with AN; one study also included participants with Bulimia Nervosa, however clear subgroup analysis was provided [38]. Eight studies identified their participants by diagnostic subtype or included only one subtype. Studies included participants across a spectrum of stage and severity of AN, and included inpatient and outpatients cohorts. Studies varied in their exclusion criteria, however all excluded participants with other serious conditions, e.g. neurological or developmental disorders. Most studies did not exclude participants using psychopharmacological medication.

Power is an issue for AN research. Five studies had a sample size of under 25 participants; four of these were studies which included only children and/or adolescents, one was an adult cohort [36]. Some studies where analysis was undertaken by subtype or stage of illness also had low numbers of participants per group.

Studies included a variety of measures of set-shifting and central coherence, summarized in Table 3. Neurocognitive predictor measures were all performance-based, except the Detail and Flexibility Questionnaire (DFlex). The Wisconsin Card Sort Task (WCST) was the most common set-shifting measure, used in nine studies (however, note [67] use as a measure of general executive function). The Rey Osterreith Complex Figure Test (ROCFT) Central Coherence Index (CCI) was the most common measure of central coherence, also used in nine studies.

Studies included a variety of functional outcome measures, summarized in Table 4. Six studies included measures of social function, three of which were social cognition measures. Six studies used measures designed to assess executive function in daily life. Two studies assessed ED-specific functional impairment and two studies measured quality of life. Functional outcome measures in five studies were self-report only. Two studies included a parent-reported measure and two included a clinician-reported measure. Four studies included a performance-based function measure; three of these were the tests of social cognition and one was a measure of executive function in daily life.

Table 1 Summary of studies included in the review

Author (year)	*Sample*	*Cognitive measures*	*Function measures*	*Results*
Oldershaw, Lavender & Schmidt [60]	AN ($n = 71$) Outpatients. Age over 18 years, *M* age = 26	WCST, Brixton, TMT, GEFT	CIA	Cognitive tests did not predict CIA scores.
Bentz et al. [9]	AN ($n = 71$) 43 first episode *M* age = 16, 28 recovered *M* age = 18. HC ($n = 41$) Age 14–22 years.	D-KEFS: Composite set-shifting measure (shift conditions of Verbal Fluency, Design Fluency and Trail Making), GEFT	ADOS	Composite SS and GEFT did not predict ADOS social function.
Hamatani et al. [36]	AN ($n = 21$: AN-BP = 13, AN-R = 8). 14 outpatients, 7 inpatients. Adults, *M* age = 32 years. HC ($n = 25$).	KWCST, ROCFT	SF-36	Greater KWCST DMS associated with lower scores on SF-36 PCS ($r = -0.658$, $p = < .05$). ROCFT CCI 30-min delay recall score associated with SF-36 MCS ($r = 0.610$, $p = < .05$).
Westwood, Mandy & Tchanturia [94]	AN ($n = 99$) Inpatients and outpatients. Age 12–47 years.	WCST, ROCFT, D-Flex	ADOS	Greater WCST %PE associated with increased ASD symptoms, Welch's F (2,59.77) = 3.77, $p = .029$. D-flex increase in cognitive rigidity scores between no vs. high ASD symptoms, $p = .018$ ROCFT not associated with increased ASD symptoms.
Renwick et al. [67]	AN ($n = 100$; AN-R = 44, AN-BP = 33, EDNOS-AN = 23) Outpatients. Adults, *M* age = 24.7 years.	WCST, Brixton, ROCFT	CIA Reading the Mind in Films Task	Cluster (17% of participants) show poor performance on WCST, ROCFT CCI and RMIF emotional ToM. No effect of cluster for ROCFT, but overall poor performance. No effect of cluster for CIA.
Talbot, Hay & Touyz [79]	AN ($n = 49$; 24 acute, 10 weight-recovered, 15 fully recovered) HC ($n = 43$) Age 19–27 years.	WCST, ROCFT, MFFT	EDQOL, IIP-32	WCST PE higher scaled scores (better performance) associated with higher IIP-32 'Too dependent' ($r = .305$, $p = .033$), 'Too aggressive' ($r = .401$, $p = .004$), 'Hard to be involved' ($r = .313$, $p = .029$) and 'Hard to be supportive' ($r = .294$, $p = .040$). WCST CC associated with higher IIP-32 'Too dependent' ($r = .354$, $p = .013$), 'Too aggressive' ($r = .334$, $p = .019$) and better financial QOL ($r = -.393$, $p = .007$). ROCFT lower CCI and OCI associated with higher IIP-32 'Hard to be supportive' (CI: $r = -.336$, $p = .020$; OCI: ($r = -.413$, $p = .004$) and lower OCI associated with higher IIP-32 'Hard to be involved' ($r = -.343$, $p = .017$).
Calderoni et al. [14]	AN-R ($n = 23$) HC ($n = 46$) Age 9–16 years.	NEPSY-II Attention and EF: Auditory response set, Inhibition shifting	NEPSY-II Social Perception: ToM verbal, ToM contextual and Affect recognition	NEPSY-II Attention and EF no group differences on overall domain but response set shifting test worse in AN vs. HC ($t_{67} = -2.17$, $p = .033$). No group differences on NEPSY-II inhibition shifting or NEPSY-II social perception domain.
Harrison, Tchanturia, Naumann & Treasure [38]	AN ($n = 85$; 35 AN-R, 15 AN-BP, 35 recovered) HC ($n = 90$) Age 18–55 years.	WCST, Brixton, ROCFT, GEFT, FPT	Reading the Mind in the Eyes test	Higher WCST PE associated with lower Reading the Mind in the Eyes emotion recognition ($r_s = -.281$, $p = .05$), but not significant after Bonferroni correction.

Table 1 Summary of studies included in the review *(Continued)*

Author (year)	*Sample*	*Cognitive measures*	*Function measures*	*Results*
Executive function in daily life				
Spitoni, Aragonaa, Bevacqua, Cotugno & Antonucci [75]	AN-R ($n = 62$) HC ($n = 70$) Age 16–42 years.	WCST, TMT, ROCFT	BADS	AN WCST PE higher (partial $\eta^2 = .03$) and TMT-B slower (partial $\eta^2 = .10$) than HC. AN lower ROCFT CCI than HC at 30s (partial $\eta^2 = .13$) and 20 min recall (partial $\eta^2 = .11$). AN BADS accuracy similar, but AN slower than HC across tasks (Rule shift cards time: partial $\eta^2 = .14$; Key search time: partial $\eta^2 = .83$, Zoo map planning time: partial $\eta^2 = .18$; Zoo Map execution time partial $\eta^2 = .12$)
Herbrich, Kappel, van Noort & Winter [39]	AN ($n = 111$; AN-R = 90, AN-BP = 21) HC ($n = 63$) Age 9–17 years.	WCST, TMT, ROCFT, GEFT	BRIEF-SR	AN-R TMT-4 faster than HC ($d = .39$) No group differences for WCST, ROCFT or GEFT. BRIEF-SR: 'Shift' subscale both subtypes higher than HC (AN-R; $d = -.89$) and (AN-BP; $d = -1.41$) and AN-BP higher than AN-R ($d = .57$).
van Noort, Kraus, Pfeiffer, Lehmkuhl & Kappel [89]	AN ($n = 20$) 15 inpatients, 5 outpatients. HC ($n = 20$) Age 12–18 years.	TMT, ROCFT	BRIEF-SR	No group differences for TMT or ROCFT at baseline. Irrespective of time point, AN less flexible than HC on BRIEF-SR subscales 'Cognitive shift' (partial $\eta^2 = -.207$), 'Behavioral shift' (partial $\eta^2 = -.230$).
Stedal & Dahlgren [76]	AN ($n = 20$, AN-R = 18, AN-BP = 2). 10 in-, 10 outpatients Age 13–18 years.	D-KEFS: TMT-4, Color-word interference test-4 and verbal fluency-3, Brixton, ROCFT	BRIEF-SR BRIEF-PF	All neurocognitive test scores, BRIEF-SR and BRIEF-PF were within normal range.
McAnarney et al. [54]	AN-R ($n = 24$) HC ($n = 37$) Age 14–20 years.	WCST, CANTAB ID/ED	BRIEF-SR BRIEF-PF	AN-R no significant differences in WCST PE or CANTAB ID/ED. AN-R greater set-shifting difficulties than HC on BRIEF-PF ($M = 54.5$ vs. 47, $p = <.008$) and BRIEF-SR ($p = .057$). BRIEF-SR 'Behavioral Shift' sub-scale scores show larger difference ($M = 64.1$ vs. 48.5, $p = <.008$) than 'Cognitive Shift' ($M = 54.9$ vs. 48.7, $p = <.008$).

Abbreviations: ADOS Autism Diagnostic Observation Schedule, *BADS* Behavioral Assessment of Dysexecutive Syndrome, *BRIEF-PF* Behavior Rating Inventory of Executive Function Parent Form, *BRIEF-SR* Behavior Rating Inventory of Executive Function Self-Report, *Brixton* Brixton Spatial Anticipation Test, *CANTAB ID/ED* Intra/Extradimensional Set Shift subtest of the Cambridge Neuropsychological Automated Battery, *CCI* Central Coherence Index, *CIA* Clinical Impairment Assessment, *D-KEFS* Delis-Kaplan Executive Function System, *DFlex* Detail and Flexibility questionnaire, *EDQoL* Eating Disorder Quality of Life scale, *FPT* Fragmented Pictures Task, *GEFT* Group Embedded Figures Test, *IIP-32* Inventory of Interpersonal Problems, *KWCST* Wisconsin Card Sort Test Keio version, *KWCST DMS* Wisconsin Card Sort Test Keio version Difficulty Maintaining Set, *MFFT* Matching Familiar Figures Test, *ROCFT* Rey-Osterreith Complex Figure Task, *ROCFT OCI* Rey-Osterreith Complex Figure Task Order of Construction Index, *SF-36* Short Form Health Survey, SF-36 PCS Short Form Health Survey Physical Component Summary, *SF-36 MCS* Short Form Health Survey Mental Component Summary, *TMT* Trail Making Test, *ToM* Theory of Mind, *WCST* Wisconsin Card Sort Task, *WCST CC* Wisconsin Card Sort Task Categories Completed, *WCST PE* Wisconsin Card Sort Task Perseverative Errors, *WCST %PE* Wisconsin Card Sort Task percentage Perseverative Errors. See Tables 2 and 3 for details of included measures

Table 2 Amended Down's and Black Quality Index scores for included studies

	Reporting					*Power*	
	Aim described?	**Main outcomes described?**	**Participant characteristics described?**	**Main findings described?**	**Estimates of random variability?**	**Probability values reported?**	**Power calculation?**
Oldershaw et al. [60]	✓	✓	✓	✓	✓	x	x
Bentz et al. [9]	✓	✓	✓	✓	✓	✓	x
Hamatani et al. [36]	✓	✓	✓	✓	✓	x	x
Westwood et al. [94]	✓	✓	✓	✓	✓	✓	x
Renwick et al. [67]	✓	✓	✓	✓	✓	✓	x
Talbot et al. [79]	✓	✓	✓	✓	✓	✓	x
Calderoni et al. [14]	✓	✓	✓	✓	✓	✓	x
Harrison et al. [38]	✓	✓	✓	✓	✓	✓	x
Spitoni et al. [75]	✓	✓	✓	✓	✓	✓	✓
Herbrich et al. [39]	✓	✓	✓	✓	✓	✓	✓
Van Noort et al. [89]	✓	✓	✓	✓	✓	✓	x
Stedal & Dahlgren [76]	✓	✓	✓	✓	✓	x	x
McAnarney et al. [54]	✓	✓	✓	✓	✓	✓	x

	External validity			*Internal validity*				
	Invited participants representative of population?	**Final participants representative of population?**	**Staff and facilities representative of population?**	**"Data dredging" made clear?**	**Statistical tests appropriate?**	**Measures valid and reliable?**	**Adjustment for confounds?**	**Total**
Oldershaw et al. [60]	✓	✓	✓	✓	✓	✓	✓	12
Bentz et al. [9]	✓	?	✓	✓	✓	✓	✓	12
Hamatani et al.	✓	✓	✓	✓	✓	✓	✓	12
Westwood et al.	✓	?	?	✓	✓	✓	✓	11
Renwick et al. [67]	✓	?	✓	✓	✓	✓	✓	12
Talbot et al. [79]	✓	✓	✓	✓	✓	✓	x	12
Calderoni et al.	✓	?	✓	✓	✓	✓	✓	12
Harrison et al. [38]	✓	?	✓	✓	✓	✓	✓	12
Spitoni et al. [75]	✓	✓	✓	✓	✓	✓	x	13
Herbrich et al. [39]	✓	?	?	✓	✓	✓	✓	12
Van Noort et al.	✓	✓	✓	✓	✓	✓	✓	13
Stedal & Dahlgren [76]	✓	?	✓	✓	✓	✓	x	10
McAnarney et al.	✓	?	?	✓	✓	✓	✓	11

Table 3 Cognitive measures in included studies

Assessment	*Type*	*Brief description*
Set-shifting		
Brixton Spatial Anticipation Test (Brixton; [13])	Performance	Participant must learn and apply rules to guess where a shape will appear next based on feedback from preceding trials.
Delis-Kaplan Executive Function System (DKEFS; [19]) Color-word interference test-4	Performance	Participants required to name the color ink in which a list of color names is printed (as Stroop task).
D-KEFS: TMT-4	Performance	As Trail Making Test below.
D-KEFS: Verbal fluency-3	Performance	Participant asked to say words from two designated semantic categories as quickly as possible while switching between categories.
Detail and Flexibility Questionnaire (DFlex; [68])	Self-report	24 items assessing cognitive rigidity and attention to detail in daily life.
Intra/Extradimensional Set Shift (IED) subtest of the Cambridge Neuropsychological Automated Battery (CANTAB) [71]	Performance	Participants must learn and apply rules guided by feedback. *Intra-dimensional shifts* - applying previous rule to a new stimulus set, are followed by *extra-dimensional shifts* - applying a new rule which was previously irrelevant. Rule changes after six consecutive correct responses.
NEPSY-II Attention and EF: Auditory response set, Inhibition shifting [44]	Performance	*Auditory response set*: Participants required to switch between matching (select blue circle when "blue" is said) and contrasting (select red when "yellow" said) response to verbal instruction. *Inhibition shifting*: Participants switch between responding to color or shape of bivalent stimuli.
Trail Making Test (TMT-A, TMT-B; [12])	Performance	TMT part B assesses shifting ability. Participant must draw lines to connect 25 circles containing numbers (1–13) and letters (A-L) in ascending order while alternating between numbers and letters (1-A-2-B) without lifting pencil. Timed.
Wisconsin Card Sort Test (WCST; [32])	Performance	Participants sort a target card to a stack of cards which match the color, shape or number of the target card guided only by feedback. Category (usually) changes every 10 trials.
Central Coherence		
Fragmented pictures task (FPT; [74])	Performance	Computerized task where a picture forms from fragments, frame by frame until participant correctly identifies the picture.
Group embedded figures test (GEFT; [98, 99])	Performance	Timed task where participants need to find simple shapes embedded in a more complex figure.
Matching Familiar Figures Test (MFFT; [41, 42])	Performance	Timed task where the participant must select the figure which matches a familiar object from an array of eight very similar figures.
Rey Osterreith Complex Figure Task (ROCFT; [61])	Performance	Participants copy a complex geometric figure. Central coherence index is calculated based on the order (global or local elements) and style of construction (continuous or fragmented).

Are poor set-shifting and central coherence associated with everyday function in anorexia nervosa?

Overall there were more associations between set-shifting and functional outcome measures than between central coherence and functional outcome measures. Seven studies reported a direct or indirect association between a set-shifting and a function measure, and three studies reported an association between a central coherence measure and a function measure. Interpretations based on grouping these associations by neurocognitive measures are very limited due to the wide range of functional outcome measures used, therefore results are grouped according to functional outcome.

Social function measures

Three studies used social cognition tasks to measure social functioning. In an adult sample with current AN, Harrison et al. [38] report higher WCST perseverative errors were associated with lower emotion recognition on the Reading the Mind in the Eyes test, however the association was not significant after Bonferroni correction.

Renwick et al. [67] tested adult participants with current AN on cognitive (WCST, Brixton Spatial Anticipation Test, ROCFT) and social cognitive (Reading the Mind in Films; RMIF) tests and used discriminant function analysis to identify three clusters representing a social-cognitive profile of high, mixed and poor performance. The cluster with poor overall performance is noted to have increased perseverative errors on the WCST, poor ROCFT copy trial scores and poor RMIF emotional theory of mind, which is interpreted as an indirect association between poor set-shifting, weak central coherence, and poor social-cognitive function.

Calderoni et al. [14] tested children/adolescents with AN-R using the full NEPSY-II battery which includes

Table 4 Functional outcome measures in included studies

Assessment	*Type*	*Brief description*
Autism Diagnostic Observation Schedule (ADOS; [51])	Observer-rated	Semi-structured assessment where participant is observed in social interaction, communication, play and imaginative use of materials.
Behavioral Assessment of Dysexecutive syndrome (BADS; [97])	Performance	Six performance tests which assess everyday problem-solving: Rule Shift Cards test (shifting), Action Program test (problem-solving), Key Search (problem-solving), Temporal Judgement, Zoo Map (planning), Modified Six Elements (time-management).
Behavior Rating Inventory of Executive Function self-report (BRIEF-SR; [31])	Self-report	Assesses executive function impairment for participants aged 11–18 years. Two summary scores: *Behavior Regulation Index* (Inhibit, Shift and Emotional Control subscales) and *Metacognitive Index* (Initiate, Working Memory, Plan/Organize, Organization of Materials and Monitor subscales) and a *Global Executive Composite Score* (summary of all subscales).
Behavior Rating Inventory of Executive Function Parent Form (BRIEF-PF; [31])	Other-report	Assesses executive function impairment for participants aged 5–18 years.
Clinical Impairment Assessment (CIA; [10])	Self-report	16-items assessing psychosocial impairment secondary to ED symptoms. Global score and 3 subscale scores: personal, social and cognitive.
Eating Disorders Quality of Life (EDQoL; [25])	Self-report	25-item ED-specific health-related quality of life scale. Subscales: psychological, physical/cognitive, financial and work/school.
Inventory of Interpersonal problems (IIP-32; [6])	Self-report	32-items assessing interpersonal difficulties; things that are "too hard" to do and things done "too much" in relationships.
NEPSY-II [44] Social Perception: ToM verbal, ToM contextual and Affect recognition	Performance	*ToM verbal*: Participants answer questions requiring understanding of the point of view of a character in a verbal/pictorial vignette. *ToM contextual*: Participants match emotions to social situations. *Affect recognition*: Participants identify basic emotions in facial expressions.
Reading the Mind in the Eyes Test [7]	Performance	Participant views the eyes of facial photos only and selects a description of the emotion expressed from four options.
Short-Form Health Survey (SF-36; [91, 92])	Self-report	36-items. *Physical health summary*: physical functioning, limitations due to physical health, pain, general health. *Mental health summary*: vitality, social function, limitations due to emotional health, mental health.

two shifting tests in the domain of attention and executive function, and three social perception tests. Direct associations between the set-shifting and social cognition tests were not included, however there were no differences between the AN-R patients and a healthy control group on the social perception tests (verbal theory of mind, contextual theory of mind and affect recognition). There were also no group differences on the overall domain of attention and executive function or the test of inhibition shifting, however performance on the response set-shifting test was marginally worse in the AN-R group.

Two studies used the Autism Diagnostic Observation Schedule (ADOS) as a measure of social functioning. Bentz et al. [9] tested an adolescent/young adult cohort comprised of individuals with first episode AN and those recovered from adolescent AN. A composite set-shifting score included the shift conditions from three Delis-Kaplan Executive Function System (D-KEFS) subtests: verbal fluency, design fluency and trail making. Composite set-shifting scores did not predict social function according to the ADOS total scores.

Westwood et al. [94] used ADOS Social Affect and Restricted and Repetitive Behavior scores to allocate a mixed age (12–47) cohort of participants with current AN into high vs. sub-clinical vs. no Autism Spectrum Disorder (ASD) symptoms groups. Participants were also tested on the WCST and the ROCFT. An increase in the percentage of perseverative errors on the WCST was associated with increased ASD symptoms, but the ROCFT was not associated with increased ASD symptoms.

One study used the Inventory of Interpersonal Problems (IIP-32). Talbot et al. [79] tested an adult cohort across stages of AN, including currently ill, weight-restored and fully recovered participants. A number of associations between WCST perseverative error (PE) scores and the IIP-32 are reported, however they are in the opposite direction to what may be expected. WCST PE scaled scores (where higher scores indicate better performance) were associated with higher scores on IIP-32 scores (which indicate greater interpersonal problems), in the subscales 'Too dependent', 'Too aggressive', 'Hard to be involved' and 'Hard to be supportive'. Talbot et al. [79] also report two further associations in the opposite direction expected, between higher WCST Categories Completed (CC) and higher IIP-32 'Too dependent' and 'Too aggressive'. However, WCST CC is a measure of runs of 10 correct trials (when rule changes after 10 trials) and may be more indicative of general abstract reasoning, or the ability to learn how to 'play the game' [48]. Participants also completed the ROCFT, which demonstrated some relation to the IIP-32 in the predicted direction. Lower ROCFT Central Coherence Index and Order of Construction Index (OCI) were associated with greater endorsement of IIP-32 'Hard to be supportive', and lower OCI was associated with higher IIP-32 'Hard to be involved'.

Measures of executive function in daily life

Six studies used assessments of executive functioning in daily life. Four studies utilized the self–report version of the Behavior Rating Inventory of Executive Function (BRIEF-SR) in younger cohorts, and two of those also included the parent form (BRIEF-PR).

Herbrich et al. [39] found no group differences between children/ adolescents with AN and healthy controls for the WCST, ROCFT or the Group Embedded Figures Test (GEFT). Participants with AN-R were faster on the Trail Making Test (TMT) than controls. BRIEF-SR scores for both AN subtypes and controls were all within normal range, however scores on the "Shift" subscale were graded, with AN-R participants indicating more issues with shifting than the controls, and AN-BP participants indicating more problems than AN-R.

van Noort, Kraus, Pfeiffer, Lehmkuhl, and Kappel [89] tested adolescents with AN and healthy control participants on the TMT, ROCFT and BRIEF-SR before and after Cognitive Remediation Therapy. There were no group differences for TMT or ROCFT at baseline. Irrespective of time point, participants with AN reported less flexibility than controls with medium-high effect on the BRIEF-SR subscales "Cognitive shift" and "Behavioral shift".

Stedal and Dahlgren [76] tested adolescents with AN with the 'Ravello Profile' battery which includes the Brixton, ROCFT, and the shift trials from the Delis-Kaplan Executive Functioning System (D-KEFS) TMT, colour-word interference and verbal fluency tests. Participants also completed the BRIEF-SR, and their parents completed BRIEF-PF. Scores for all performance-based test scores and the BRIEF-SR and BRIEF-PF were within normal range.

McAnarney et al. [54] tested adolescents and young adults with AN-R (14–20 years) on the WCST, CANT AB Intra-Extra Dimensional Set Shift Test (IED), BRIEF-SR and BRIEF-PF. Participants with AN-R scored more poorly than a control group on WCST total errors, but perseverative error scores were not significantly worse. There were no significant group differences on the IED. Self and parent-reported difficulties with shifting were greater for AN-R participants than controls. At the subscale level, differences between AN-R participants and controls were greater for the BRIEF-SR Behavioral Shift than BRIEF-SR Cognitive Shift.

One study tested a mixed age cohort of participants with AN using the BADS and the WCST, TMT and ROCFT. Spitoni, Aragonaa, Bevacqua, Cotugno, and Antonucci [75] found perseverative errors on the WCST were higher for participants with AN than a control group, though the effect size was small. Performance on the TMT-B was slower than controls with small to medium effect. Participants with AN had a lower ROCFT Central Coherence Index (CCI) than controls with small to medium effects at 30 s and 20 min recall, however, the direct copy trial is the preferred CCI measure [46], and there was no group difference on direct copy trial performance. On the BADS battery, participants with AN performed similarly to controls in accuracy, however AN participants were slower than controls across most tasks with medium to very large effect sizes.

One study used the Detail and Flexibility Questionnaire (DFlex), a self-report measure of cognitive rigidity and attention to detail in daily life. Westwood et al. [94] found no significant difference in DFlex scores across high vs. sub-clinical vs. no ASD symptom groups, however on the cognitive rigidity subscale scores were significantly higher (more rigidity) in the high than the no ASD symptoms group.

Clinical impairment assessment

Two studies used the Clinical Impairment Assessment (CIA) to assess functional impairment secondary to ED symptoms. Renwick et al. [67] administered the CIA to an adult cohort with AN alongside the WCST, Brixton, and ROCFT (and social cognition measures, as described above), however a discriminant function analysis found no effect of cluster on CIA scores. Also in an adult cohort, Oldershaw et al. [60] found cognitive tests (WCST, Brixton, TMT, GEFT) did not predict CIA scores.

Quality of life measures

Two studies used QoL measures. In a cohort of adults with AN, Hamatani et al. [36] found greater Difficulty Maintaining Set (DMS) on the WCST Keio version was associated with lower scores on SF-36 Physical Component Summary (PCS). However, PCS scores for AN participants were not significantly different from a healthy control group, and DMS is not a standard set-shifting measure. DMS is the number of times an incorrect response occurs after 2–5 consecutive correct responses and may be more indicative of distractibility, as failing to maintain set has been inversely associated with performance on a vigilance task [29]. In the same group of participants, ROCFT central coherence index 30-min delayed recall was positively associated with SF-36 Mental Component Summary, however, as mentioned previously, the direct copy trial is considered to be best measure [46].

Talbot et al. [79] report an association between higher WCST Categories Completed (CC) and better financial

QoL. However, as mentioned above, WCST CC is not a standard set-shifting measure and may be more indicative of general abstract reasoning or the ability to learn the task-rule.

Discussion

The current review synthesizes the existing evidence of associations between tests of set-shifting and central coherence and function measures in AN. Overall, the review highlights that this question has received little empirical focus, and of the studies which have assessed the question directly or indirectly, only a limited number of associations have been identified. Differences in the methodologies, measures and samples in the included studies complicate interpretation of the results, however it is possible to make a few general conclusions.

Firstly, the impact of set-shifting and central coherence deficits on functional outcomes in AN appears to be limited, and specific in nature. Levels of functional impairment have been compared to schizophrenia [4], however in schizophrenia neurocognitive deficits appear to exert a substantial general effect on overall functional outcome. The pattern of effect in AN represented by the current review is very different; associations between the cognitive tasks and functional outcomes were inconsistent, with many studies finding no association, and those noted were mostly at the subscale level, indicating a specific impact.

A second general conclusion is that the associations between set-shifting and central coherence deficits and functional outcome identified by the current review were in the adult samples, not the child/adolescent samples. There was generally little evidence of set-shifting and central coherence deficits on performance measures in the younger samples, which is largely consistent with meta-analytic results [40, 47]. However, significant differences between adolescents with AN and control participants were identified by the Behavior Rating Inventory of Executive Function (BRIEF).

Which is the third general conclusion; results of the current review suggest assessments of executive functioning in everyday life may be more sensitive to the cognitive-behavioral flexibility issues experienced by individuals with AN. This is particularly clear for the studies with child/adolescent participants where there were no group differences on the cognitive performance measures, but those that utilized the BRIEF identified that young people with AN report more difficulties with shifting in their daily lives than controls. These differences were noted using both the self-report and parent-report versions of the BRIEF. Results also suggest that behavioral shifting may be more problematic than cognitive shifting. This is consistent with neuroimaging research that suggests rigidity in AN may be secondary to impairments in behavioral response shifting rather than cognitive set-shifting [101].

Additionally, the one adult study which used a measure of executive functioning in everyday life, the Behavioral Assessment of Dysexecutive Syndrome (BADS), was the only study to find a general effect across measures. The BADS is comprised of tasks which are more complex and less structured than standard cognitive tests, involving not only the execution of a task, but planning, organizing, initiation and decision-making that is more similar to real-life task completion. Spitoni et al. [75] found adults with AN were just as accurate, but generally slower across most tasks, and concluded this may be due to perfectionism related to a detail-oriented processing style. The results are also consistent with a large synthesis of studies which questioned the nature of this general 'slow-down' effect seen in ED cohorts, which showed speed of information processing in simple reaction-time tasks was not impaired, but choice reaction time was slower [27].

Both the BRIEF and the BADS are test batteries designed to improve the ecological validity of executive function testing, an issue that has been extensively debated in the clinical and general population literature (see [16] for a review). Researchers in the eating disorder field have called for the use of more ecologically-valid measures to assess cognitive functioning in everyday tasks [15, 62, 76]. Objective performance tests with a specific focus on ecological validity have not been widely utilized in ED research, however measures of self-reported executive function are increasingly used, including ED-specific measures such as the Detail and Flexibility Questionnaire (D-flex; see Table 2), and a measure which encompasses both general and ED-specific flexibility, the Eating Disorder Flexibility Index (EDFLIX; [17]).

Although the current review suggests the nature of the impact of set-shifting and central coherence issues on functional outcome is specific, it is unable to identify which area of function is most affected. The review identified more associations with social function than other areas, however, it is not possible to conclude that social function is most impacted because many of the included studies were more focused on social difficulties than work or everyday activities. A focus on interpersonal problems is valid; patients with AN often experience reduced motivation for, and pleasure from, social interaction, and social-emotional avoidance is a key maintenance factor in the Cognitive-Interpersonal Maintenance Model for AN [72]. However, in terms of the question of possible associations with everyday function, investigations in other disorders suggest a focus on social impact may be an issue. Although results in schizophrenia suggest a general effect of neurocognitive performance on functional outcomes, there is a greater impact on occupational than social function [34]. And in obsessive-compulsive disorder, a more specific relationship has been identified; a retrospective in-patient study found poor set-shifting, measured by the Trail Making Test part B predicted poorer vocational outcome, but not social outcome or independent living status [64]. This raises the question: Could the use of outcome measures that are heavily weighted towards social items mean that the potential impact of cognitive difficulties is being missed by the outcome measure? Answering this question will require further systematic assessment of everyday function across social, workplace and everyday activities.

Although the quality of the studies included in the current review was generally high, the quality of the evidence regarding associations between the cognitive tests and functional outcome measures may be limited by several measurement and sample issues. For the majority of the included studies, associations with functional outcomes was not the primary outcome measure, therefore these issues are discussed not as criticisms of the studies, but rather to highlight methodological issues which may be addressed in future research.

Measurement issues

Studies included in the review primarily used the Wisconsin Card Sort Task (WCST) as the set-shifting measure. Nine studies used the WCST, and in three cases [36, 79, 94] the WCST was the only set-shifting measure. Seven studies reported an association between a set-shifting and a function measure, and in five cases the measure was the WCST. This may be an issue, because the WCST has a limited ability to isolate set-shifting ability from other areas of executive function, known as the *task impurity problem*. The problem arises because performance on even a simple behavioral task will involve cognitive processes outside the variable of interest [56]. Executive function broadly encompasses three areas: *shifting* flexibly between mental sets, *updating* working memory, and *inhibition* of a prepotent response [57]. The WCST dependent variable for set-shifting ability is number of perseverative errors, or errors in sorting where enough information to derive the correct sorting rule has been given. However, perseverative errors could occur due to difficulties with monitoring or updating working memory or inhibiting a response. In particular, the ability to inhibit a previously rewarded response, or reversal learning ability, has been raised as a problematic confound for ED research which uses the WCST [96]. Overall, these issues mean the WCST is best taken as a general measure of executive function, as it was used in one included study [67]. Concurrent measurement of working memory and inhibition, or a composite set-shifting measure to reduce task-related variability may improve the measurement of shifting-specific variance. One study included in the review [9] used a composite measure comprised of the shift conditions of verbal fluency, design fluency and trail making tests from the D-KEFS.

Included studies primarily used the Rey Osterreith Complex Figure Test (ROCFT) as the central coherence measure. Nine of the twelve studies which assessed central coherence used the ROCFT, and in six studies the ROCFT was the only central coherence measure [36, 67, 75, 76, 89, 94]. To provide a more comprehensive assessment of central coherence, utilizing both a global processing measure and a detail-oriented processing measure to demonstrate a bias away from global and towards local processing is useful. Three studies reported an association between a central coherence measure and a function measure, in all cases the measure was the ROCFT, however only one of these studies calculated central coherence index using the direct copy trial, which is the preferred measure [46].

A wide variety of functional outcome measures were used in the included studies and differences in their sensitivity to detect the impact of cognitive inefficiencies may account for the inconsistent findings. A meta-analysis of the associations between cognitive tests and everyday function in Bipolar Disorder notes the strength of correlations varied more due to functional measurement than cognitive domain [20]. General measures may be designed for populations where deficits are of greater magnitude or are more global in nature, and may therefore lack sensitivity to the level or pattern of impairment experienced by individuals with AN. Disorder-specific function measures such as the CIA may be more sensitive to functional impairments than general measures, however significant associations were not found using the CIA in this review. Null results may be partly explained by the general finding that associations between performance-based and self-report measures are low [52, 76], and most included studies used performance measures of set-shifting and central coherence, and many used self-report measures of functional outcome.

Four studies included a performance-based function measure, however, three of these were tests of social cognition only. The Reading the Mind in the Eyes test is a common test of social cognition, however it may be more strongly related to vocabulary than to emotion recognition or theory of mind ability [59].

Sample issues

Null effects may also be due to small sample sizes, or to the heterogeneity of the sample. Sample sizes in AN research are often low, and therefore it is usually only possible to avoid one of these issues. Significant differences in set-shifting and central coherence have been suggested between adults and children, by AN subtype, and between currently ill and recovered individuals, therefore investigating these groups separately is important. However, the power to detect effects was limited in the studies included in this review which sampled only children and/or adolescents, or split their analyses by diagnostic subtype. One study included a particularly wide age range of 12–47 years [94] which may be an issue because although maximum development in executive function occurs between 7 and 12 years old [65], executive function continues to develop until the early 20s, and age has been associated with performance on set-shifting and detail processing tasks [43]. However, age was included as a covariate in the analysis, and the WCST was the primary measure of set-shifting, on which performance is estimated to reach an adult level by around 12 years [65].

Finally, it is important to measure depression, anxiety and IQ (or an estimate of premorbid IQ) alongside cognitive measures. Evidence of the extent to which these factors affect performance on cognitive tasks is somewhat inconsistent in the general psychiatric literature, but results of a review in AN suggest set-shifting performance is negatively impacted by depression [2]. Most studies measured depression and anxiety, however three did not [75, 76, 79]. One study measured depression, but not anxiety [54]. An estimate of premorbid IQ was reported in all but one study [60].

There are also strengths and limitations to the current review. The database search included published conference abstracts and was supplemented by a dissertations and theses search. However, unpublished data and data not available in English was not included, and the review was not pre-registered. Although this may have biased the results, many of the studies included in the review report non-significant findings. To maximize the breadth of studies included and provide a rich analysis of the existing evidence in this area, the review included a broad range of functional outcome measures. However, differences in the methodologies employed in the included studies limit the conclusions which can be drawn from the review.

Extending beyond the scope of the current review, there may be issues related to the limited focus on set-shifting and central coherence deficits when investigating the possible impact of cognitive predictors on functional outcomes. A focus on these two deficits is not without reason - these are the areas where performance difficulties are consistently noted for participants with AN. However, the result is a very narrow measurement of potentially determining factors which does not consider the effects of areas of cognitive strength, or the possibility of compensatory strategy use. For example, individuals with AN show superior performance to control groups in verbal fluency and verbal category switching [77, 80], and verbal memory has been shown to be a strong predictor of everyday function in schizophrenia [34]. Data from one of the studies included in the current review showed performance on set-shifting and central coherence tasks did not predict ADOS social function – but higher verbal memory scores did [9]. Tests of specific cognitive processes may underestimate the ability to function in daily life if strong compensatory strategies like these are used [53]. Recent research found adolescent participants with weight-restored AN showed superior performance to a control group on a verbal and visual-motor set-shifting task, but when inhibition was controlled for in the analyses, their performance was worse, demonstrating strong inhibitory control was used as a compensatory mechanism [93]. Results such as this highlight that to understand the impact of neuropsychological tests on everyday life, a cognitive profile of not only deficits, but also the strengths which could compensate for them is needed. Research in this area could provide support for future cognitive strengths-based approaches to support functional recovery in AN, as has recently been suggested for first-episode psychosis [3].

Conclusion

Despite increasing interest in the assessment of possible links between cognitive impairments and clinical symptoms in AN, very little empirical work has been undertaken to explore whether there is relationship with everyday function. The current review synthesized research which has noted direct or indirect associations between set-shifting and central coherence tests and functional outcome measures in AN across a broad range of samples, measures and methodologies. The results of the review suggest that poor set-shifting and central coherence as measured by performance on standard cognitive tests has only a limited and specific effect on functional outcome, but that measures of executive functioning in daily life may be more sensitive to functional difficulties experienced by individuals with AN. Although the quality of the included studies was high, functional outcome was often a secondary measure, and associations between cognitive performance and functional outcome have not been as systematically assessed as is evident in other psychiatric disorders. However, as mentioned by Green [33], although cognitive research 'looks inwards', the studies included in this review also attempt to 'look outwards' to understand how cognitive inefficiencies impact functional outcomes for individuals with AN. This is important, because functional improvements are milestones of recovery which may increase patient engagement with therapy in AN. Future research in this area could improve current cognition-focused therapies by identifying broader therapeutic targets, and functional milestones by which the therapies can be evaluated.

Abbreviations

ADOS: Autism Diagnostic Schedule; AN: Anorexia Nervosa; AN-BP: Anorexia Nervosa Binge-Purge subtype; AN-R: Anorexia Nervosa Restricting subtype; ASD: Autism Spectrum Disorder; BADS: The Behavioral Assessment of Dysexecutive Syndrome; BMI: Body Mass Index; BRIEF: Behavior Rating Inventory of Executive Function; CC: Categories Completed; CCI: Central Coherence Index; CIA: Clinical Impairment Assessment; CRT: Cognitive Remediation Therapy; DKEFS: Delis-Kaplan Executive Function System; DMS: Difficulty Maintaining Set; DFlex: Detail and Flexibility Questionnaire; ED: Eating Disorder; GEFT: Group Embedded Figures Test; IED: Intra-Extra Dimensional set shift test; IIP: Inventory of Interpersonal Problems; IQ: Intelligence Quotient; OCI: Order of Construction Index; PCS: Physical Component Summary; PE: Perseverative Errors; PRISMA: Preferred Reporting Items for Systematic Reviews; QoL: Quality of Life; TMT: Trail Making Test; ROCFT: Rey Osterreith Complex Figure Test; WCST: Wisconsin Card Sort Task

Acknowledgements

Not applicable.

Authors' contributions

KD, PH and ST conceptualized the review. KD conducted the literature search and wrote the manuscript. KD and ST screened studies for inclusion. All authors reviewed drafts of the manuscript. All authors contributed to, and have approved, the final manuscript.

Competing interests

PH has prepared a report under contract for (July 2017) and received honoraria for education of psychiatrists from Takeda (formerly Shire) Pharmaceuticals.
ST has received travel grants, research grants and honoraria from Takeda for commissioned reports, public speaking and consultant work. He chairs their Australian Clinical Binge Eating Advisory Board.
KD has no conflict of interest.

Author details

[1]School of Psychology, University of Sydney, Sydney, Australia. [2]School of Medicine, Western Sydney University, Sydney, Australia. [3]InsideOut Institute and School of Psychology, University of Sydney, Sydney, Australia.

References

1. American Psychiatric Association. Diagnostic and statistical manual of mental disorders, fifth edition (DSM-5) (5th ed). Arlington: American Psychiatric Publishing; 2013.
2. Abbate-Daga G, Buzzichelli S, Marzola E, Aloi M, Amianto F, Fassino S. Does depression matter in neuropsychological performances in anorexia nervosa? A descriptive review. Int J Eat Disord. 2015;48(6):736–45. https://doi.org/10.1002/eat.22399.
3. Allott K, Steele P, Boyer F, de Winter A, Bryce S, Alvarez-Jimenez M, Phillips L. Cognitive strengths-based assessment and intervention in first-episode psychosis: a complementary approach to addressing functional recovery? Clin Psychol Rev. 2020;79:101871. https://doi.org/10.1016/j.cpr.2020.101871.
4. Arkell J, Robinson P. A pilot case series using qualitative and quantitative methods: biological, psychological and social outcome in severe and enduring eating disorder (anorexia nervosa). Int J Eat Disord. 2008;41(7): 650–6. https://doi.org/10.1002/eat.20546.
5. Bamford B, Barras C, Sly R, Stiles-Shields C, Touyz S, Le Grange D, et al. Eating disorder symptoms and quality of life: where should clinicians place their focus in severe and enduring anorexia nervosa? Int J Eat Disord. 2015; 48(1):133–8. https://doi.org/10.1002/eat.22327.
6. Barkham M, Hardy GE, Startup M. The IIP-32: a short version of the inventory of interpersonal problems. Br J Clin Psychol. 1996;35(1):21–35. https://doi.org/10.1111/j.2044-8260.1996.tb01159.x.
7. Baron-Cohen S, Wheelwright S, Hill J, Raste Y, Plumb I. The "Reading the mind in the eyes" test revised version: a study with Normal adults, and adults with Asperger syndrome or high-functioning autism. J Child Psychol Psychiatry. 2001;42(2):241–51. https://doi.org/10.1111/1469-7610.00715.
8. Benau EM, Orloff NC, Janke EA, Serpell L, Timko CA. A systematic review of the effects of experimental fasting on cognition☆. Appetite. 2014;77:52–61. https://doi.org/10.1016/j.appet.2014.02.014.
9. Bentz M, Jepsen JRM, Kjaersdam Telléus G, Moslet U, Pedersen T, Bulik CM, Plessen KJ. Neurocognitive functions and social functioning in young females with recent-onset anorexia nervosa and recovered individuals. J Eat Disord. 2017;5(1). https://doi.org/10.1186/s40337-017-0137-3.
10. Bohn K, Doll HA, Cooper Z, O'Connor M, Palmer RL, Fairburn CG. The measurement of impairment due to eating disorder psychopathology. Behav Res Ther. 2008;46(10):1105–10. https://doi.org/10.1016/j.brat.2008.06.012.
11. Brockmeyer T, Friederich H-C. Comprehending and fostering cognitive-behavioural flexibility in anorexia nervosa; 2015. p. 92–108.
12. Bucks RS. Trail-Making Test. In: Gellman MD, Turner JR, editors. Encyclopedia of behavioral medicine. New York: Springer New York; 2013. p. 1986–7.
13. Burgess PW, Shallice T. The hayling and brixton tests. London: Pearson; 1997.
14. Calderoni S, Muratori F, Leggero C, Narzisi A, Apicella F, Balottin U, et al. Neuropsychological functioning in children and adolescents with restrictive-type anorexia nervosa: an in-depth investigation with NEPSY-II. J Clin Exp Neuropsychol. 2013;35(2):167–79. https://doi.org/10.1080/13803395.2012.760536.
15. Carral-Fernández L, González-Blanch C, Goddard E, González-Gómez J, Benito-González P, Bustamante-Cruz E, Gómez Del Barrio A. Planning abilities in patients with anorexia nervosa compared with healthy controls. Clin Neuropsychol. 2016;30(2):228–42. https://doi.org/10.1080/13854046.2016.1147603.
16. Chaytor N, Schmitter-Edgecombe M. The ecological validity of neuropsychological tests: a review of the literature on everyday cognitive skills. Neuropsychol Rev. 2003;13(4):181–97. https://doi.org/10.1023/B:NERV.0000009483.91468.fb.
17. Dahlgren CL, Hage TW, Wonderlich JA, Stedal K. General and eating disorder specific flexibility: development and validation of the eating disorder flexibility index (EDFLIX) questionnaire. Front Psychol. 2019;10(663). https://doi.org/10.3389/fpsyg.2019.00663.
18. Dakanalis A, Alix Timko C, Colmegna F, Riva G, Clerici M. Evaluation of the DSM-5 severity ratings for anorexia nervosa in a clinical sample. Psychiatry Res. 2018;262:124–8. https://doi.org/10.1016/j.psychres.2018.02.009.
19. Delis DC, Kaplan E, Kramer JH. Delis-Kaplan executive function system; 2001.
20. Depp CA, Mausbach BT, Harmell AL, Savla GN, Bowie CR, Harvey PD, Patterson TL. Meta-analysis of the association between cognitive abilities and everyday functioning in bipolar disorder. Bipolar Disord. 2012;14(3):217–26. https://doi.org/10.1111/j.1399-5618.2012.01011.x.
21. Diamond A. Executive Functions. Annu Rev Psychol. 2013;64(1):135–68. https://doi.org/10.1146/annurev-psych-113011-143750.
22. Dingemans AE, Danner UN, Donker JM, Aardoom JJ, van Meer F, Tobias K, et al. The effectiveness of cognitive remediation therapy in patients with a severe or enduring eating disorder: a randomized controlled trial. Psychother Psychosom. 2014;83(1):29–36. https://doi.org/10.1159/000355240.
23. Downs SH, Black N. The feasibility of creating a checklist for the assessment of the methodological quality both of randomised and non-randomised studies of health care interventions. J Epidemiol Community Health. 1998; 52(6):377–84. https://doi.org/10.1136/jech.52.6.377.
24. Elliott H, Jones PJ, Schmidt U. Central symptoms predict Posttreatment outcomes and clinical impairment in anorexia nervosa: a network analysis. Clin Psychol Sci. 2019;8(1):139–54. https://doi.org/10.1177/2167702619865958.
25. Engel SG, Wittrock DA, Crosby RD, Wonderlich SA, Mitchell JE, Kolotkin RL. Development and psychometric validation of an eating disorder-specific health-related quality of life instrument. Int J Eat Disord. 2006;39(1):62–71. https://doi.org/10.1002/eat.20200.
26. Evans V, Iverson G, Yatham L, Lam R. The relationship between neurocognitive and psychosocial functioning in major depressive disorder. J Clin Psychiatry. 2014;75(12):1359–70. https://doi.org/10.4088/JCP.13r08939.
27. Ferraro FR, Kramer R, Weigel S. Speed of processing time slowing in eating disorders. J Gen Psychol. 2018;145(1):79–92.
28. Ferro MA, Speechley KN. Depressive symptoms among mothers of children with epilepsy: a review of prevalence, associated factors, and impact on children. Epilepsia. 2009;50(11):2344–54. https://doi.org/10.1111/j.1528-1167.2009.02276.x.
29. Figueroa, I., & Youmans, R. (2013). Failure to maintain set. Proceedings of the Human Factors and Ergonomics Society Annual Meeting, 57, 828-832. doi:https://doi.org/10.1177/1541931213571180

30. Franko, D., Keshaviah, A., Eddy, K., Krishna, M., Davis, M., Keel, P., & Herzog, D. (2013). A Longitudinal Investigation of Mortality in Anorexia Nervosa and Bulimia Nervosa 170(8), 917–925. doi:https://doi.org/10.1176/appi.ajp.2013.12070868.
31. Gioia GA, Isquith PK, Roth RM. Behavior rating inventory for executive function. In: Kreutzer JS, DeLuca J, Caplan B, editors. Encyclopedia of clinical neuropsychology. Cham: Springer International Publishing; 2018. p. 532–8.
32. Grant DA, Berg E. A behavioral analysis of degree of reinforcement and ease of shifting to new responses in a Weigl-type card-sorting problem. J Exp Psychol. 1948;38(4):404–11. https://doi.org/10.1037/h0059831.
33. Green MF. What are the functional consequences of neurocognitive deficits in schizophrenia? Am J Psychiatr. 1996;153(3):321–30.
34. Green MF, Llerena K, Kern RS. The "right stuff" revisited: what have we learned about the determinants of daily functioning in schizophrenia? Schizophrenia Bull. 2015;41(4):781–5. https://doi.org/10.1093/schbul/sbv018.
35. Hagan KE, Christensen KA, Forbush KT. A preliminary systematic review and meta-analysis of randomized-controlled trials of cognitive remediation therapy for anorexia nervosa. Eat Behav. 2020:37:101391.
36. Hamatani S, Tomotake M, Takeda T, Kameoka N, Kawabata M, Kubo H, et al. Influence of cognitive function on quality of life in anorexia nervosa patients. Psychiatry Clin Neurosci. 2017;71(5):328–35. https://doi.org/10.1111/pcn.12491.
37. Happé F. Autism: cognitive deficit or cognitive style? Trends Cogn Sci. 1999; 3(6):216–22. https://doi.org/10.1016/S1364-6613(99)01318-2.
38. Harrison A, Tchanturia K, Naumann U, Treasure J. Social emotional functioning and cognitive styles in eating disorders. Br J Clin Psychol. 2012; 51(3):261–79. https://doi.org/10.1111/j.2044-8260.2011.02026.x.
39. Herbrich L, Kappel V, van Noort BM, Winter S. Differences in set-shifting and central coherence across anorexia nervosa subtypes in children and adolescents. Eur Eat Disord Rev. 2018. https://doi.org/10.1002/erv.2605.
40. Hirst RB, Beard CL, Colby KA, Quittner Z, Mills BM, Lavender JM. Anorexia nervosa and bulimia nervosa: a meta-analysis of executive functioning. Neurosci Biobehav Rev. 2017;83:678–90. https://doi.org/10.1016/j.neubiorev.2017.08.011.
41. Kagan J. Reflection-impulsivity: the generality and dynamics of conceptual tempo. J Abnorm Psychol. 1966;71(1):17.
42. Kagan J, Rosman BL, Day D, Albert J, Phillips W. Information processing in the child: significance of analytic and reflective attitudes. Psychol Monogr Gen Appl. 1964;78(1):1.
43. Kalkut EL, Han SD, Lansing AE, Holdnack JA, Delis DC. Development of set-shifting ability from late childhood through early adulthood. Arch Clin Neuropsychol. 2009;24(6):565–74. https://doi.org/10.1093/arclin/acp048.
44. Kemp SL. NEPSY-ii. In: Kreutzer JS, DeLuca J, Caplan B, editors. Encyclopedia of clinical neuropsychology. New York: Springer New York; 2011. p. 1732–6.
45. Lang K, Lopez C, Stahl D, Tchanturia K, Treasure J. Central coherence in eating disorders: an updated systematic review and meta-analysis. World J Biol Psychiatry. 2014a;15(8):586–98. https://doi.org/10.3109/15622975.2014.909606.
46. Lang K, Roberts M, Harrison A, Lopez C, Goddard E, Khondoker M, et al. Central coherence in eating disorders: a synthesis of studies using the Rey Osterrieth complex figure test. Plos One. 2016;11(11).
47. Lang K, Stahl D, Espie J, Treasure J, Tchanturia K. Set shifting in children and adolescents with anorexia nervosa: an exploratory systematic review and meta-analysis. Int J Eat Disord. 2014b;47(4):394–9. https://doi.org/10.1002/eat.22235.
48. Lange F, Kip A, Klein T, Müller D, Seer C, Kopp B. Effects of rule uncertainty on cognitive flexibility in a card-sorting paradigm. Acta Psychol. 2018;190: 53–64. https://doi.org/10.1016/j.actpsy.2018.07.002.
49. Leppanen J, Adamson J, Tchanturia K. Impact of Cognitive Remediation Therapy on Neurocognitive Processing in Anorexia Nervosa. 2018;9(96). https://doi.org/10.3389/fpsyt.2018.00096.
50. Lopez C, Tchanturia K, Stahl D, Treasure J. Central coherence in eating disorders: a systematic review. Psychol Med. 2008;38(10):1393–404. https://doi.org/10.1017/S0033291708003486.
51. Lord C, Risi S, Lambrecht L, Cook EH, Leventhal BL, DiLavore PC, et al. The autism diagnostic observation schedule—generic: a standard measure of social and communication deficits associated with the Spectrum of autism. J Autism Dev Disord. 2000;30(3):205–23. https://doi.org/10.1023/A:1005592401947.
52. Lounes N, Khan G, Tchanturia K. Assessment of cognitive flexibility in anorexia nervosa-self-report or experimental measure? A brief report. J Int Neuropsychol Soc, 2011;17(5):925-928. https://doi.org/10.1017/S1355617711000671.
53. Marcotte TD, Scott JC, Kamat R, Heaton RK. Neuropsychology and the prediction of everyday functioning Neuropsychology of everyday functioning. New York: The Guilford Press; 2010. p. 5–38.
54. McAnarney ER, Zarcone J, Singh P, Michels J, Welsh S, Litteer T, et al. Restrictive anorexia nervosa and set-shifting in adolescents: a biobehavioral Interface. J Adolesc Health. 2011;49(1):99–101. https://doi.org/10.1016/j.jadohealth.2010.11.259.
55. Mitchison D, Morin A, Mond J, Slewa-Younan S, Hay P. The bidirectional relationship between quality of life and eating disorder symptoms: a 9-year community-based study of Australian women. PLoS One. 2015;10(3): e0120591. https://doi.org/10.1371/journal.pone.0120591.
56. Miyake A, Friedman NP. The nature and organization of individual differences in executive functions: four general conclusions. 2012;21(1):8–14. https://doi.org/10.1177/0963721411429458.
57. Miyake A, Friedman NP, Emerson MJ, Witzki AH, Howerter A, Wager TD. The Unity and Diversity of executive functions and their contributions to complex "frontal lobe" tasks: a latent variable analysis. Cogn Psychol. 2000; 41(1):49–100. https://doi.org/10.1006/cogp.1999.0734.
58. Mond JM, Owen C, Hay PJ, Rodgers B, Beumont PJV. Assessing quality of life in eating disorder patients. Qual Life Res. 2005;14(1):171–8. https://doi.org/10.1007/s11136-004-2657-y.
59. Olderbak S, Wilhelm O, Olaru G, Geiger M, Brenneman MW, Roberts RD. A psychometric analysis of the reading the mind in the eyes test: toward a brief form for research and applied settings. Front Psychol. 2015;6:1503. https://doi.org/10.3389/fpsyg.2015.01503.
60. Oldershaw A, Lavender T, Schmidt U. Are socio-emotional and neurocognitive functioning predictors of therapeutic outcomes for adults with anorexia nervosa? Eur Eat Disord Rev. 2018;26(4):346–59. https://doi.org/10.1002/erv.2602.
61. Osterrieth P. The test of copying a complex figure: a contribution to the study of perception and memory. Arch Psychol. 1944;30:206–356.
62. Øverås M, Kapstad H, Brunborg C, Landrø NI, Lask B. Are poor set-shifting abilities associated with a higher frequency of body checking in anorexia nervosa? J Eat Disord. 2015;3(1). https://doi.org/10.1186/s40337-015-0053-3.
63. Pender S, Gilbert S, Serpell L. The neuropsychology of starvation: set-shifting and central coherence in a fasted nonclinical sample. *PLoS ONE, 9*(10), e110743-undefined. 2014. https://doi.org/10.1371/journal.pone.0110743.
64. Perna G, Cavedini P, Harvey PD, Di Chiaro NV, Daccò S, Caldirola D. Does neuropsychological performance impact on real-life functional achievements in obsessive-compulsive disorder? A preliminary study. Int J Psychiatry Clin Pract. 2016;20(4):224–31. https://doi.org/10.1080/13651501.2016.1223856.
65. Peters S, Crone E. Cognitive flexibility in childhood and adolescence. In Grange J, Houghton G, editors. Task Switching and Cognitive Control. New York: Oxford University Press; 2014.
66. Reas DL, Ro O. Less symptomatic, but equally impaired: clinical impairment in restricting versus binge-eating/purging subtype of anorexia nervosa. Eat Behav. 2018;28:32–7. https://doi.org/10.1016/j.eatbeh.2017.12.004.
67. Renwick B, Musiat P, Lose A, DeJong H, Broadbent H, Kenyon M, et al. Neuro- and social-cognitive clustering highlights distinct profiles in adults with anorexia nervosa. Int J Eat Disord. 2015;48(1):26–34. https://doi.org/10.1002/eat.22366.
68. Roberts ME, Barthel FM, Lopez C, Tchanturia K, Treasure JL. Development and validation of the detail and flexibility questionnaire (DFlex) in eating disorders. Eat Behav. 2011;12(3):168–74. https://doi.org/10.1016/j.eatbeh.2011.04.001.
69. Roberts ME, Tchanturia K, Treasure JL. Exploring the neurocognitive signature of poor set-shifting in anorexia and bulimia nervosa. J Psychiatric Res. 2010;44(14):964–70. https://doi.org/10.1016/j.jpsychires.2010.03.001.
70. Roberts ME, Tchanturia K, Treasure JL. Is attention to detail a similarly strong candidate endophenotype for anorexia nervosa and bulimia nervosa? World J Biol Psychiatry. 2013;14(6):452–63. https://doi.org/10.3109/15622975.2011.639804.
71. Sahakian BJ, Owen AM. Computerized assessment in neuropsychiatry using CANTAB: discussion paper. J R Soc Med. 1992;85(7):399–402.
72. Schmidt U, Treasure J. Anorexia nervosa: valued and visible. A cognitive-interpersonal maintenance model and its implications for research and practice. 2006;45(3):343–66. https://doi.org/10.1348/014466505x53902

73. Smith KE, Mason TB, Johnson JS, Lavender JM, Wonderlich SA. A systematic review of reviews of neurocognitive functioning in eating disorders: the state-of-the-literature and future directions Int J Eat Disord, no pagination specified. 2018. https://doi.org/10.1002/eat.22929.
74. Snodgrass JG, Vanderwart M. A standardized set of 260 pictures: norms for name agreement, image agreement, familiarity, and visual complexity. J Exp Psychol Hum Learn Mem. 1980;6(2):174.
75. Spitoni GF, Aragonaa M, Bevacqua S, Cotugno A, Antonucci G. An ecological approach to the behavioral assessment of executive functions in anorexia nervosa. Psychiatry Res. 2018;259:283–8. https://doi.org/10.1016/j.psychres.2017.10.029.
76. Stedal K, Dahlgren CL. Neuropsychological assessment in adolescents with anorexia nervosa – exploring the relationship between self-report and performance-based testing. J Eat Disord. 2015;3(1):27. https://doi.org/10.1186/s40337-015-0062-2.
77. Stedal K, Landro NI, Lask B. Verbal fluency in anorexia nervosa. Eat Weight Disord. 2013;18(2):151–6. https://doi.org/10.1007/s40519-013-0024-0.
78. Stedal K, Rose M, Frampton I, Landro NI, Lask B. The neuropsychological profile of children, adolescents, and young adults with anorexia nervosa. Arch Clin Neuropsychol. 2012;27(3):329–37. https://doi.org/10.1093/arclin/acs032.
79. Talbot A, Hay P, Touyz S. Exploring the relationship between cognitive style and daily functioning in patients with anorexia nervosa. Adv Eat Disord. 2015;3(3):300–10. https://doi.org/10.1080/21662630.2015.1057858.
80. Tamiya H, Ouchi A, Chen R, Miyazawa S, Akimoto Y, Kaneda Y, Sora I. Neurocognitive impairments are more severe in the binge-eating/purging anorexia nervosa subtype than in the restricting subtype. Front Psychiatry. 2018;9(APR). https://doi.org/10.3389/fpsyt.2018.00138.
81. Tchanturia K, Davies H, Reeder C, Wykes T. Cognitive remediation programme for anorexia nervosa: a manual for practitioners. London: Institute of Psychiatry; 2010.
82. Tchanturia K, Giombini L, Leppanen J, Kinnaird E. Evidence for cognitive remediation therapy in young people with anorexia nervosa: systematic review and meta-analysis of the literature. Eur Eat Disord Rev. 2017;25(4):227–36. https://doi.org/10.1002/erv.2522.
83. Tchanturia K, Hambrook D, Curtis H, Jones T, Lounes N, Fenn K, et al. Work and social adjustment in patients with anorexia nervosa. Compr Psychiatry. 2013;54(1):41–5. https://doi.org/10.1016/j.comppsych.2012.03.014.
84. Tchanturia K, Harrison A, Davies H, Roberts M, Oldershaw A, Nakazato M, et al. Cognitive flexibility and clinical severity in eating disorders. Plos One. 2011;6(6). https://doi.org/10.1371/journal.pone.0020462.
85. Tchanturia K, Lounes N, Holttum S. Cognitive remediation in anorexia nervosa and related conditions: a systematic review. Eur Eat Disord Rev. 2014;22(6):454–62. https://doi.org/10.1002/erv.2326.
86. Touyz S, Le Grange D, Lacey H, Hay P, Smith R, Maguire S, et al. Treating severe and enduring anorexia nervosa: a randomized controlled trial. Psychol Med. 2013;43(12):2501–11. https://doi.org/10.1017/S0033291713000949.
87. Uznadze DN. The psychology of set; 1966.
88. Van Autreve S, Vervaet M. Are there differences in central coherence and set shifting across the subtypes of anorexia nervosa?: a systematic review. J Nervous Ment Dis. 2015;203(10):774–80. https://doi.org/10.1097/NMD.0000000000000366.
89. van Noort BM, Kraus MKA, Pfeiffer E, Lehmkuhl U, Kappel V. Neuropsychological and Behavioural short-term effects of cognitive remediation therapy in adolescent anorexia nervosa: a pilot study. Eur Eat Disord Rev. 2016;24(1):69–74. https://doi.org/10.1002/erv.2383.
90. van Passel B, Danner UN, Dingemans AE, Aarts E, Sternheim LC, Becker ES, et al. Cognitive remediation therapy does not enhance treatment effect in obsessive-compulsive disorder and anorexia nervosa: a randomized controlled trial. Psychother Psychosom. 2020:1–14. https://doi.org/10.1159/000505733.
91. Ware, J. E. (2000). SF-36 Health Surv Update 25(24), 3130–3139.
92. Ware JE, Sherbourne CD. The MOS 36-item short-form health survey (SF-36): I. conceptual framework and item selection. Med Care. 1992;30(6):473–83.
93. Weinbach N, Bohon C, Lock J. Set-shifting in adolescents with weight-restored anorexia nervosa and their unaffected family members. J Psychiatr Res. 2019;112:71–6. https://doi.org/10.1016/j.jpsychires.2019.02.022.
94. Westwood H, Mandy W, Tchanturia K. The association between symptoms of autism and neuropsychological performance in females with anorexia nervosa. Psychiatry Res. 2017, *258*:531–7. https://doi.org/10.1016/j.psychres.2017.09.005.
95. Westwood H, Stahl D, Mandy W, Tchanturia K. The set-shifting profiles of anorexia nervosa and autism spectrum disorder using the Wisconsin card sorting test: a systematic review and meta-analysis. Psychol Med. 2016;46(9):1809–27. https://doi.org/10.1017/S0033291716000581.
96. Wildes JE, Forbes EE, Marcus MD. Advancing research on cognitive flexibility in eating disorders: the importance of distinguishing attentional set-shifting and reversal learning. Int J Eat Disord. 2014;47(3):227–30. https://doi.org/10.1002/eat.22243.
97. Wilson BA, Evans JJ, Emslie H, Alderman N, Burgess P. The development of an ecologically valid test for assessing patients with a Dysexecutive syndrome. Neuropsychol Rehabil. 1998;8(3):213–28. https://doi.org/10.1080/713755570.
98. Witkin H, Oltman P, Raskin E, Karp S. Group embedded figures test manual. Redwood City: Mind Garden, Inc.; 2002.
99. Witkin HA. A manual for the embedded figures tests. Palo Alto: Consulting Psychologists Press; 1971.
100. Wu M, Brockmeyer T, Hartmann M, Skunde M, Herzog W, Friederich HC. Set-shifting ability across the spectrum of eating disorders and in overweight and obesity: a systematic review and meta-analysis. Psychol Med. 2014;44(16):3365–85. https://doi.org/10.1017/S0033291714000294.
101. Zastrow A, Kaiser S, Stippich C, Walther S, Herzog W, Tchanturia K, et al. Neural correlates of impaired cognitive-behavioral flexibility in anorexia nervosa. Am J Psychiatry. 2009;166(5):608–16. https://doi.org/10.1176/appi.ajp.2008.08050775.

Permissions

All chapters in this book were first published by BioMed Central; hereby published with permission under the Creative Commons Attribution License or equivalent. Every chapter published in this book has been scrutinized by our experts. Their significance has been extensively debated. The topics covered herein carry significant findings which will fuel the growth of the discipline. They may even be implemented as practical applications or may be referred to as a beginning point for another development.

The contributors of this book come from diverse backgrounds, making this book a truly international effort. This book will bring forth new frontiers with its revolutionizing research information and detailed analysis of the nascent developments around the world.

We would like to thank all the contributing authors for lending their expertise to make the book truly unique. They have played a crucial role in the development of this book. Without their invaluable contributions this book wouldn't have been possible. They have made vital efforts to compile up to date information on the varied aspects of this subject to make this book a valuable addition to the collection of many professionals and students.

This book was conceptualized with the vision of imparting up-to-date information and advanced data in this field. To ensure the same, a matchless editorial board was set up. Every individual on the board went through rigorous rounds of assessment to prove their worth. After which they invested a large part of their time researching and compiling the most relevant data for our readers.

The editorial board has been involved in producing this book since its inception. They have spent rigorous hours researching and exploring the diverse topics which have resulted in the successful publishing of this book. They have passed on their knowledge of decades through this book. To expedite this challenging task, the publisher supported the team at every step. A small team of assistant editors was also appointed to further simplify the editing procedure and attain best results for the readers.

Apart from the editorial board, the designing team has also invested a significant amount of their time in understanding the subject and creating the most relevant covers. They scrutinized every image to scout for the most suitable representation of the subject and create an appropriate cover for the book.

The publishing team has been an ardent support to the editorial, designing and production team. Their endless efforts to recruit the best for this project, has resulted in the accomplishment of this book. They are a veteran in the field of academics and their pool of knowledge is as vast as their experience in printing. Their expertise and guidance has proved useful at every step. Their uncompromising quality standards have made this book an exceptional effort. Their encouragement from time to time has been an inspiration for everyone.

The publisher and the editorial board hope that this book will prove to be a valuable piece of knowledge for researchers, students, practitioners and scholars across the globe.

List of Contributors

Inger Halvorsen
Regional Department for Eating Disorders, Division of Mental Health and Addiction, Oslo University Hospital - Ullevål Hospital, Nydalen, N-0424 Oslo, Norway

Øyvind Rø
Regional Department for Eating Disorders, Division of Mental Health and Addiction, Oslo University Hospital - Ullevål Hospital, Nydalen, N-0424 Oslo, Norway
Division of Mental Health and Addiction, Institute of Clinical Medicine, University of Oslo, Oslo, Norway
Institute of Clinical Medicine, Faculty of Medicine, University of Oslo, 0318 Oslo, Norway

Jessica Aradas and Diana Sales
University of Western Sydney, Locked Bag 1797, Penrith 2751, Australia

Louise Bezzina, Sarah Young and Sloane Madden
University of Sydney, Sydney, Australia

Nasim Foroughi
School of Medicine, Western Sydney University, Sydney, Australia

Stacy Clemes
Loughborough University, Loughborough, UK

Caroline Meyer
University of Warwick, Coventry, UK

Jon Arcelus
University of Nottingham, Nottingham, UK

Kathleen M. Pike
Columbia University, New York, USA

Phillipa Hay
Translational Health Research Institute, School of Medicine, Western Sydney University, Locked Bag 1797, Penrith, South NSW 2715, Australia

Ella Wufong, Paul Rhodes and Janet Conti
Western Sydney University, Locked Bag 1797, Penrith 2751, Australia

Thomas Blikshavn
Regional Department for Eating Disorders, Division of Mental Health and Addiction, Oslo University Hospital, N-0424 Oslo, Norway
Department of Child and Adolescent Mental Health, Akershus University Hospital, Lørenskog, Norway

Tone Seim Fuglset
Division of Mental Health and Addiction, Møre and Romsdal Hospital Trust, Parkvegen 84, 6412 Molde, Norway

Dennis Gibson and Ashlie Watters
ACUTE Center for Eating Disorders at Denver Health, 723 Delaware St, Pav M 3rd floor, Denver, CO 80204, USA
Department of Medicine, University of Colorado School of Medicine, 13001 E 17th Pl, Aurora, CO 80045, USA

Jeana Cost
ACUTE Center for Eating Disorders at Denver Health, 723 Delaware St, Pav M 3rd floor, Denver, CO 80204, USA
Eating Recovery Center, 7351 E Lowry Blvd, Denver, CO 80230, USA

Margherita Mascolo
Department of Medicine, University of Colorado School of Medicine, 13001 E 17th Pl, Aurora, CO 80045, USA

Philip S. Mehler
ACUTE Center for Eating Disorders at Denver Health, 723 Delaware St, Pav M 3rd floor, Denver, CO 80204, USA
Department of Medicine, University of Colorado School of Medicine, 13001 E 17th Pl, Aurora, CO 80045, USA
Eating Recovery Center, 7351 E Lowry Blvd, Denver, CO 80230, USA

Liv Nilsen
Division of Mental Health and Addiction, Oslo University Hospital, Nydalen, Oslo, Norway

Veronica Lockertsen and Jan Ivar Røssberg
Division of Mental Health and Addiction, Oslo University Hospital, Nydalen, Oslo, Norway
Institute of Clinical Medicine, Faculty of Medicine, University of Oslo, 0318 Oslo, Norway

Lill Ann Wellhaven Holm
Oslo, Norway

Linn May Burger
Drammen, Norway

Morgane Marion, Sylvie Lacroix, Emmanuelle Caldagues and Marylène Caquard
CHU de Nantes, Department of adolescent medicine, Pédiatrie générale, 7 quai Moncousu, 44000 Nantes, France

Laurence Dreno
CHU de Nantes Department of child psychiatry, University of Hospital Nantes, Nantes, France

Pauline Scherdel
CHU de Nantes, Centre d'Investigation Clinique (CIC004), Nantes, France

Christèle Gras Le Guen
CHU de Nantes, Centre d'Investigation Clinique (CIC004), Nantes, France
CHU de Nantes, Department of Pediatrics, Nantes, France

Elise Launay
CHU de Nantes, Department of Pediatrics, Nantes, France

Melanie Rylander
Departments of Internal Medicine and Psychiatry, Denver Health Medical Center, University of Colorado School of Medicine, 777 Bannock St, Denver, CO 80204, USA

Gillian Taylor, Susan Bennett and Christopher Pierce
Department of Psychiatry, Denver Health Medical Center, University of Colorado School of Medicine, Denver, CO 80204, USA

Angela Keniston
Department of Internal Medicine, University of Colorado School of Medicine, Denver, CO 80204, USA

Mouna Hanachi
Clinical Nutrition Unit, Raymond Poincaré Hospital (AP-HP), Garches, France
Université de Versailles, Saint-Quentin-en-Yvelines, Montigny-le-Bretonneux, Versailles, France

Annabel Pleple, Marika Dicembre, Emilie Latour and Maeva Duquesnoy
Clinical Nutrition Unit, Raymond Poincaré Hospital (AP-HP), Garches, France

Caroline Barry
France INSERM, U1178 Paris, VI, France

Jean-Claude Melchior
Clinical Nutrition Unit, Raymond Poincaré Hospital (AP-HP), Garches, France
Université de Versailles, Saint-Quentin-en-Yvelines, Montigny-le-Bretonneux, Versailles, France
France INSERM, U1178 Paris, VI, France

Abdallah Fayssoil
Institut de Myologie, Groupe Hospitalier Pitié-Salpêtrière, APHP, Paris, France

Michitaka Funayama, Taketo Takata and Shin Kurose
Department of Neuropsychiatry, Ashikaga Red Cross Hospital, 284-1 Yobe, Ashikaga-city, Tochigi 326-0843, Japan

Yu Mimura
Department of Neuropsychiatry, Ashikaga Red Cross Hospital, 284-1 Yobe, Ashikaga-city, Tochigi 326-0843, Japan
Department of Neuropsychiatry, Keio University School of Medicine, Shinjuku, Tokyo, Japan

Akihiro Koreki
Department of Neuropsychiatry, Ashikaga Red Cross Hospital, 284-1 Yobe, Ashikaga-city, Tochigi 326-0843, Japan
Department of Neuropsychiatry, National Hospital Organization Shimofusa Psychiatric Medical Center, Chiba, Japan

Satoyuki Ogino
Department of Neuropsychiatry, Ashikaga Red Cross Hospital, 284-1 Yobe, Ashikaga-city, Tochigi 326-0843, Japan
Department of Trauma and Critical Care Medicine, Kyorin University School of Medicine, Mitaka, Tokyo, Japan

Anne Bargiacchi, Coline Stordeur, Grégor Mamou and Richard Delorme
Child and Adolescent Psychiatry Department, Assistance Publique-Hôpitaux de Paris, Robert Debré University Hospital, Paris, France

Julia Clarke
Child and Adolescent Psychiatry Department, Assistance Publique-Hôpitaux de Paris, Robert Debré University Hospital, Paris, France
Université de Paris, Institute of Psychiatry and Neuroscience of Paris, INSERM U1266, Paris, France

Hugo Peyre
Child and Adolescent Psychiatry Department, Assistance Publique-Hôpitaux de Paris, Robert Debré University Hospital, Paris, France
Université de Paris, INSERM UMR 1141, Paris, France

Marianne Alison
Radiology Department, Assistance Publique-Hôpitaux de Paris, Robert Debré University Hospital, Pediatric, Paris, France

Priscilla Boizeau
Unit of Clinical Epidemiology, Assistance Publique-Hôpitaux de Paris, Robert Debré University Hospital, Paris, France

Sophie Guilmin Crépon
Radiology Department, Assistance Publique-Hôpitaux de Paris, Robert Debré University Hospital, Pediatric, Paris, France
Department of Pediatric Endocrinology and Diabetology & Reference centre for Growth and Development Endocrine diseases, Assistance Publique-Hôpitaux de Paris, Robert Debré University Hospital, Paris, France
INSERM UMR-S 1123 ECEVE and CIC-EC 1426, Paris, France

Corinne Alberti
INSERM UMR-S 1123 ECEVE and CIC-EC 1426, Paris, France

Juliane Léger
Université de Paris, INSERM UMR 1141, Paris, France
Department of Pediatric Endocrinology and Diabetology & Reference centre for Growth and Development Endocrine diseases, Assistance Publique-Hôpitaux de Paris, Robert Debré University Hospital, Paris, France

Denise Kästner, Angelika Weigel, Bernd Löwe, Ines Buchholz and Antje Gumz
Department of Psychosomatic Medicine and Psychotherapy, University Medical Centre, Hamburg-Eppendorf, Martinistr. 52, W37, 20246 Hamburg, Germany

Ulrich Voderholzer
Schön Clinic Roseneck, Prien am Chiemsee, Germany
Department of Psychiatry and Psychotherapy, University Hospital Freiburg, Freiburg, Germany
Department of Psychiatry and Psychotherapy, University of Munich (LMU), Munich, Germany

Jenni Leppanen
Department of Neuroimaging, Institute of Psychology, Psychiatry and Neuroscience, King's College London, London, UK
Department of Psychological Medicine, Institute of Psychology, Psychiatry and Neuroscience, King's College London, 103 Denmark Hill, London SE5 8AF, UK

Steven Williams
Department of Neuroimaging, Institute of Psychology, Psychiatry and Neuroscience, King's College London, London, UK

Lara Tosunlar and Rachael Blackburn
Department of Psychological Medicine, Institute of Psychology, Psychiatry and Neuroscience, King's College London, 103 Denmark Hill, London SE5 8AF, UK

Kate Tchanturia
Department of Psychological Medicine, Institute of Psychology, Psychiatry and Neuroscience, King's College London, 103 Denmark Hill, London SE5 8AF, UK
South London and Maudsley NHS Foundation Trust National Eating Disorder Service, London, UK
Psychology Department, Illia State University, Tbilisi, Georgia

Felicity Sedgewick
School of Education, University of Bristol, Bristol, UK

Maya Dalack
New York State Psychiatric Institute, 1051 Riverside Drive, Unit 98, New York, NY 10032, USA

Nathaniel Daw
Princeton Neuroscience Institute, Department of Psychology, Princeton University, Princeton, NJ 08540, USA

Daphna Shohamy
Psychology Department and Zuckerman Mind Brain and Behavior Institute, Columbia University, 3227 Broadway, New York, NY 10027, USA

Deborah R. Glasofer, Alexandra F. Muratore, Hillary Minkoff, B. Timothy Walsh, Karin Foerde and Joanna E. Steinglass
Department of Psychiatry, Columbia University Irving Medical Center, New York State Psychiatric Institute, 1051 Riverside Drive, Unit 98, New York City, NY 10032, USA

Evelyn Attia
Department of Psychiatry, Columbia University Irving Medical Center, New York State Psychiatric Institute, 1051 Riverside Drive, Unit 98, New York City, NY 10032, USA
Center for Eating Disorders, Weill Cornell Medical College, 21 Bloomingdale Road, White Plains, NY 10605, USA

Peng Wu and Yuanjia Wang
Department of Biostatistics, Mailman School of Public Health, 722 West 168th Street, New York, NY 10032, USA

Teresa Rufin
Harvard T.H. Chan School of Public Health, 677 Huntington Avenue, Boston, MA 02115, USA

Hanne Weie Oddli
Department of Psychology, University of Oslo, Oslo, Norway

Jan-Vegard Nilsen
Department of Psychology, University of Oslo, Oslo, Norway
Regional Department for Eating Disorders, Division of Mental Health and Addiction, Oslo University Hospital, Oslo, Norway

Martina Isaksson, Caisa Öster and Mia Ramklint
Department of Neuroscience, Psychiatry, Uppsala University, Entrance 10, Floor 3B, SE-751 85 Uppsala, Sweden

Ata Ghaderi
Division of Psychology, Department of Clinical Neuroscience, Karolinska Institutet, SE-171 77 Stockholm, Sweden
Stockholm Centre for Eating Disorders, Stockholm Health Care Services, Stockholm County Council, SE-171 77 Stockholm, Sweden

Martina Wolf-Arehult
Department of Neuroscience, Psychiatry, Uppsala University, Entrance 10, Floor 3B, SE-751 85 Uppsala, Sweden
Psychiatry Northwest, Region Stockholm, Clinical Management, SE-191 22 Sollentuna, Sweden

Bethan Dalton, Jessica McClelland, Savani Bartholdy, Maria Kekic and Iain C. Campbell
Section of Eating Disorders, Department of Psychological Medicine, Institute of Psychiatry, Psychology & Neuroscience, King's College London, London SE5 8AF, UK

Ulrike Schmidt
Section of Eating Disorders, Department of Psychological Medicine, Institute of Psychiatry, Psychology & Neuroscience, King's College London, London SE5 8AF, UK
South London and Maudsley NHS Foundation Trust, Maudsley Hospital, Denmark Hill, London SE5 8AZ, UK

Kelly M. Dann
School of Psychology, University of Sydney, Sydney, Australia

Stephen Touyz
Inside Out Institute and School of Psychology, University of Sydney, Sydney, Australia

Index

www.ingramcontent.com/pod-product-compliance
Lightning Source LLC
LaVergne TN
LVHW081033210926
848485LV00004B/1013